The Founders of Operative Surgery

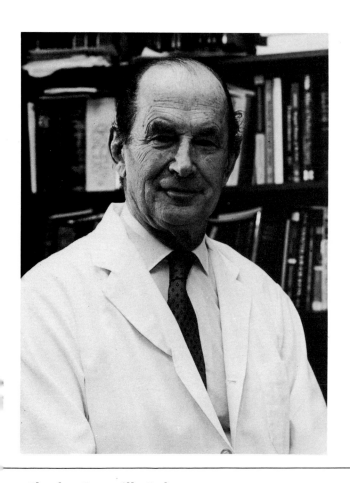

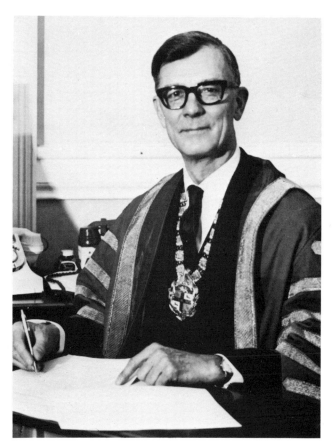

Charles Granville Rob MC, MChir, MD, FRCS, FACS
Professor of Surgery, Department of Surgery, Uniformed
Services University of the Health Sciences, F. Edward Hébert
School of Medicine, Bethesda, Maryland
Quondam: Professor of Surgery, St Mary's Hospital Medical
School, London 1950–1960;
Professor and Chairman, Department of Surgery, University of
Rochester, New York, 1960–1978;
Professor of Surgery, East Carolina University, 1978–1983

Lord Smith of Marlow KBE, MS, FRCS, Hon DSc
(Exeter and Leeds), Hon MD (Zurich), Hon FRACS,
Hon FRCS(Ed), Hon FACS, Hon FRCS(Can), Hon FRCSI,
Hon FCS(SA), Hon FDS
Honorary Consulting Surgeon, St George's Hospital, London
Quondam: Surgeon, St George's Hospital, London,
1946–1978;
President of the Royal College of Surgeons of England,
1973–1977

Rob & Smith's
Operative Surgery

Thoracic Surgery

Fourth Edition

Rob & Smith's
Operative Surgery

General Editors

Hugh Dudley ChM, FRCS(Ed), FRACS, FRCS
Professor of Surgery, St Mary's Hospital, London, UK

David C. Carter MD, FRCS(Ed), FRCS(Glas)
St Mungo Professor of Surgery, University of Glasgow;
Honorary Consultant Surgeon, Royal Infirmary, Glasgow, UK

Rob & Smith's
Operative Surgery

Thoracic Surgery
Fourth Edition

Edited by

John W. Jackson MCh, FRCS
Formerly Consultant Thoracic Surgeon, Harefield Hospital, Middlesex, UK

and

D. K. C. Cooper PhD, FRCS, FACC
Associate Professor, Department of Cardiothoracic Surgery, University of Cape Town Medical School and Groote Schuur Hospital, Cape Town, South Africa

Butterworths
London   Boston   Durban   Singapore   Sydney   Toronto   Wellington

© Butterworths 1986

First edition published in eight volumes 1956–1958
Second edition published in fourteen volumes 1968–1971
Third edition published in nineteen volumes 1976–1981
Fourth edition published 1983–

British Library Cataloguing in Publication Data

Rob, Charles
    Rob & Smith's operative surgery. — 4th ed.
    Thoracic Surgery
    1. Surgery
    I. Title   II. Smith, Rodney Smith, *Baron*
    III. Rob, Charles. Operative Surgery
    IV. Jackson, John W.   V. Cooper, D.K.C.
    617   RD31

    ISBN 0-407-00661-3

Library of Congress Cataloging in Publication Data
(Revised for volume 6)

Rob & Smith's operative surgery.

    Rev. ed. of: Operative surgery. 3rd ed. 1976–.
    Includes bibliographies and indexes.
    Contents; [1] Alimentary tract and abdominal wall.
1. General principles, oesophagus, stomach, duodenum,
small intestine, abdominal wall, hernia/edited by
Hugh Dudley – [6] Thoracic surgery/edited
by John W. Jackson and D. K. C. Cooper.
    1. Surgery, Operative.   I. Rob, Charles.
II. Smith of Marlow, Rodney Smith, Baron, 1914–
III. Dudley, Hugh A. F. (Hugh Arnold Freeman)
IV. Pories, Walter J. V. Carter, David C. (David Craig)
VI. Jackson, John W. (John Walter)   VII. Cooper, D. K. C.
1939–   .   VIII. Operative surgery. [DNLM·
1. Surgery, Operative. WO 500 061 1982]
RD32.06   1983   617'.91   83-14465
ISBN 0-407-00651-6 (v. 1)

Photoset by Butterworths Litho Preparation Department
Printed by Blantyre Printing Ltd, London & Glasgow
Bound by Robert Hartnoll Ltd, Bodmin, Cornwall

Volumes and Editors

Alimentary Tract and Abdominal Wall

1 **General Principles · Oesophagus · Stomach · Duodenum · Small Intestine · Abdominal Wall · Hernia**

Hugh Dudley ChM, FRCS(Ed), FRACS, FRCS
Professor of Surgery, St Mary's Hospital, London, UK

2 **Liver · Portal Hypertension · Spleen · Biliary Tract · Pancreas**

Hugh Dudley ChM, FRCS(Ed), FRACS, FRCS
Professor of Surgery, St Mary's Hospital, London, UK

3 **Colon, Rectum and Anus**

Ian P. Todd MS, MD(Tor), FRCS, DCH
Consulting Surgeon, St Bartholomew's Hospital, London;
Consultant Surgeon, St Mark's Hospital and
King Edward VII Hospital for Officers, London, UK

L. P. Fielding MB, FRCS
Chief of Surgery, St Mary's Hospital, Waterbury, Connecticut, USA;
Associate Professor of Surgery, Yale University, Connecticut, USA

Cardiac Surgery

Stuart W. Jamieson MB, FRCS, FACS
Professor and Head, Cardiothoracic Surgery,
University of Minnesota, Minneapolis, Minnesota, USA

Norman E. Shumway MD, PhD, FACS, FRCS
Professor and Chairman, Department of Cardiovascular Surgery,
Stanford University School of Medicine, California, USA

The Ear

John C. Ballantyne CBE, FRCS, HonFRCSI, DLO
Consultant Ear, Nose and Throat Surgeon,
Royal Free and King Edward VII Hospital for Officers, London, UK

Andrew Morrison FRCS
Senior Surgeon, Ear, Nose and Throat Department, The London
Hospital, UK

General Principles, Breast and Extracranial Endocrines

Hugh Dudley ChM, FRCS(Ed), FRACS, FRCS
Professor of Surgery, St Mary's Hospital, London, UK

Walter J. Pories MD, FACS
Professor and Chairman, Department of Surgery, School of Medicine,
East Carolina University, Greenville, North Carolina, USA

Gynaecology and Obstetrics

J. M. Monaghan MB, FRCS(Ed), MRCOG
Consultant Surgeon, Regional Department of Gynaecological
Oncology,
Queen Elizabeth Hospital, Gateshead, UK

Plastic Surgery

T. L. Barclay ChM, FRCS, FRCS(Ed)
Formerly Consultant Plastic Surgeon, Bradford Royal Infirmary and
St Luke's Hospital, Bradford, West Yorkshire, UK

Desmond A. Kernahan MD, FRCS(C), FACS
Chief, Division of Plastic Surgery,
Children's Memorial Hospital, Chicago;
Professor of Surgery, North Western University
Medical School, Chicago, Illinois, USA

Thoracic Surgery

John W. Jackson MCh, FRCS
Formerly Consultant Thoracic Surgeon, Harefield Hospital,
Middlesex, UK

D. K. C. Cooper PhD, FRCS, FACC
Associate Professor, Department of Cardiothoracic Surgery,
University of Cape Town Medical School and Groote Schuur Hospital,
Cape Town, South Africa

Trauma

John V. Robbs FRCS
Associate Professor of Surgery,
Department of Surgery, University of Natal, South Africa

Howard R. Champion FRCS
Chief, Trauma Service;
Director, Surgery Critical Care Services,
The Washington Hospital Center, Washington DC, USA

Donald Trunkey MD
Chairman, Department of Surgery, University of Portland, Portland,
Oregon, USA

Urology

W. Scott McDougal MD
Professor and Chairman, Department of Urology, Vanderbilt
University, Nashville, Tennessee, USA

Vascular Surgery

James A. DeWeese MD
Professor and Chairman, Division of Cardiothoracic Surgery,
University of Rochester Medical Center, Rochester, New York, USA

Contributors

I. Barnnet Angorn FRCS(Ed), FRCS
Professor of Surgery, Natal University Medical School, Durban, South Africa

S. R. Benatar FFA, FRCP
Professor and Head, Department of Medicine, University of Cape Town Medical School and Groote Schuur Hospital, Cape Town, South Africa

D. K. C. Cooper PhD, FRCS, FACC
Associate Professor, Department of Cardiothoracic Surgery, University of Cape Town Medical School and Groote Schuur Hospital, Cape Town, South Africa

Joel D. Cooper MD, FACS, FRCS(C)
Head, Division of Thoracic Surgery, Toronto General Hospital and University of Toronto, Toronto, Ontario, Canada

A. H. K. Deiraniya FRCS
Consultant Cardiothoracic Surgeon, Wythenshawe Hospital, Manchester, UK

J. E. Dussek FRCS
Consultant Thoracic Surgeon, Guy's Hospital and The Brook Hospital, London, UK

E. Ginzberg MD
Professor of Thoracic Surgery, Military Medical Academy, Belgrade, Yugoslavia

Peter Goldstraw FRCS, FRCS(Ed)
Consultant Thoracic Surgeon, Brompton Hospital, Middlesex Hospital, and University College Hospital, London, UK

R. P. Hewitson FRCS, FRCS(Ed)
Associate Professor of Thoracic Surgery, Groote Schuur Hospital and University of Cape Town Medical School, Cape Town, South Africa

Lucius D. Hill MD
Head, Section of General, Thoracoesophageal and Vascular Surgery, Virginia Mason Medical Center, Seattle, Washington, USA

Raymond Hurt FRCS
Thoracic Surgeon, Regional Thoracic Surgical Centre, North Middlesex Hospital, Edmonton, London, and St Bartholomew's Hospital, London, UK

John J. Jackson MCh, FRCS
Formerly Consultant Thoracic Surgeon, Harefield Hospital, Harefield, Middlesex, UK

A. W. Jowett FRCS
Consultant Thoracic Surgeon, The Royal Hospital, Wolverhampton, UK

G. Keen MS, FRCS
Consultant Cardiothoracic Surgeon, United Bristol Hospitals and Frenchay Hospital, Bristol, UK

W. F. Kerr FRCS(Ed)
Formerly Consultant Thoracic Surgeon, Norfolk and Norwich Hospital, Norwich, UK

R. E. Lea FRCS
Consultant Thoracic Surgeon, Southampton General Hospital, Southampton, UK

Stuart C. Lennox MB, FRCS
Surgeon, The Brompton Hospital, London; Senior Lecturer, Cardiothoracic Institute, University of London, UK

Werner Maassen MD
Professor and Head, Ruhrlandclinic for Pneumonology and Thoracic Surgery, Essen, Federal Republic of Germany

I. K. R. McMillian FRCS
Thoracic Surgeon, Wessex Regional Cardiothoracic Unit, Southampton General Hospital, and Southampton University Hospitals, Southampton, UK

Hugoe R. Matthews FRCS
Consultant Thoracic Surgeon, East Birmingham Hospital, Birmingham, UK

Mark B. Orringer MD, FACS
Professor and Head, Section of Thoracic Surgery, University of Michigan, Ann Arbor, Michigan, USA

K. Michael Pagliero FRCS
Thoracic Surgeon, Royal Devon and Exeter Hospital; Clinical Tutor, Exeter University Postgraduate Medical School, Exeter, Devon, UK

W. Spencer Payne MD
Consultant, Section of Thoracic, Cadiovascular, Vascular and General Surgery, Mayo Clinic and Mayo Foundation; James C. Masson Professor of Surgery, Mayo Medical School, Rochester, Minnesota, USA

F. G. Pearson MD, FRCS(C), FACS
Professor of Surgery, University of Toronto; Surgeon-in-Chief, Toronto General Hospital, Toronto, Ontario, Canada

Melvin R. Platt MD
Clinical Associate Professor and Former Chairman, Division of Cardiothoracic Surgery, Southwestern Medical School, Dallas, Texas, USA

Keith D. Roberts ChM, FRCS
Consultant Paediatric Cardiothoracic Surgeon, The Children's Hospital, Birmingham; Senior Clinical Lecturer in Surgery, University of Birmingham, UK

Sir Keith Ross MS, FRCS
Consultant Cardiac Surgeon, Wessex Cardiac and Thoracic Centre, Southampton General Hospital, Southampton, UK

Colin O. H. Russell FRACS
Prince Henry's Hospital, Melbourne, Australia

Mary P. Shepherd MS, FRCS
Consultant Thoracic Surgeon, Harefield Hospital, Harefield, Middlesex, UK

Lewis Spitz PhD, FRCS
Nuffield Professor of Paediatric Surgery, Institute of Child Health, University of London; Honorary Consultant Paediatric Surgeon, Hospital for Sick Children, Great Ormond Street, London, UK

Rex De L. Stanbridge MRCP, FRCS
Consultant Cardiothoracic Surgeon, St Mary's Hospital, and Hammersmith Hospital, London, UK

M. F. Sturridge MS, FRCS
Consultant Thoracic Surgeon, The Middlesex Hospital, London; Consultant Surgeon, London Chest Hospital; Honorary Consultant Surgeon, The National Hospital for Nervous Diseases, London, UK

Vernon C. Thompson FRCS
Consultant Thoracic Surgeon, The London Hospital and The London Chest Hospital, London, UK

Kjell Thor MD, PhD
Associate Professor of Surgery, Karolinska Institute, Ersta Hospital, Stockholm, Sweden

E. R. Townsend FRCS
Consultant Thoracic Surgeon, North West Thames Regional Health Authority and Oxford Regional Health Authority and Harefield Hospital, Middlesex, UK

J. Kent Trinkle MD
Professor and Head of Cardiothoracic Surgery, University of Texas Health Science Center, San Antonio, USA

Nicolas Velasco MD
Virginia Mason Medical Center, Seattle, Washington, USA

Contributing Medical Artists

Sue Abraham

Leslie Arwin
University of Michigan, Ann Arbor, USA

Peter Drury

Patrick Elliott
Senior Medical Artist, Department of Medical Illustration, Royal Hallamshire Hospital, Glossop Road, Sheffield, UK

Susan W. Evans
3838 Windom Place NW, Washington DC, 20016, USA

Peter Jack
21 Acorn Close, Marchwood, Southampton SO4 7YN, UK

Jenny Halstead
The Red House, 85 Christchurch Road, Reading Berkshire, UK

Barbara Hyams MA, AMI
Medical Illustrator, Poynings, Northchurch Common, Northchurch, Berkhamsted, Hertfordshire, UK

N. Krstić
Artist, Military Medical Academy, Belgrade, Yugoslavia

Robert N. Lane
Medical Illustrator, Studio 19a, Edith Grove, London SW10, UK

Gillian Lee AIMBI, MMAA
Medical Illustrator, 15 Little Plucketts Way, Buckhurst Hill, Essex IG9 5QU, UK

Margot B. Mackay
Medical Illustrator, Department of Art as Applied to Medicine, University of Toronto, Toronto, Ontario, Canada

Kevin Marks
Illustrator, 3 Hilltop Court, Grange Road, Upper Norwood, London SE19 3BQ, UK

John J. Martini

Medical Graphics Department
Mayo Clinic, Rochester, Minnesota, USA

Raith Overhill
61 Arbury Road, Cambridge, UK

Michael P. Schenk MSMI
Clinical Assistant Professor in Biomedical Communications, Southwestern Graduate School of Biomedical Sciences, U.T.H.S.C.D., Dallas, Texas 75235, USA

Lesley Skeates BA(Hon)
Medical Artist, University of Birmingham, UK

Cathy Slater
Medical Illustrator, 16 Gravel Path, Berkhamsted, Hertfordshire, UK

P. Somerset BA
Medical Artist, Wythenshawe Hospital, Manchester, UK

Kathleen E. Sweeney
University of Michigan, Ann Arbor, USA

Christopher Tyrrell

Charles Wood
Biomedical Illustrations, 1117 Minor, Seattle, Washington, USA

Contents

Tribute to John Jackson

Sadly, John Jackson, the senior editor of this volume, did not live to see it published. He had accomplished the preparation of this edition despite the increasing ill-health and pain which required him to undergo numerous operative and therapeutic procedures; his cheerful fortitude during this time was remarkable. The third-edition volume, covering both cardiac and thoracic surgery and this present volume remain as tributes to his editorial capabilities.

To those who knew him personally, however, he will not be remembered solely for his undoubted expertise as a thoracic surgeon. Rather, he will be remembered for the human qualities he possessed and demonstrated to the full — his concern for both patients and junior colleagues, his kindness, sensitivity and generosity, his delightful sense of humour. John Jackson will be sadly missed by all who were fortunate enough to know him — patients, colleagues, and friends.

D. K. C. Cooper

Preface

Those readers familiar with earlier editions of the series 'Operative Surgery' will note a major change in this current (fourth) edition, namely, the division of cardiac and thoracic surgery into two separate volumes. Hitherto, cardiothoracic operations have been described in a single volume – the third edition being edited by my late colleague John Jackson. There has been a tendency for surgeons to concentrate their practices increasingly in either cardiac of thoracic work, and it was felt that the preparation of separate volumes in these two fields would be timely. Though there will be those who deplore this further small step in the division of cardiothoracic surgery into two subspecialties, there will equally be many others who will applaud. Both the general editors and those involved with the preparation of the two volumes hope that the resulting texts will be easier to consult, and will even more adequately satisfy the needs of the reader.

In this particular volume on thoracic surgery, the requirements of the surgeon in training have been to the fore in the minds of the editors and authors, and it is hoped that the text and figures provide clear guidance for those inexperienced in the performance of certain operations.

The arrangement of the chapters, though now confined largely to mediastinal, pulmonary, and oesophageal operative topics, has largely followed that of the previous edition. The more complicated and less common operations follow minor and investigatory procedures in a more or less logical manner so that it should be possible for the reader to locate any one chapter without continual reference to the index. Where possible, each chapter follows the same pattern – an outline of investigations and indications followed by the operation, and finally aspects of postoperative care. All of the operations are well-tried standard procedures, and each surgeon has been encouraged to describe his own method, to include pitfalls and complications, and to mention or describe alternative procedures where appropriate.

Greater attention has been paid to investigatory procedures, and the chapters on rigid and flexible bronchoscopy, bronchography, aspiration of the chest, pleural biopsy and needle biopsy of the lung, mediastinoscopy, and oesophagoscopy, have been considerably expanded. Blunt and penetrating chest trauma has also been given greater attention, as have certain conditions not seen commonly in the United Kingdom or North America, such as pulmonary hydatid cysts.

The international flavour of the contributions has been increased further, and chapters are included from surgeons in the UK, the USA, Canada, South Africa, Yugoslavia and Germany. The text therefore reflects operative techniques practised and accepted worldwide.

D. K. C. Cooper

Congenital diaphragmatic hernia and eventration

Lewis Spitz PhD, FRCS
Nuffield Professor of Paediatric Surgery, Institute of Child Health, University of London;
Honorary Consultant Paediatric Surgeon, The Hospital for Sick Children, Great Ormond Street, London, UK

DIAPHRAGMATIC HERNIA

History

Ambroise Paré reported the first diaphragmatic hernia, which was of traumatic origin, in 1597. In 1848, Vincent Alexander Bochdalek published his description of the congenital diaphragmatic hernia that now bears his name. The defect as described by Bochdalek was a triangular slit between the lumbar portion of the diaphragm and the apex of the twelfth rib. He attributed the herniation to rupture of a previously intact membrane in the lumbocostal triangle.

1a & b

Types of hernia

The various areas in the diaphragm (excluding the oesophageal hiatus) through which hernias may occur are shown.

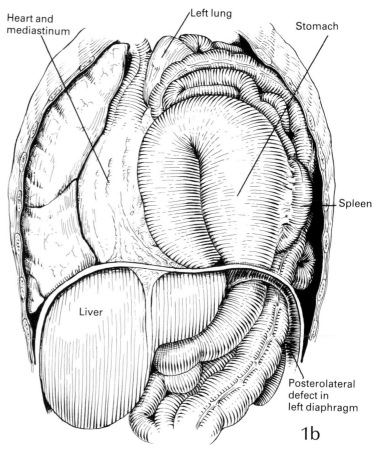

Parasternal (Morgagni) hernia

IVC

Oesophageal hiatus

Aorta

Agenesis of diaphragm (septum transversum defect)

Posterolateral (Bochdalek) hernia

Heart and mediastinum

Left lung

Stomach

Spleen

Liver

Posterolateral defect in left diaphragm

1a

1b

1

Diagnosis

Diaphragmatic hernia through the patent pleuro-peritoneal canal, generally referred to as the foramen of Bochdalek, usually presents as an acute emergency in the neonatal period. The classical diagnostic triad consists of respiratory distress, apparent dextrocardia and a flat 'scaphoid' abdomen. Breath sounds are diminished on the affected side and borborygmi may be auscultated in the chest. The presenting symptoms in cases manifesting at a later stage include recurrent respiratory infections, dyspnoea, especially after meals, and vomiting. The left side is affected in 85–90 per cent of cases. This has been attributed to the later closure of the left pleuroperitoneal canal during the eighth week of intrauterine development. Bilateral hernias are rare.

2

A chest radiograph, which should always include the abdomen, is usually diagnostic. The affected hemithorax is filled with gas-containing loops of intestine, the mediastinum is displaced to the opposite side, and there is a decrease in the amount of intraperitoneal intestinal gas shadows.

The presence of a normal intestinal gas configuration with an apparently intact diaphragm is suspicious of congenital lobar emphysema or adenoid cystic malformation of the lung. Contrast studies of the gastrointestinal tract may be required to differentiate these two primary pulmonary conditions from a true diaphragmatic hernia.

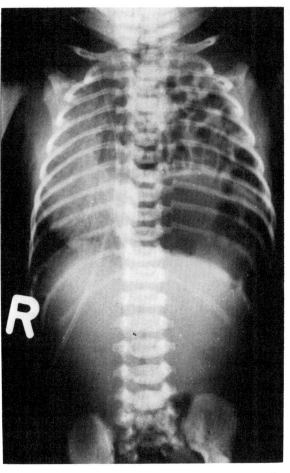

2

Resuscitative measures

As soon as the diagnosis is suspected, a large calibre (No. 10 gauge) nasogastric tube should be introduced into the stomach and all swallowed contents evacuated. The infant is nursed in 100 per cent oxygen and if this fails to improve the respiratory embarrassment, ventilatory assistance is administered via an endotracheal tube. Ventilation with a face mask is strictly contraindicated as this forces air into the stomach and intestines, further embarrassing the respiration. Sudden deterioration during resuscitation may be due to a tension pneumothorax. This is relieved by inserting a hypodermic needle (No. 21 gauge) into the affected pleural space. An intercostal drain with underwater seal can then be formally introduced in a relatively stable patient. Correction of acidosis should be attempted with extreme caution.

Transportation

Where possible, transfer of the infant to a paediatric surgical centre should be carried out promptly while all resuscitative measures continue. This implies attendance by experienced medical and nursing personnel ensuring as far as possible that the infant remains normothermic and adequately oxygenated and that the intestines remain decompressed.

Anaesthesia

This consists of standard neonatal anaesthesia with preoxygenation and awake endotracheal intubation (if this was not required during resuscitation) followed by hand ventilation with an Ayre's T-piece. Gentle ventilation, using inspiratory pressures of up to 25 cm H_2O with 5 cm H_2O end-respiratory pressure to maintain the functional residual capacity, is maintained throughout the operative period. Monitoring of electrocardiogram, core temperature (rectal probe), central venous and arterial pressures, blood gases and blood loss is carried out intraoperatively.

The operation

The incision

The abdominal approach is preferred for all left-sided congenital posterolateral diaphragmatic hernias. Correction of the associated intestinal malrotation and enlargement of the peritoneal cavity to accommodate the displaced viscera are more easily achieved through an abdominal incision.

A transthoracic approach may be used for the right-sided hernia where liver may be the only contents, or for recurrent hernias where adhesions prevent simple reduction of the herniated contents.

3

The abdominal approach is via a left upper abdominal transverse muscle-cutting (or alternatively a left oblique subcostal) incision placed 2 cm above the umbilical cord and extending from the midline to the tip of ninth costal cartilage.

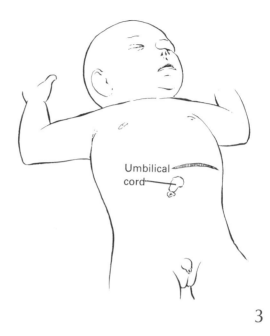

3

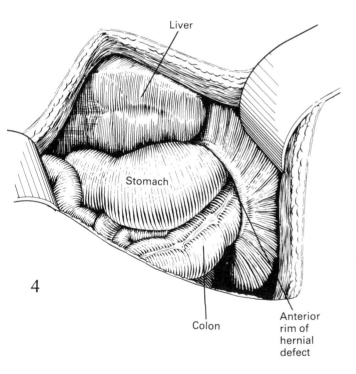

4

4

Exposure of the diaphragmatic defect

The cranial part of the wound is retracted upwards to reveal the anterior well-muscularized diaphragm and the posteriorly located defect through which most of the abdominal viscera have herniated into the pleural cavity. The peritoneal cavity is relatively empty.

5

Definition of the diaphragmatic defect

The herniated contents, which may include the entire small intestine together with a variable amount of the right colon, stomach, spleen and left lobe of liver, are gently withdrawn. The anterior rim of the defect is usually well defined and easily identifiable. The posterior rim is frequently adherent to the posterior abdominal wall in close proximity to the left adrenal and kidney. Occasionally the posterior rim is completely deficient but more commonly it gradually fades out laterally, where the margin of the defect merges with the chest wall.

Exposure of the margins of the defect may be facilitated by retracting the left lobe of the liver medially after dividing the left triangular ligament. A careful search is now made for a sac which is present in 10–15 per cent of cases. The sac may be extremely thin and closely applied to the pleura. The sac should be excised up to the margins of the diaphragmatic defect. A plastic drainage tube is inserted into the pleural cavity via the ninth intercostal space in the mid-axillary line. Some surgeons prefer not to drain the pleural space; others prophylactically insert catheters into both sides of the chest.

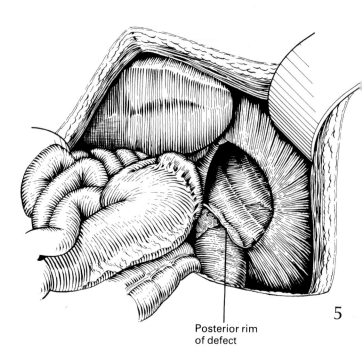

5

Posterior rim
of defect

Repair of the defect

The hernial orifice is closed in two layers by approximating the margins of the defect with interrupted non-absorbable suture material (2/0 or 3/0 silk or braided polyamine).

6

The first row consists of horizontal mattress sutures inserted 5 mm from the edge of the defect.

6

7

The second row approximates the everted rim.

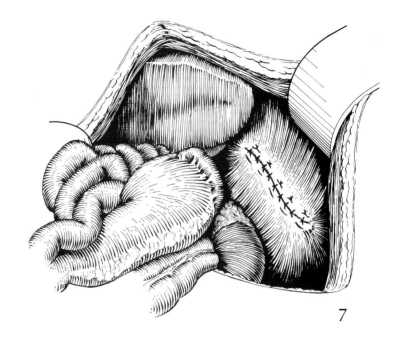

7

Where the posterior rim is partially or totally absent, the sutures should be placed around the adjacent rib to achieve a secure repair. Direct apposition of the hernial margins is occasionally impossible. In these cases the defect is best closed with a prosthetic patch (Dacron, Teflon). Alternatively a flap of anterior abdominal wall may be rotated into the opening and sutured in position.

Additional manoeuvres

The intestinal malrotation is corrected by dividing abnormal bands and splaying the root of the mesentery. The duodenal loop is straightened, and the small intestine placed in the right side of the abdomen with the caecum in the left upper quadrant. The peritoneal cavity is enlarged by forcibly stretching the muscles of the anterior abdominal wall.

Closure of the abdomen

The abdominal incision is closed *en masse* or in layers with 3/0 polyglycolic acid sutures. A subcuticular 4/0 polyglycolic acid suture approximates the skin edges. In the very rare case closure of the abdominal wall cannot be achieved without profound tension which will further embarrass respiration. In these cases the establishment of a ventral hernia or accommodation of the intestine temporarily in a pouch fashioned with Silastic sheeting may be required.

The intercostal drain is connected to an underwater seal with 2–3 cm H_2O of negative pressure. We prefer to clamp the drainage tube, releasing it for a short period only every 6 hours. This manoeuvre allows gentle expansion of the ipsilateral lung while extreme to-and-fro shifting of the mediastinum is prevented. The intercostal drain is removed when full expansion of the lung has occurred or when a stable state has been achieved. No attempt at rapid re-expansion of the lung should be made.

Postoperative care

All neonates presenting within 12 hours of birth are electively ventilated postoperatively. Monitoring consists of electrocardiogram, temperature, central venous pressure (via internal jugular vein catheter) and arterial pressure (via the right radial artery). Transcutaneous arterial P_{O_2} is measured in the upper part of the abdomen to give an early indication of ductal shunting of blood arising from increased pulmonary vascular resistance.

Fifteen per cent of infants are at risk of developing a transitional circulation (right-to-left shunting at ductal and atrial level) due to the pulmonary vascular resistance rising above systemic pressures. Such patients may respond dramatically to pulmonary vasodilators (e.g. tolazoline 1–2 mg/kg bodyweight per hour as an intravenous infusion). Dopamine (5–15 µg/kg/min) may be required in addition to improve the systemic circulation by its direct inotropic effect. Owing to the vasodilatory effects of both these drugs, large volumes of plasma expanders may be required. These requirements are best assessed by monitoring the central venous pressure.

Weaning of the infant from ventilatory assistance is accomplished slowly using intermittent mandatory ventilation once cardiopulmonary stability has been achieved. Prolonged ileus, particularly in the infant requiring ventilatory support, may indicate the need for parenteral nutrition for a variable period during the postoperative course.

Results

The mortality rate is directly proportional to the degree of pulmonary hypoplasia. Infants presenting within 6–12 hours of birth usually have advanced pulmonary hypoplasia, whereas those infants in whom the diagnosis is not evident before 12–24 hours have little impairment of pulmonary development. The survival rate for infants presenting within 12 hours of birth is between 45–60 per cent, while few deaths should occur in infants older than 12 hours at the time of diagnosis. At the Hospital for Sick Children, London, 92 infants with diaphragmatic hernia were treated between 1979 and 1981. The overall survival rate was 74 per cent (68 infants). All the deaths, 24 cases, occurred in those infants presenting within 6 hours of birth (overall survival rate in this group 61 per cent, i.e. 37 of 61 patients).

EVENTRATION OF THE DIAPHRAGM

This refers to an abnormally high position of one or both leaflets of the intact diaphragm as a result of paralysis, hypoplasia or atrophy of the muscle fibres. It is poorly tolerated by the young infant especially if bilateral. If there is a possibility that the damage to the phrenic nerve is reversible, the condition can be successfully managed with continuous positive airway pressure ventilation for a period of 4–6 weeks. Where the phrenic nerve injury is thought to be permanent or where there is a relapse following a trial of conservative management, surgery is recommended. The aim of surgery in eventration is to fix the paralysed diaphragm in the inspiratory position, thereby minimizing paradoxical movement and preventing shift of the mediastinum with respiration.

The operation

The incision

A thoracic or abdominal approach may be used. In bilateral eventration, an upper abdominal transverse muscle-cutting incision is performed, while in unilateral cases, especially when the right hemidiaphragm is involved, a thoracic approach affords easier access and allows identification of the branches of the phrenic nerve. The lateral thoracotomy is via the unresected bed of the eighth rib.

8

Exposure of the diaphragm

The inferior pulmonary ligament is divided and the distribution of the branches of the phrenic nerve defined.

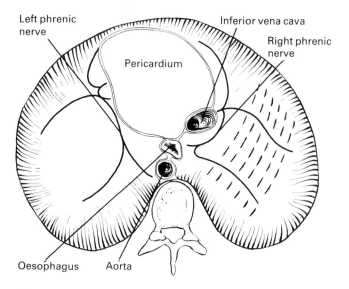

Left phrenic nerve · Inferior vena cava · Right phrenic nerve · Pericardium · Oesophagus · Aorta

9–11

Technique of plication

Four to six rows of 2/0 or 3/0 non-absorbable sutures (silk or braided polyamine) are inserted into the diaphragm from anterolateral to posteromedial. Each row comprises five to six pleats, avoiding the branches of the phrenic nerve. The suture should not pass through the full thickness of the diaphragm as underlying adjacent viscera may be traumatized. The sutures are left untied until all the rows are in position.

An intercostal drain with underwater seal may be inserted and removed when full expansion of the lung has been shown to have occurred. No special postoperative measures are necessary. Recovery is rapid and uneventful and complications rarely occur.

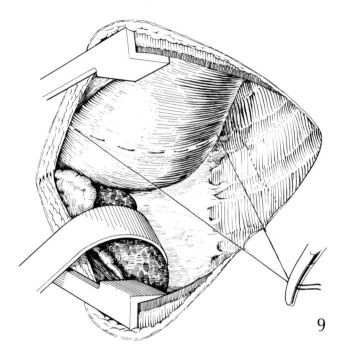

9

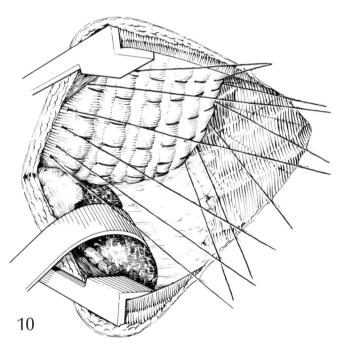

10

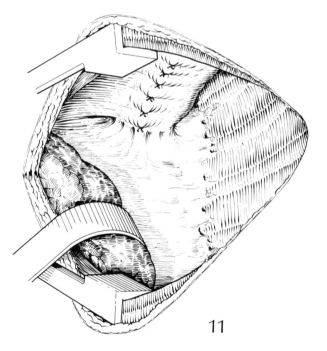

11

Further reading

Bloss, R. S., Aranda, J. V., Beardmore, H. E. Congenital diaphragmatic hernia: pathophysiology and pharmacologic support. Surgery 1981; 89: 518–524

Carter, R. E. B., Waterston, D. J., Aberdeen, E. Hernia and eventration of the diaphragm in childhood. Lancet 1962; 1: 656–659

Haller, J. A., Pickard, L. R., Tepas, J. J., Rogers, M. C., Robotham, J. L., Shorter, N., Shermata, D. W. Management of diaphragmatic paralysis in infants with special emphasis on selection of patients for operative plication. Journal of Pediatric Surgery 1979; 14: 779–785

Schwartz, M. Z., Filler, R. M. Plication of the diaphragm for symptomatic phrenic nerve paralysis. Journal of Pediatric Surgery 1978; 13: 259–263

Sumner, E., Frank, J. D. Tolazoline in the treatment of congenital diaphragmatic hernia. Archives of Diseases in Childhood 1981; 56: 350–353

Pectus excavatum

I. K. R. McMillan   FRCS
Thoracic Surgeon, Wessex Regional Cardiothoracic Unit, Southampton General Hospital, and
Southampton University Hospitals, Southampton, UK

Preoperative

Indications

1a & b

Pectus excavatum (funnel chest) presents with a varying degree of depression of the sternum and costal cartilages in the front of the chest, and is usually associated with kyphotic posture and a protruberant abdomen.

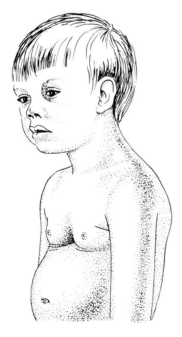

1a

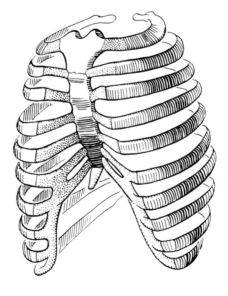

1b

This is a fairly common deformity, but in many patients it is so mild as not to warrant any operative procedure. Operation is only undertaken in patients in whom there is adequate reason. In spite of the degree of deformity, which may be associated with considerable shift of the heart to the left, relatively few patients have obvious respiratory embarrassment. The deformity may be brought to light by the occurrence of an associated infection, such as enlarged adenoids in infants which decrease the airway, or by abdominal space-occupying conditions such as pregnancy, and these may be enough to tip the patient over into respiratory difficulty. There are cases where the deformity is sufficiently gross to produce respiratory difficulty on its own, as evidenced by a decrease in exercise tolerance. It is, however, true that many patients claim very considerable subjective improvement after operation, and the mothers of children, in particular, claim that they suffer from fewer respiratory infections and recover from these more quickly than before the operation. Many patients remark how their chests felt tight before the operation, but they experience a feeling of freedom postoperatively.

Cardiorespiratory embarrassment is very rare but again does occur occasionally, and these patients usually have an outflow systolic murmur and minor ECG changes.

The deformity is congenital and is usually first noted in infancy, when it tends to be relatively mild, but it is nearly always progressive. If the deformity is deep, or if the patient has any respiratory disturbance, or after observation over a period of months the deformity is obviously progressing, then operation at any age can be advised. In the normal course of events, it is best to watch the child and, in severe deformities, to carry out the operation ideally at age 3–4 years before the child goes to school. However, many children are not referred until after they have reached school age and there is no difficulty in operating on the patient at any age up until the early 20s. The majority of patients therefore fall into the age range of 3–18 years and only rarely is operation required in adults. Whatever the age of the patient at the time of operation, the principles and technique are the same, except that fixation in infants may be modified.

The deformity is the common presenting symptom, the parents saying that their child, in particular boys, gets severely teased by his fellows at school, and this tends to make the child withdrawn and uncooperative. One of the most satisfying results of the operation is to find, once the deformity is corrected, that the child becomes very much more open and active and takes part in school life, like any other normal child.

The indications for operation are, therefore, the presence of a severe deformity which is causing disturbance to the patient, and, in the case of young children, to their parents, and the firm desire on the part of the patient or the parents that this should be corrected after the matter has been carefully explained to them. The operation must be regarded in most cases as being purely cosmetic and, therefore, no mortality is acceptable. A second, and rare indication is for the correction of physiological disturbance, mainly respiratory.

Contraindications

If the patient is otherwise fit, there is no contraindication to operation except in cases of Marfan's syndrome, where the correction of the deformity must be balanced against future prognosis and need for cardiac surgery.

Choice of technique

Operations have been devised for the correction of pectus excavatum for the last 50 years, but all modern techniques are based largely on the pioneer work of Ravitch[1] who established the principles on which this operation should be carried out.

The object of the operation is to correct the deformity and this means resection of the abnormal costal cartilages and maintaining the sternum in a corrected and normal position. Failure to disconnect the costal cartilages and, more importantly, the perichondrium from the sternum will result in recurrence. External fixation of the sternum is difficult and unnecessary; either an autoplastic method or metal fixation with bars or pins is employed.

Earlier results in our unit using the original Ravitch technique[2] without metallic fixation resulted in a high incidence of recurrence[3]; so, for the last 20 years, we have used a metal strut for fixation of the sternum[4]. A suitable strut of the right size can be employed in any patient aged 3–30 years. In infants it is sometimes technically difficult to use this form of fixation and, if freeing of the costal cartilages to the sternum is not sufficient, then fixation with wire or a pin vertically through the sternum is usually adequate.

Anaesthesia

As the patients are all fit, anaesthesia presents no special problems. The operation is done under general anaesthesia; endotracheal intubation and control of respiration is the usual technique employed.

The operation

Position of patient

The patient is placed supine and the surgeon stands on the right-hand side of the patient to carry out the incision and resect the costal cartilages. As in thyroid surgery, changing to the left side may make operating easier on this side.

The incision

2a & b

The incision in adults is midline and vertical from the second costal cartilage downwards, extending over the xiphoid into the epigastrium (a). In a smaller deformity it may be possible to start a little lower down, but in high deformities a better scar can be produced by curving the top few centimetres or so to the right or left, so enabling the patient to wear a 'V' neck without the scar showing. It can also be bowed a little way to the left or right as it comes down over the sternum so that in thin people the skin scar is not directly over the sternum. In girls, a transverse submammary incision may be used (b) but this necessitates mobilization of the skin flaps separately from the underlying muscle and is therefore more likely to present problems in skin healing, particularly in the centre of the incision, as the vascular supply to the edge of the upper flap may not be as satisfactory. Many surgeons prefer the transverse incision, but this is a matter of personal choice.

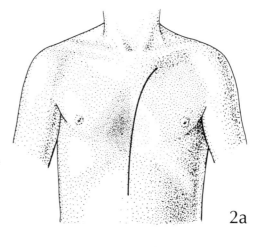

2a

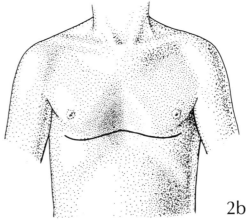

2b

Exposure of costal cartilages

3

Vertical incision

The incision is made straight down to the midline of the sternum, and the flaps are then dissected laterally to include skin, subcutaneous tissue and muscle in one piece so as to expose the sternum and the whole of the costal cartilages on each side, until the front ends of ribs are visible. Care should be taken when doing this to secure the perforating branches of the internal mammary artery. At the lower end it is necessary to open the sheath of the rectus abdominis muscle and free part of this muscle so that all of the cartilages down to the costal margin are visible. The upper cartilages are exposed to the level of the first apparently 'normal' cartilage, but not above the second.

Transverse incision

The same technique is employed after the skin flaps have been raised, the pectoralis major muscle being dealt with separately.

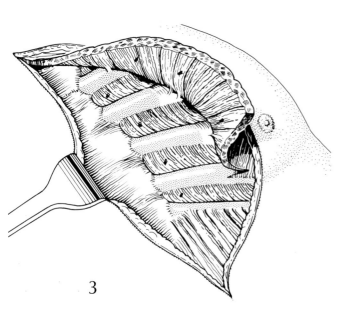

3

4

Resection of deformed costal cartilages

There are many ways of doing this, but it is easiest to make an incision along the length of the costal cartilage through the perichondrium with a scalpel or diathermy. The perichondrium can then be separated from the costal cartilage with a periosteal elevator. When the costal cartilage is free over the whole of the abnormal curvature, the cartilages are divided laterally and this may be at the costochondral junction. Next, a large towel clip is applied to the cartilage and, as the assistant pulls it upwards and medially, the posterior perichondrium can be gently stripped from the costal cartilage. When the cartilage is free it is divided at the sternocostal joint with a knife and removed.

All the abnormal cartilages on each side, usually the third to the seventh, are dealt with in this way. The second costal cartilage is seldom involved and, in the author's experience, it never needs to be resected. Thus, all the abnormal costal cartilages will have been removed from the sternum laterally. As perichondrium is difficult to strip in older patients, it may only be possible to leave a posterior strip in these cases.

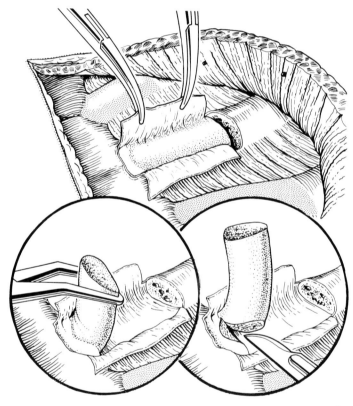

4

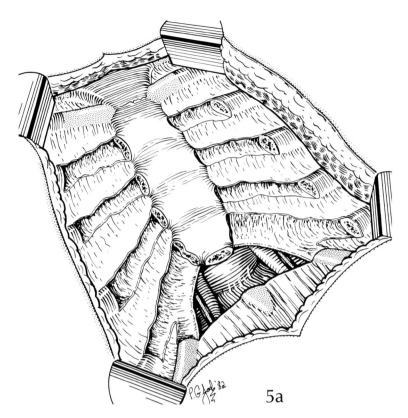

5a

5a & b

Division of the xiphoid process

The xiphoid process is separated from the sternum and usually removed, to stop the pull of the rectus abdominis muscle on the sternum, which is thought to be one of the possible causes of this deformity. The internal mammary artery divides to become the superior epigastric and musculophrenic arteries which, at this point, should be looked for and avoided or, if necessary, ligated and divided.

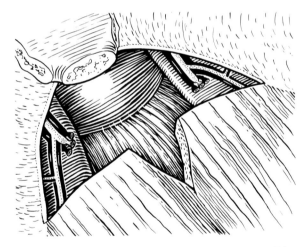

5b

Freeing the sternum

6

Once the xiphoid has been removed, a finger can be inserted into the anterior mediastinum and the retrosternal space mobilized upwards as far as is necessary, so that the whole of the back of the sternum can be freed to the point where the sternal osteotomy will be performed. This maneouvre allows the pleura to retract laterally on each side. The pleura should not normally be opened.

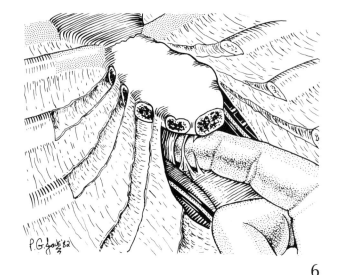

6

7

The sternum is now freed by dividing the perichondrium and the intercostal muscles of the sternochondral junction on each side to the level of the proposed osteotomy. Care should be taken to avoid damaging the internal mammary arteries and some bleeding from small side branches can usually be controlled by diathermy coagulation. If the main artery on one side is damaged, it may be ligated without undue worry, but it is preferable to leave both arteries.

Occasionally an artery will be found entering directly into the back of the body of the sternum and, if this is so, should be carefully preserved. Sternal vessels come from the internal mammary arteries.

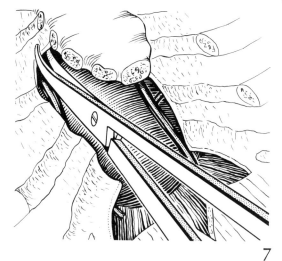

7

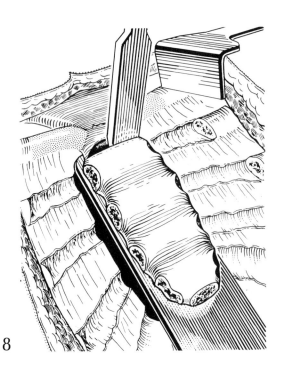

8

8

Sternal osteotomy

In most cases the manubrium is normal so the position of the osteotomy depends on where the deformity of the body of the sternum commences; this is usually at the level of the third costal cartilage, where the posterior bend of the sternum begins. A partial wedge osteotomy is carried out by dividing, with a chisel, the periosteum and anterior table of the sternum transversely below the lowest normal costal cartilage. The posterior periosteum should be left intact. The sternum can now be hinged forwards to the corrected position.

9

Insertion of metal strut and fixation of sternum

The metal strut is placed behind the sternum to lie comfortably on the ribs laterally, so that it maintains the correct position of the sternum by counterpressure on the ribs. To achieve this the strut must have been carefully moulded to fit the curve of the ribs laterally. In the middle it is concave so that it lies comfortably behind the sternum and is maintained in a normal anatomical position.

Great care must be taken to ensure that the strut lies comfortably under the pectoral muscles on each side and in front of the ribs, without protruding under the skin laterally. It may take a considerable amount of adjustment using orthopaedic bar benders to get the curve exactly right. The sternum, ribs and bar must lie in a good position so that no outward sign is visible at the end of the operation. The bar has a notch at each end and once the best position has been achieved these are fixed by a catgut stitch (No. 2 chromic) to the ribs or periosteum on each side as illustrated. This position will become firm after a few weeks, once a fibrous pocket has developed around the bar. Additional fixation may be achieved by passing a catgut suture around the bar and through the sternum on one or both sides. It does not matter if the bar is not perfectly horizontal as long as the position of the bony skeleton is good.

Very occasionally, in adults with a large, shallow deformity, it may be necessary to use two bars and these are inserted in exactly the same way.

In infants it may not be possible to use a strut and in these cases we employ a Kirschner wire driven up the centre of the body of the sternum across the oesteotomy and into the upper fragment. This is not a satisfactory procedure in older children and adults.

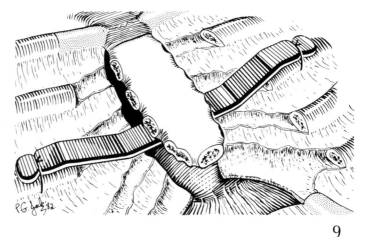

9

The strut can be left in indefinitely, but, in our experience and practice, removal of the bar at the end of a year to 18 months, when the correction is firm and will not recur, is easily accomplished by a small lateral incision. This seems to us more desirable than leaving a strut or pin indefinitely.

Drainage

At this stage of the operation it is important to check meticulously for haemostasis in the retrosternal space and along the internal mammary vessels. It is necessary to drain the retrosternal space, where fluid invariably collects. A retrosternal vacuum drain is placed behind the sternum through a separate small stab incision in the epigastrium; if the pleura has been opened, it is safer to use an intercostal drain as well.

Meticulous haemostasis before closure of the wound is vital to avoid haematomas or fluid collecting, which will prejudice wound healing.

10

Closure

Once the position of the sternum and bar is deemed satisfactory, the pectoralis muscles are sutured together in the midline with No. 1 chromic catgut, so as to provide muscle cover over the front of the sternum. At the lower end this is more difficult owing to the freeing of the rectus abdominis muscle. One of the advantages of using the retrosternal strut is that the rectus muscle can be reattached to the lower costal cartilages or to any adjacent muscle and the chest wall, provided the xiphisternum is not reattached, thus filling this rather awkward gap. The subcutaneous tissues, if thick, should be carefully sutured to avoid any pockets and finally the skin should be very carefully sutured with interrupted non-absorbable sutures. Great care should be taken during this final part of the operation as it is essential to obtain good wound healing in this difficult area, made more difficult by forward pressure of the corrected sternum on the skin.

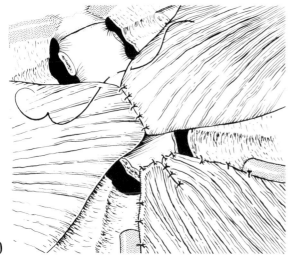

10

Postoperative care

Once the operation is completed it is very important to avoid any lateral pull on the skin incision, and we find that putting two lengths of elastic strapping over the sides of the chest and drawing the skin from the side towards the midline to produce some loose skin in the middle in the region of the incision, and holding it in place for 2–3 days, helps wound healing.

The wound should be watched carefully and if there is any evidence of fluid collection, either subcutaneously or deep to the sternum, it should be aspirated immediately as this may delay wound healing.

A chest X-ray is taken postoperatively to exclude a pneumothorax or effusion and to check the bar position. The drainage tube is normally removed in 24 hours.

The patient can sit up as soon as sufficiently recovered from the anaesthetic and should be encouraged to get out of bed the following day.

There is usually no need for blood transfusion in children, but blood should be available, as in larger teenagers or young adults it may be necessary.

The skin stitches are removed after 8–10 days and, if the wound is satisfactory, the patient is allowed home, being warned to take care to avoid any undue risk of trauma to the front of the chest for the first month.

The patient should be X-rayed at least twice before leaving the hospital to make sure that the bar position remains constant, and is usually seen a month after discharge. By this time most children are able to return to school.

During the time the retrosternal strut is left in, for about a year, patients may live an entirely normal life and normally do not complain of its presence at all, but they are advised to avoid contact sport because of the small risk of a blow on the bar. The patient returns at the end of a year, either as a day case or for overnight stay, and the bar is removed through a 13 mm incision over whichever end is most easily palpable. It can be simply pulled out of its sheath and, from then on, no further treatment is required.

With strut fixation, as the repair is firm, no patient has had any respiratory trouble from paradox and postoperative morbidity has been minimal.

Keloid scars are an annoying complication and may take time to resolve.

Conclusion

In out experience, recurrence is extremely rare with this method of fixation and in the last 200 cases we have only seen 1 case where reoperation was needed. This was in a girl who had her bar removed at 4 months rather than after the full year. There is no contraindication to reoperation.

Even though it is not always possible to achieve a perfect result, and the surgeon may wish he could have done better, the patients themselves are often most grateful for what has been achieved.

References

1. Ravitch, M. M. Congenital deformities on the chest wall and their operative correction. Philadelphia: W. B. Saunders, 1977

2. Chin, E. F. Surgery of funnel chest and congenital sternal prominences. British Journal of Surgery 1957; 44: 360–376

3. Moghissi, K. Long-term results of surgical correction of pectus excavatum and sternal prominence. Thorax 1964; 19: 350–354

4. McMillan, I. K. R. Surgical correction of pectus excavatum and pectus carinatum. In: Williams, W. G., Smith, R. E. eds. Oesophageal and other thoracic problems. Bristol: John Wright and Sons, 1982: 46–64

Pectus carinatum

I. K. R. McMillan   FRCS
Thoracic Surgeon, Wessex Regional Cardiothoracic Unit, Southampton General Hospital, and
Southampton University Hospitals, Southampton, UK

Introduction

1

Pectus carinatum (pigeon chest) is a much more variable deformity than pectus excavatum, and, while it would seem that the principal disturbance is due to the sternum, in practice it is much more commonly due to the congenital deformity of the costal cartilages on either side of the sternum. The sternum is secondarily moved forward as a result of this, giving the classic prominence that is often associated with a tilt backwards of the lower end of the sternum and xiphoid.

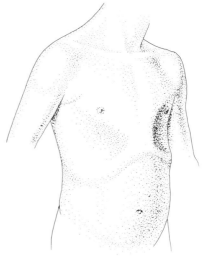

1

2a & b

While the deformity is classically a bilateral one (a), and associated with well-developed bilateral Harrison's sulci, frequently it can be a unilateral deformity (b) which leads secondarily to a prominent sternum which is also tilted upwards towards the side of maximum protuberance of the costal cartilages. Every operation on pectus carinatum must therefore be planned to meet the particular circumstances. There is no one guideline to be followed.

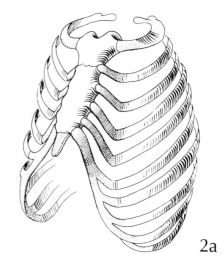

2a

Pectus carinatum is also associated with other congenital abnormalities, notably absence of the pectoralis major, on one or other side, and with unequal development of the two sides of the chest, or even of the body as a whole. So, again, the amount of surgery required has to be guided by this, as the deformity may be more prominent simply because of absence of structures on the opposite side to the maximum protuberance.

The reasons for surgery in this condition are nearly always cosmetic: the patient dislikes his appearance, is often extremely embarrassed by it, and is unwilling to appear with a bare chest. It is therefore not so likely to cause trouble in infants and young children. Patients tend to appear complaining of this deformity in later childhood and particularly in the second decade of life. Respiratory embarrassment is virtually unknown in this condition unless it coincides with other respiratory disease, such as asthma. Therefore, the justification for surgery is purely on appearance.

However, as in pectus excavatum, many patients complain of a feeling of tightness in the chest and a number of rather vague pains behind the sternum, particularly on exercise. Postoperatively the symptoms disappear entirely and patients are more active afterwards, claiming that their exercise tolerance has increased. They tend to be extremely satisfied with the results of surgery. It must be emphasized however, that, owing to the variability of the deformity – which can be very severe – it is not always possible to achieve a perfect correction. Removal of the main protuberance usually produces such an improvement in the patient's appearance that he will be satisfied, even if the surgeon himself is not entirely pleased with the end-result.

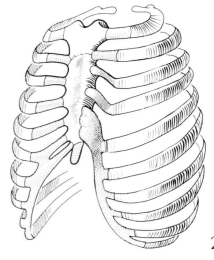

2b

The operation

The incision

A vertical incision over the midline usually provides the best exposure for this condition, as in pectus excavatum. However, if it is decided beforehand that the condition is unilateral and that the sternum does not need to be mobilized, the incision can be carried laterally and over the maximum protuberance. This has the advantage of better healing, as the incision will then be over the muscle rather than the sternum itself.

Occasionally a transverse incision can be used where the protuberance is localized to the lower end, but, in our experience, this is not common. As the protuberance is removed and the sternum transposed backwards in this operation, there is no need for the insertion of struts or pins, and there is less tension on the skin. Usually there is no problem with healing of the sternal wound. The upper end can also be curved laterally, as in the pectus excavatum incision, to provide the patient with a scar-free 'V' neck area.

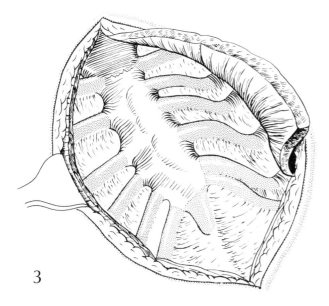

3

Reflection of muscles

3

The incision is carried down to the muscles. These are reflected laterally off the costal cartilages, as in the operation for pectus excavatum (see chapter on 'Pectus excavatum', pp. 9–16). The upper ends of the recti abdominis are also freed and reflected inferiorly to expose, as in the previous operation, the whole of the affected portion of the sternum and the costal cartilages. Even if it is only planned to do one side, it is better to expose the whole area. The deformity of the sternum may be much more obvious once this dissection is completed, and it will enable the sternum to be dealt with without any further trouble.

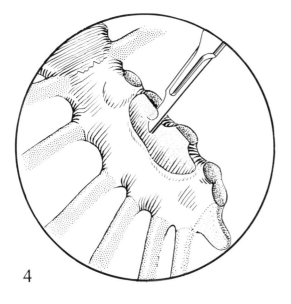

4

4

Resection of the cartilages

The deformed costal cartilages are resected subperichondrially, as in the pectus excavatum operation. There is no need to remove the whole cartilage; only as much as necessary to enable the forward bulge to be removed and for the cartilage to lie in good position in relation to the sternum.

Resection of the cartilage nearly always needs to be carried right up to the sternum. Even if the sternum does not need correcting, there may well be protuberances at the sternochondral junction which can almost always be shaved off with a chisel, taking part of the anterior table of the sternum, in order to achieve a flat, smooth anterior surface to the sternum.

Correction of the sternum

If the sternum can be corrected by the previous simple manoeuvres, no further action is required. However, in the severest deformities, where the sternum is angulating sharply forwards and, in particular, when it is angled upwards to the side of the deformity, it is best to carry out an anterior osteotomy (*see* chapter on 'Pectus excavatum', pp. 9–16), to replace the sternum in the normal position. This is carried out in precisely the same way, but does not need a strut to maintain its position. As the sternum has to be freed to carry out this manoeuvre, obviously the perichondrium has to be divided on each side of the sternum as before, but it can be resutured at the end of the procedure before the closure.

In our experience, in both pectus excavatum and pectus carinatum, if the perichondrium is left lying in the right place, there is no need for reattachment as this appears to occur quite rapidly on its own. In neither condition have we had any trouble with paradoxical chest movement and, in the course of a few weeks, the chest wall is completely firm. This is confirmed by the occasional case where reoperation may be required. If the distal end of the sternum is angulated very sharply backwards, then a further wedge osteotomy may be made at this level and maintained with mattress sutures between the upper and lower fragments.

Closure

5

Once the sternum has been correctly placed and, if required, the perichondrium resutured, the closure will be the same as for the pectus excavatum in that the muscles are apposed with interrupted catgut stitches in front of the sternum. The rectus abdominis muscle tends to keep the deformity corrected.

The subcutaneous skin layers are very carefully closed, maintaining careful haemostasis and using interrupted sutures, particularly fine ones to the skin.

There is normally no need for drainage except in large adults and if the wound appears to be rather oozy afterwards. Transfusion is not usually required. Of course, if the pleura has been opened on either side, and if it cannot be sutured at the time of operation, it should be left open and an intercostal drain inserted. Routine postoperative chest X-ray should be taken to make sure there is no residual pneumothorax.

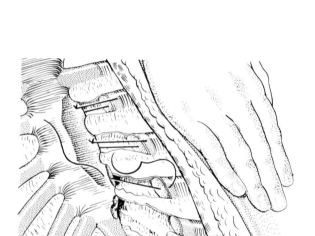

5

Postoperative care

6

As the chest wall has some mobility postoperatively and is not fixed by a strut, the patient is nursed supine for the first 48 hours. A sandbag placed longitudinally on the front of the chest provides sufficient downward pressure to maintain the correction and is well tolerated by the patients, causing no respiratory embarrassment. Sandbags should weigh about 0.7 kg (1.5 lb), depending on the size of the patient. Obviously, if a sandbag is too heavy, it can be removed at any time.

At the end of this period the patient is mobilized as quickly as possible. He should be able to return home in 7–9 days and can rapidly resume normal life, but should avoid games of contact for 2–3 months until the correction has become firm.

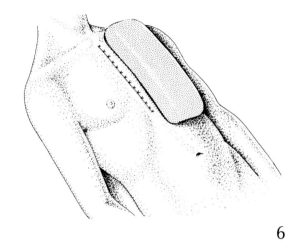

6

Results

The pectus carinatum defect, unlike the pectus excavatum, occasionally involves the second costal cartilage. We do not resect this at the time of operation but if, later, a protuberant residual knob is found at the top or bottom, this can be resected as a minor procedure, if the patient desires it. An overnight stay only is required and further scarring can be avoided by utilizing part of the old incision.

It should not be forgotten that in both pectus excavatum and pectus carinatum a perfect result cannot always be achieved by correcting the bony deformity. In some cases a planned procedure, in conjunction with plastic surgeons, could lead to a more satisfactory end-result. This is particularly true in women with associated maldevelopment of one of the breasts. In severe cases of pectus excavatum the position of the breasts may be so altered that the nipples point inwards towards each other. If these are not corrected by dealing with the bony deformity, plastic surgery can be extremely helpful.

Pre- and postoperative clinical photographs are helpful in assessing results. Pectus carinatum has no recurrence rate except for minor tailoring of residual knobs if they were not sufficiently dealt with at the first operation. There has been no serious morbidity in any of the cases in our series.

Further reading

McMillan, I. K. R. Surgical correction of pectus excavatum and pectus carinatum. In: Williams, W. G., Smith, R. E., eds. Oesophageal and other thoracic problems. Bristol: John Wright and Sons, 1982: 46–64

Ravitch, M. M. Congenital deformities of the chest wall and their operative correction. Philadelphia: W. B. Saunders, 1977

Management of blunt thoracic injuries

J. Kent Trinkle MD
Professor and Head of Cardiothoracic Surgery, University of Texas Health Science Center, San Antonio, Texas, USA

Introduction

In the Western World trauma ranks only behind cardiovascular disease and cancer as a cause of death. For example, in the United States it is the leading cause of death in people under the age of 37 years and claims over 50 000 victims per year. Thoracic injuries are the sole cause of death in 25 per cent of the victims and are a contributory cause in another 50 per cent[1]. Thus, it is important for every physician and surgeon to be familiar with the basic principles of management of the thoracic trauma victim. The initial resuscitation of a patient with a thoracic injury includes attention to the ABCs – Airway, Bleeding and Circulation. Next the vital signs are obtained, a Foley catheter is inserted in the bladder and chest X-rays are obtained. If possible, the X-rays should be taken upright, posteroanterior, and in full inspiration to delineate clearly possible intrathoracic injuries.

Initial monitoring

1

A central venous catheter is inserted via the subclavian vein for pressure monitoring and rapid infusion of intravenous fluids. The patient is placed in a 20° head-down position. The vein is punctured by inserting a 14 gauge needle just inferior to the midpoint of the clavicle and directed toward the suprasternal notch.

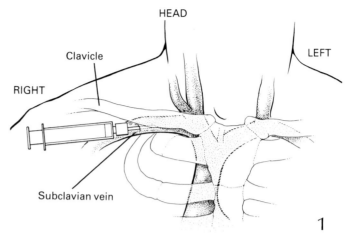

2

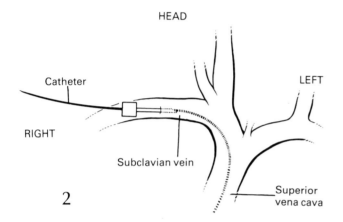

After blood is withdrawn for typing, crossmatching and measurement of haematocrit, a 17 gauge catheter is inserted. The needle is then withdrawn from the vein, leaving the catheter in place.

3

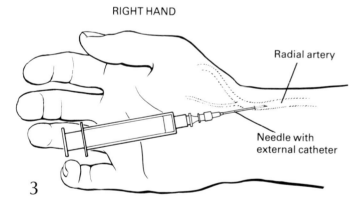

A percutaneous arterial line is established by puncturing the radial artery with a 21 gauge needle with an external plastic sheath catheter.

4

After blood is aspirated, the sheath is advanced into the artery and the needle withdrawn. This line is used for arterial blood gas determinations and pressure monitoring.

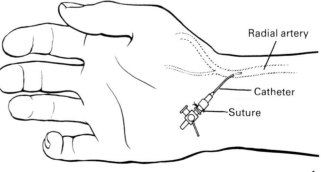

5

In patients who are haemodynamically unstable, a triple lumen Swan-Ganz catheter with a thermodilution probe is inserted. The internal jugular vein is punctured with an 18 gauge needle three finger's breadths above the head of the clavicle at the anterior edge of the sternocleidomastoid muscle.

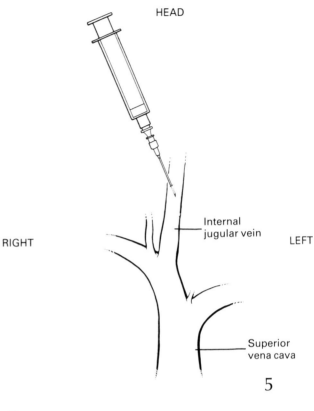

5

6

A guide-wire is threaded into the superior vena cava.

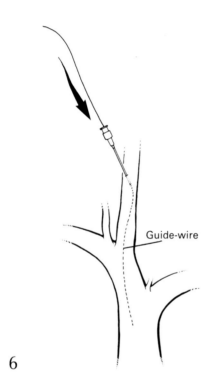

6

7

The skin puncture site is enlarged to about 4 mm with a scalpel. A blunt-tip dilator with an outer hollow sheath is passed over the wire and into the vein for 5 or 6 cm.

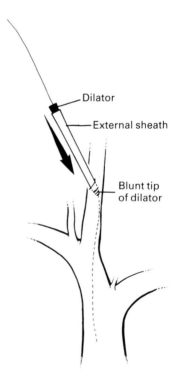

7

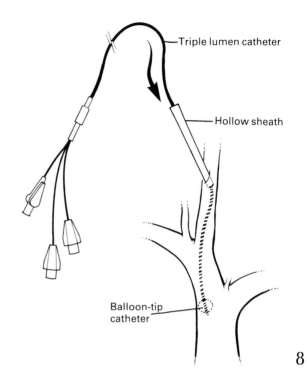

- Triple lumen catheter
- Hollow sheath
- Balloon-tip catheter

8

8

When the dilator is removed a triple lumen, balloon-tip catheter is inserted and passed into the superior vena cava.

CV pressure
PA pressure
Wedge pressure
Cardiac output
Mixed venous O_2

9

9

The balloon is inflated and the catheter is advanced until pulmonary artery pressures are obtained. The balloon is then deflated and advanced a few centimetres until reinflation produces a lower 'wedge' pressure, which reflects the pressure in the pulmonary veins and left atrium.

If respiratory distress is clinically obvious, an endotracheal tube is inserted for mechanical ventilation. An endotracheal tube is quicker and safer than emergency tracheostomy. Our initial ventilator settings for an adult are 12/min, with a tidal volume of 10–12 ml/kg, peak inspiratory pressure of 20 cm H_2O, and 100 per cent oxygen. The settings are changed according to the arterial blood gas determinations. Positive end-expiratory pressure of 5 or 10 cm H_2O may be added if the initial blood gas determinations indicate hypoxaemia.

Tube thoracostomy

Tube thoracostomy is performed in all patients with either a haemothorax or a pneumothorax following blunt chest trauma. Other indications include severe rib fractures in patients requiring mechanical ventilation or general anaesthesia. A large (36 Fr) plastic catheter with multiple holes is inserted into the pleural space in a dependent position. Small rubber tubes should be avoided as they frequently become obstructed.

10

The patient is recumbent with the injured side slightly elevated. The lower ribs are palpated and the insertion site is chosen in the sixth or seventh intercostal space in the posterior axillary line. It is important to place the tube anterior to the latissimus dorsi muscle for ease of insertion and patient comfort. The area is prepared and draped with sterile towels and 1 per cent lignocaine (lidocaine; Xylocaine) is infiltrated into the skin and subcutaneous tissue. Additional local anaesthetic is injected over the periosteum of the ribs and adjacent pleura.

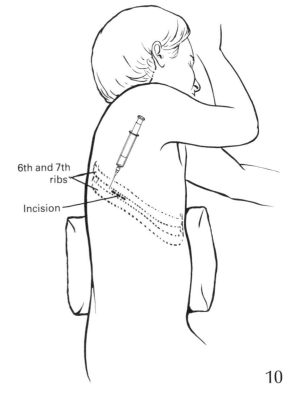

10

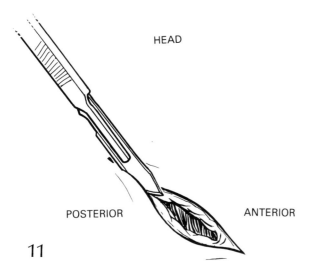

11

11

A 2 cm incision is made through only the skin and subcutaneous tissue.

12

The dissection is carried through the muscles by alternately opening and closing a surgical clamp. The pleura must be penetrated with a sharp 'jab' following which the opening in the muscles and pleura is enlarged by spreading the clamp.

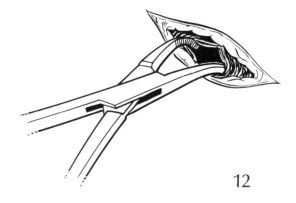

12

13

The physician's finger is inserted to enlarge the hole, break up loculations, and to ascertain that there are no pleural adhesions and that the opening is above the diaphragm.

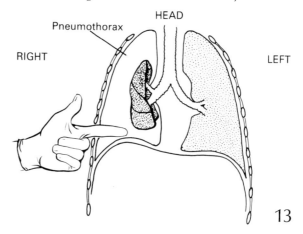

13

14

The clamp is then placed on the end of the tube which is inserted and directed superior and posterior into the pleural cavity.

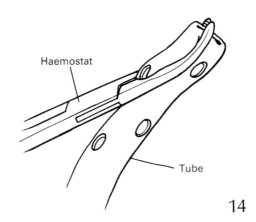

14

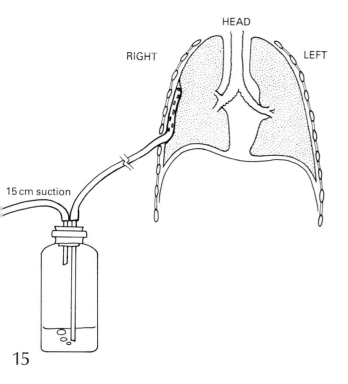

15

15

The tube is advanced until the last hole is inside the pleura and connected to an underwater seal with 15 cm suction.

Usually a single, well-positioned tube will evacuate both blood and air. A second tube is rarely necessary. The tube is then secured to the skin with a large, non-absorbable, horizontal mattress suture.

The initial bloody drainage fluid following tube thoracostomy may be frighteningly large. Bleeding from the lung parenchyma will rapidly decrease as the lung is re-expanded against the parietal pleura. Likewise, large air leaks rapidly decline with pulmonary re-expansion unless there is an underlying tracheobronchial injury. If massive blood loss and air leak continue following lung re-expansion, a thoracotomy may be necessary. Approximately 85 per cent of trauma patients with either a haemo- or pneumothorax can be treated solely by tube thoracostomy[2,3]. The chest tube is left in place until at least 48 hours after the air leak ceases and the drainage is less than 100 ml/day and becomes serosanguinous. Dark drainage fluid indicates residual lysing clot and the tube should be left in place. Occasionally a second large chest tube may be required if all air and blood is not evacuated and the lung is incompletely expanded.

Rib fractures

The so-called 'simple rib fracture' may be life-threatening. There is a 20 per cent mortality rate in the elderly patient with rib fractures as a result of pain and splinting leading to atelectasis and pneumonia[4]. A minimal haemothorax may progress to a large bloody effusion, owing to the high oncotic pressure of lysing clot, and progress to a post-traumatic empyema. Patients at high risk include the elderly and those patients with chronic obstructive pulmonary disease, underlying pulmonary contusion or depressed arterial blood gases.

Pain relief by analgesics and intercostal nerve blocks are important to allow vigorous coughing and deep breathing.

16

For performance of an intercostal nerve block the patient should sit on the side of the bed with the arms pulled forward to rotate the scapula laterally. The skin is infiltrated posteriorly, immediately lateral to the paraspinal muscles, with 1 per cent lignocaine over the neck of each affected rib. Additional pain relief may be obtained by infiltrating the actual fracture site.

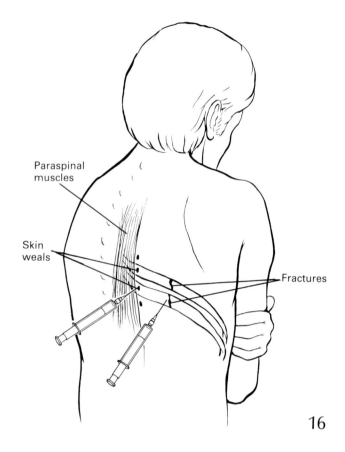

16

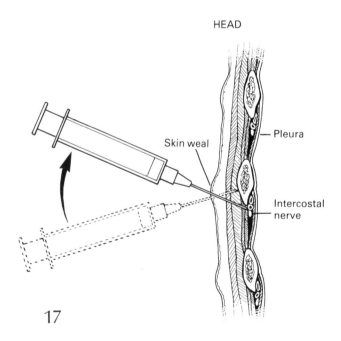

17

17

The needle is advanced until the rib is encountered and further local anaesthetic is injected over the lower edge of the rib to block the intercostal nerve. Even with a short-acting anaesthetic drug such as lignocaine, the pain relief lasts surprisingly long.

18

Nasotracheal suction may be required if the patient is unable to cough and breathe deeply. Neither the patients nor the nurses appreciate this manoeuvre but it has documented therapeutic benefits. The tongue is grasped with the patient sitting. A red rubber catheter is inserted through either nostril and advanced into the larynx until violent coughing paroxysms ensue.

Blow bottles and incentive spirometry are also beneficial. However, the value lies in the fact that the patient must take a deep breath prior to exerting positive pressure. Another technique is to have the patient blow up a balloon. This is particularly well accepted by children. Intermittent positive pressure breathing, on the other hand, has been shown to be worthless in preventing atelectasis and pneumonia. In addition to the exorbitant cost, it has the hazards of gastric dilatation and contamination of the tracheobronchial tree with pathogenic bacteria.

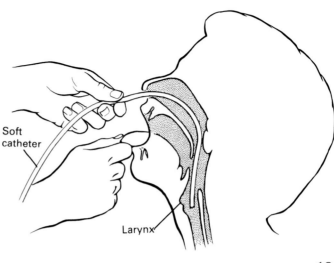

18

Sternal fractures

This injury generally occurs in the driver of a motor vehicle who is not wearing a shoulder harness or seat-belt, and strikes the steering wheel. Owing to the tremendous force required to fracture the sternum, the physician should suspect associated injuries such as myocardial contusion, cardiac chamber rupture, transection of the aorta or its major branches, pulmonary contusion, or haemo/pneumothorax[5].

Most sternal fractures are transverse and the majority occur at the sterno-manubrial joint. These fractures are extremely painful and tender.

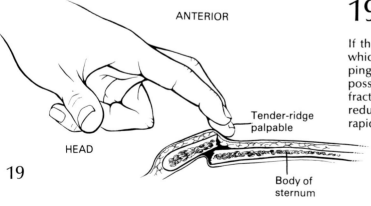

19

If the fracture is displaced there will be a palpable ridge which is exquisitively tender. If the fractures are overlapping, operation is mandatory. Closed reduction is not possible and a painful pseudoarthrosis will develop if the fracture is not realigned. It is best to perform operative reduction within one week following injury owing to the rapid formation of callus.

20

A vertical 10 cm incision is made over the fracture site. Heavy wires are passed through *both* tables of the sternum. Although it is technically easier to use only the outer table, or to screw on a compression plate, this frequently leads to recurrence. The fracture is displaced with a periosteal elevator and a sterile tablespoon is inserted under the proximal segment to catch the needle and prevent injury to the underlying structures.

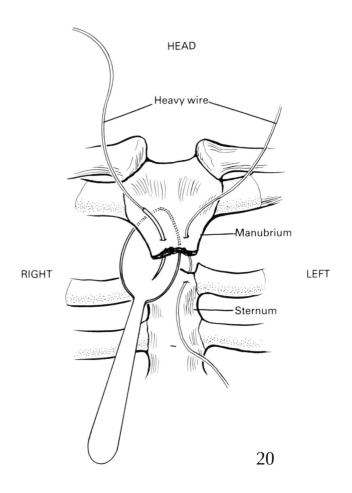

20

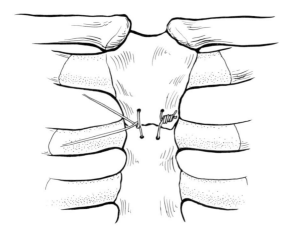

21

21

Two or three wires are inserted and twisted until the fracture site is approximated.

The skin and subcutaneous tissue are closed with absorbable sutures. Pain relief and sternal stability are immediate.

First rib fracture

22

The first rib is a short, broad structure which is well protected by overlying musculoskeletal elements. Tremendous kinetic energy is needed to fracture a first rib. The mortality rate in our experience is 36 per cent owing to the high incidence of associated injuries[6]. These include orthopaedic – 75 per cent, chest – 64 per cent, central nervous system – 53 per cent, abdominal – 33 per cent, and cardiovascular – 14 per cent. In another 22 per cent there is injury to the adjacent brachial plexus, sympathetic ganglia or subclavian vessels. No specific therapy is indicated for a first rib fracture other than an arm sling, but the physician should be aware of the high incidence of other major injuries.

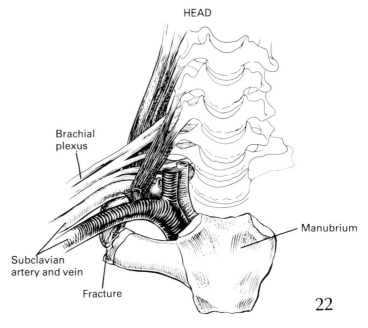

HEAD

Brachial plexus

Manubrium

Subclavian artery and vein

Fracture

22

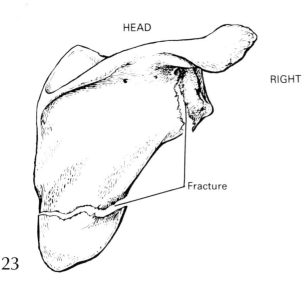

HEAD

RIGHT

Fracture

23

Scapular fracture

Like the first rib, the scapula has a high tensile strength and is well protected by the overlying musculature. Therefore, this is an indication of a major force applied to the chest wall and carries a high incidence of associated injury[7].

23

Two-thirds of the fractures are through the neck of the scapula and the remainder in the body. The main significance of scapular fractures is in the high incidence of major associated injuries. In one series, only 19 per cent of patients with a scapular fracture had no associated injuries. This lesion may be suspected because of local pain and tenderness, but is usually diagnosed by X-ray.

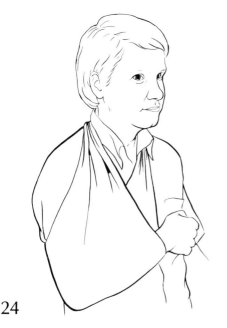

24

24

The only treatment is immobilization for a few weeks in a sling until the pain resolves.

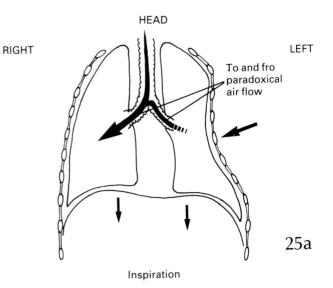

25a

Inspiration

Traumatic flail chest

25a & b

Patients with traumatic flail chest are frequently in severe respiratory distress. Various ventilatory defects have been documented – decreased vital capacity and functional residual capacity, hypoxaemia, reduced pulmonary compliance and tidal volume, and an increase in airway resistance and work or breathing. This is generally blamed on paradoxical motion of the chest wall and the unproven concept of Pendelluft – to and fro movement of air between the lungs during paradoxical respiration.

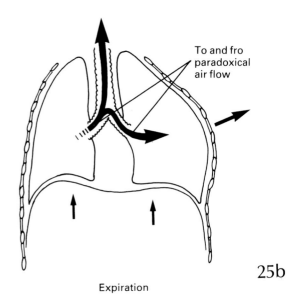

25b

Expiration

26

Therapy has frequently been directed toward stabilizing the chest wall with sandbags, towel clips and, more recently, either prolonged mechanical ventilation with a volume ventilator or operative fixation. In the author's clinic we feel that paradoxical motion of the chest wall is usually a minor part of the total pathophysiology and that underlying pulmonary contusion is the main problem[8]. Pulmonary contusion is treated with the following regimen.

1. Intravenous crystalloid solutions are restricted to 1000 ml or less during resuscitation and 50 ml/h thereafter.
2. Hypovolaemia, as evidenced by a low central venous or pulmonary wedge pressure, is treated only with colloid solutions, such as whole blood, fresh frozen plasma, or synthetic plasma.
3. Frusemide (furosemide), 20 mg intravenously, is given twice a day for several days to eliminate the crystalloid fluid overload during resuscitation.
4. Methylprednisolone, 30 mg/kg per day, is used in patients not requiring mechanical ventilation.
5. Pain relief is obtained with intercostal nerve blocks and frequent small doses of morphine sulphate.
6. Pulmonary toilet is accomplished with frequent nasotracheal suction, blow bottles, incentive spirometry, and inflating a balloon.

We have found that this regimen has decreased both morbidity and mortality rates, and the duration of hospitalization in patients with traumatic flail chest. Mechanical ventilation is instituted only if the arterial P_{O_2} is below 60 mmHg or the P_{CO_2} above 50 mmHg. Mechanical ventilation is not instituted solely on the basis of chest wall paradox. In patients undergoing endotracheal intubation and mechanical ventilation, the respirator is set on intermittent mandatory ventilation which is gradually reduced from 10 to 2 breaths per minute. At each stage arterial blood gases are obtained and the patient evaluated for tachypnoea, tachycardia and an increased respiratory effort. The patient is extubated when the respiratory rate is below 20/min with suitable arterial blood gases without ventilatory support. In patients not responding to the above regimen, a Swan-Ganz catheter is inserted to evaluate cardiac output, systemic vascular resistance and pulmonary capillary wedge pressure. If the cardiac output is depressed and the pulmonary capillary wedge pressure elevated above 15 mmHg, intravenous nitroprusside and/or dopamine are started. If a thermodilution catheter and computer is not available, a mixed venous oxygen saturation obtained from the pulmonary artery will yield a reasonable estimate of cardiac output. Mixed venous oxygen saturation above 60 per cent is indicative of an adequate cardiac output while a saturation below 40 per cent is disastrously low. This simple evaluation is useful for a clinical approximation of cardiac output and for measuring the response to various therapeutic manoeuvres.

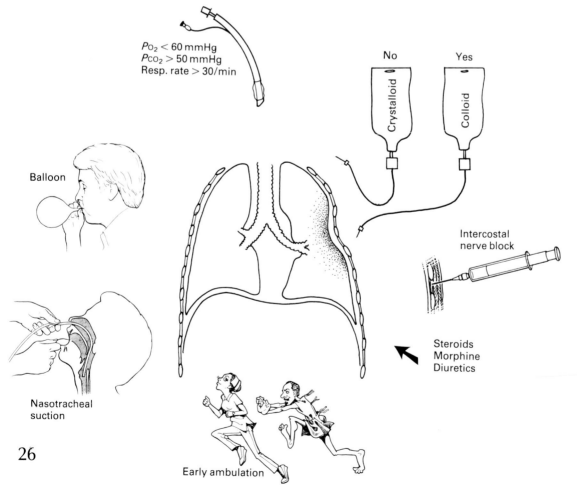

$P_{O_2} < 60$ mmHg
$P_{CO_2} > 50$ mmHg
Resp. rate > 30/min

No   Yes

Crystalloid   Colloid

Balloon

Intercostal nerve block

Nasotracheal suction

Steroids
Morphine
Diuretics

Early ambulation

26

Post-traumatic empyema

Occasionally tube thoracostomy fails to evacuate all blood and clot from the pleural space. Retained blood is an ideal culture medium and minimal contamination may lead to an infected haemothorax or empyema. This frequently occurs if the thoracostomy tube is small or not in a dependent position. Treatment of empyema has two objectives: to re-expand the underlying lung and to evacuate infected material from the pleural space.

27

As retained intrapleural clot undergoes lysis, there is an increased oncotic pressure resulting in a protein-rich, expanding effusion which leaves a fibrinous precipitate over the surface of the collapsed lung.

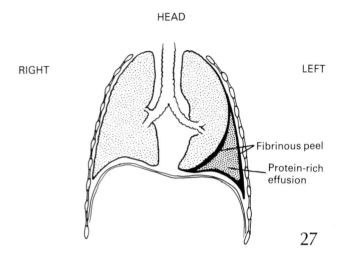

27

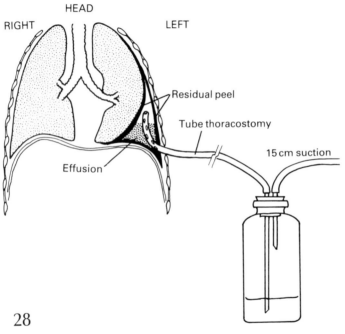

28

28

A subsequent tube thoracostomy may yield only straw-coloured fluid, but if the fibrinous peel has already formed, the tube will probably be unsuccessful in accomplishing the objectives. Generally, if the chest tube has not re-expanded the lung and cleared the pleural space within 3 or 4 days the patient is condemned to either a thoracotomy and decortication or prolonged tube drainage.

29

If decortication is chosen, the patient is placed in a direct lateral position and a lateral thoracotomy incision is made in the fifth or sixth intercostal space. The restricting purulent, fibrinous peel is removed from the lung by blunt and sharp dissection. The apical and mediastinal surfaces are usually free with the majority of the peel lying posteriorly and inferiorly. If operation is performed within the first 2 or 3 weeks, the underlying lung is easily decorticated, leaving an intact visceral pleura. Two large chest tubes are inserted and the ribs are approximated with circumferential No. 1 absorbable sutures (Vicryl). The muscles are closed in layers with continuous subcuticular 2/0 Vicryl sutures. The incidence of wound infection is surprisingly low[9].

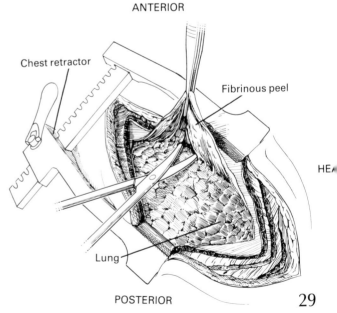

29

Diaphragmatic injuries

30

Rupture of the diaphragm as a result of blunt injury is approximately three times more frequent on the left, since the right diaphragm is protected by the underlying liver. The differential pressure between the pleural and peritoneal cavities pumps the intra-abdominal viscera through the laceration and into the pleural space. These injuries have the following three clinical stages.

1. The *acute phase* during which the signs and symptoms reflect injury to the intrathoracic and intra-abdominal contents and shift of the mediastinum.
2. The *interval phase* is generally silent and may last a few days or years.
3. In the *late stage* complications of the herniated intra-abdominal viscera develop, such as bowel obstruction, gangrene, gastric stasis with bleeding, and cardiorespiratory compression.

Recognition of a ruptured diaphragm requires immediate operation in any phase. In the acute phase the most frequent radiological appearance is an elevated diaphragm with a hazy diaphragmatic shadow and blunting of the costophrenic angle. Occasionally the injury will be discovered by the surgeon's finger during tube thoracostomy. Confirmation may be obtained by passing a nasogastric tube and observing its location above the diaphragm or, if the colon is herniated, by performing a barium enema. Operation in the acute phase generally requires a laparotomy incision. Our preference is a subcostal approach.

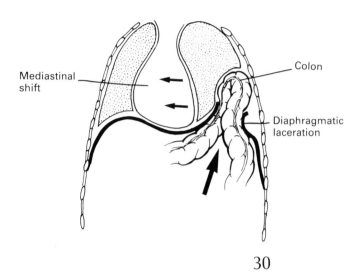

30

31

In the interval or late phase a thoracoabdominal approach is required owing to adhesions of the intra-abdominal viscera to the pleura. For this approach the patient's chest is elevated 45°–60° and an anterolateral incision is made in the eighth intercostal space.

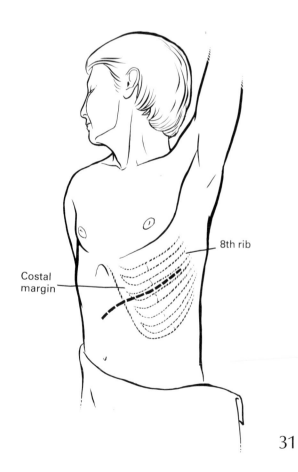

31

32

If required, the incision can be extended across the costal margin with a radial incision in the anterolateral aspect of the diaphragm. This approach allows simultaneous exposure of both the pleural and peritoneal cavities. It is important to excise a small segment of cartilage if the costal arch is transected and not to place sutures through the cartilage.

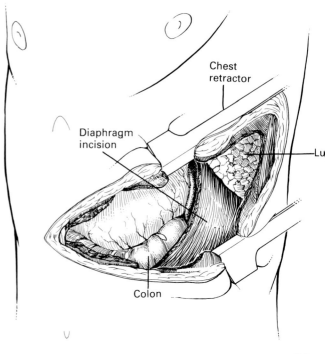

32

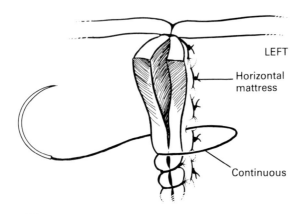

33

33

The diaphragm should be repaired in two layers with large non-absorbable sutures, interrupted horizontal mattress sutures being used for the first layer and a continuous suture for the second. Untreated diaphragmatic lacerations gradually enlarge and the repairs tend to recur if not closed very securely. The chest incision is closed as described for post-traumatic empyema and the abdominal incision as described elsewhere[10].

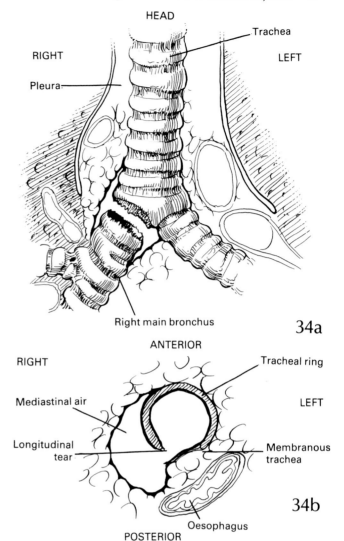

34a

Tracheobronchial injuries

34a, b & c

Injuries to the trachea and major bronchi are caused by the following mechanisms.

(a) Anteroposterior compression of the chest wall with a 'straddle' injury to a main-stem bronchus – usually the right.

(b) A sudden increase in endotracheal pressure with compression to the chest wall and a closed glottis. This produces a 'blow-out' injury where the membranous portion of the trachea is separated longitudinally from the rings, usually on the right. If the mediastinal pleura is intact there may be massive mediastinal emphysema. If the pleura is not intact, there will be a large pneumothorax and air leak.

(c) Rapid deceleration produces a shearing effect due to the firm attachment of the trachea at the level of the cricoid and the carina. This produces a transverse fracture of the trachea.

The symptoms of tracheobronchial injury generally include dyspnoea, hoarseness and haemoptysis. There may also be severe subcutaneous and/or mediastinal emphysema. A pneumothorax will be present if the mediastinal pleura and/or fascia around the main-stem bronchus has been ruptured. The most frequent clinical courses include persistent atelectasis, a massive air leak with incomplete re-expansion of the underlying lung, and mediastinal or subcutaneous emphysema. If any of these signs is present, rigid bronchoscopy and preparations for operation should be undertaken.

34b

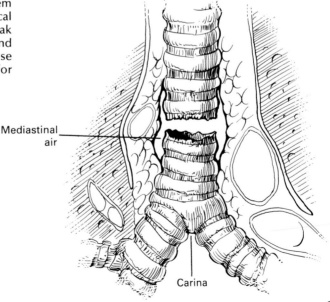

34c

35

With the patient under general anaesthesia the airway may have to be secured by ventilation through the rigid bronchoscope or an endotracheal tube guided into the distal tracheal segment over a fibreoptic bronchoscope.

A thoracotomy is used for main-stem bronchial injuries and blow-out type injuries of the trachea, as well as distal, transverse tracheal fractures. A collar neck incision with a median sternotomy may be used for cervical transverse tracheal injuries. It is important to debride all fractured cartilage and to anastomose adjacent intact rings with 3/0 monofilament interrupted sutures.

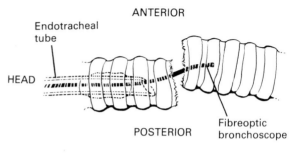

ANTERIOR

Endotracheal tube

HEAD

POSTERIOR

Fibreoptic bronchoscope

35

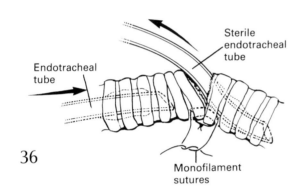

Sterile endotracheal tube

Endotracheal tube

Monofilament sutures

36

36

The distal trachea is ventilated via a sterile endotracheal tube while the posterior half of the trachea or main-stem bronchus is repaired. A second endotracheal tube is then passed through the laynx and guided digitally by the surgeon into the distal trachea or main-stem bronchus while the anterior portion of the repair is completed[11].

References

1. Accident facts. National Safety Council. Chicago, Illinois, 1978

2. Kish, G., Kozloff, L., Joseph, W. L., Adkins, P. C. Indications for early thoracotomy in the management of chest trauma. Annals of Thoracic Surgery 1976; 22: 23–28

3. Siemens, R., Polk, H. C. Jr, Gray, L. A., Jr, Fulton, R. L. Indications for thoracotomy following penetrating thoracic injury. Journal of Trauma 1977; 17: 493–500

4. Conn, J. H., Hardy, J. D., Fain, W. R., Netterville, R. E. Thoracic trauma: analysis of 1022 cases. Journal of Trauma 1963; 3: 22–40

5. Richardson, J. D., Grover, F. L., Trinkle, J. K. Early operative management of isolated sternal fractures. Journal of Trauma 1975; 15: 156–158

6. Richardson, J. D., McElvein, R. B., Trinkle, J. K. First rib fracture: a hallmark of severe trauma. Annals of Surgery 1975; 181: 251–254

7. Imatani, R. J. Fractures of the scapula: a review of 53 fractures. Journal of Trauma 1975; 15: 473–478

8. Trinkle, J. K. Flail chest and pulmonary contusion. In: Trinkle, J. K., Grover, F. L. Management of thoracic trauma victims. Philadelphia: J. B. Lippincott, 1980, 39–45

9. Arom, K. V. Post-traumatic empyema. In: Trinkle, J. K., Grover, F. L. Management of thoracic trauma victims. Philadelphia: J. B. Lippincott Co., 1980, 27–30

10. Hood, R. M. Traumatic diaphragmatic hernia (collective review). Annals of Thoracic Surgery 1971; 12: 311–324

11. Kirsh, M. M., Orringer, M. B., Behrendt, D. M., Sloan, H. Management of trancheobronchial disruption secondary to nonpenetrating trauma. Annals of Thoracic Surgery 1976; 22: 93–101

Penetrating wounds of the chest

Melvin R. Platt MD
Clinical Associate Professor and Former Chairman, Division of Cardiothoracic Surgery,
Southwestern Medical School, Dallas, Texas, USA

Editor's note

This chapter should be read in conjunction with the chapter on 'Management of blunt thoracic injuries', pp. 22–38.

Initial evaluation

1

Patients admitted with penetrating chest injuries require rapid, orderly evaluation and resuscitation to obtain maximum salvage. While vital signs are obtained, 'life-lines' are inserted as rapidly as possible, including a 14 gauge peripheral intravenous (i.v.) line and a central venous pressure (CVP) and infusion catheter, usually also 14 gauge. Though a pneumothorax is a rare complication in experienced hands, the CVP is always inserted on the side that is injured, since contralateral placement could result in bilateral pneumothoraces, depending on the injury. If the patient is in shock, two CVP lines can often be inserted more rapidly than a cutdown or a peripheral i.v. can be performed; one can use both subclavian veins or the subclavian and internal jugular veins on the same side.

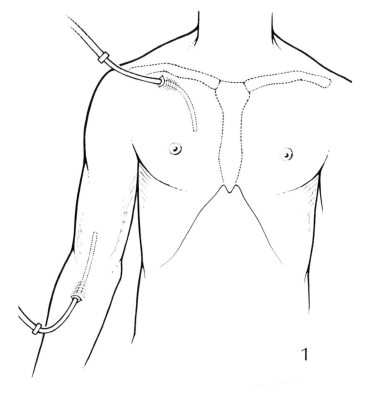

1

2

Unless physical examination reveals normal breath sounds on the injured side in a clinically stable patient, a single tube thoracostomy is placed before a chest X-ray is obtained. A 36 Fr plastic tube is placed at the sixth or seventh intercostal space, anterior axillary line, and threaded superiorly and posteriorly so that the last holes are just inside the chest wall. The tube is never placed through the injury site, because this is considered to be contaminated and also because divided vessels which have retracted and clotted may be manipulated and made to rebleed. If blood or air are not obtained with the exploring clamp used to form the tube tract, then finger exploration is performed to ensure that the tract freely communicates with the chest cavity.

The tube is connected to water seal and then 20 cm suction. If the nature of the injury lends itself to observation, then hourly chest drainage is measured. Drainage of more than $200\,ml/m^2$ that persists for more than 2 consecutive hours requires exploration under most circumstances. One must be sure that the initial haemothorax has been evacuated by the tube, so that the drainage represents active bleeding. A portable chest X-ray should indicate whether a second tube thoracostomy is required to drain residual blood or air.

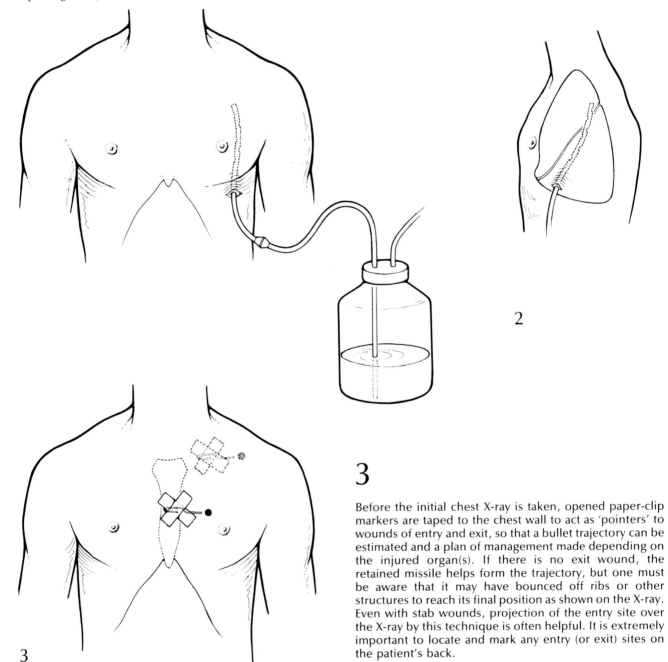

2

3

Before the initial chest X-ray is taken, opened paper-clip markers are taped to the chest wall to act as 'pointers' to wounds of entry and exit, so that a bullet trajectory can be estimated and a plan of management made depending on the injured organ(s). If there is no exit wound, the retained missile helps form the trajectory, but one must be aware that it may have bounced off ribs or other structures to reach its final position as shown on the X-ray. Even with stab wounds, projection of the entry site over the X-ray by this technique is often helpful. It is extremely important to locate and mark any entry (or exit) sites on the patient's back.

3

Chest wall and lung injuries

Most chest wall injuries do not require any debridement or local care except a dressing, unless active bleeding persists. Shotgun wounds are an exception as they are often contaminated with shotgun wadding as well as clothing, and extensive local debridement is almost always necessary. Particularly with stab wounds, if the medias-tinal structures are not involved, persistent bleeding requiring exploration is rarely due to organ injury, but is almost always caused by a torn intercostal (or internal mammary) artery. It is preferable to avoid the morbidity of a posterolateral thoracotomy for what probably requires only one suture to control.

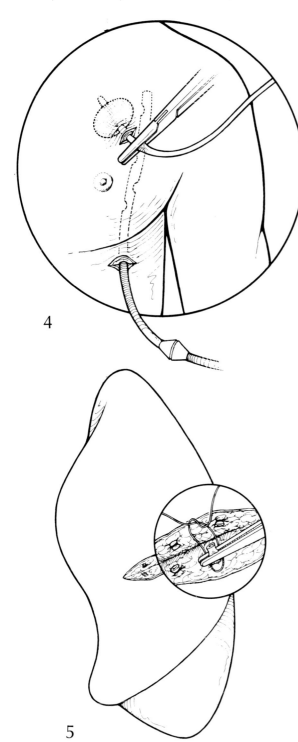

4

Foley catheter placement

In such a circumstance, and when active bleeding is occurring, placement of a Foley catheter, inflation of its 30 ml balloon, and then external traction on the catheter with a haemostat at the skin will often tamponade the bleeding site. If the wound is medial enough to have injured the internal mammary artery, exploration is still required to rule out a cardiac injury.

5

Posterolateral thoracotomy

When bleeding persists despite these measures, the chest is explored through a posterolateral thoracotomy. If the lung is actively bleeding, it is important to avoid simply oversewing the lung surface, as the bleeding is likely to continue and result in a large parenchymal haematoma. Instead, individual bleeding vessels and open bronchioles are ligated for control, and the laceration is usually not closed.

6

Wedging

In some cases, the haematoma in the injured lung makes individual vessels hard to identify, and it is often easier to use a stapling device to wedge out the affected area. A V-shaped wedge is shown, but a U-shaped wedge can be used for deeper injuries, requiring three staple lines. If the injury is near the hilum, early control of the main pulmonary artery is often life saving, and then the vessel may be sought out and sutured. Only rarely is a lobectomy required, but injuries caused by destructive, high velocity weapons may not be reparable, and lobar or more extensive resection is required.

One should always be aware of the relationship of the intra-abdominal structures to the chest wall. All penetrating wounds below the fifth interspace have the potential for intra-abdominal injury, and even without peritoneal signs, a diagnostic saline lavage is indicated. Penetration of the diaphragm does not by itself require exploration, though it obviously should be repaired during the course of thoracic or abdominal exploration, as rare cases of late visceral herniation through penetrating diaphragmatic wounds have occurred.

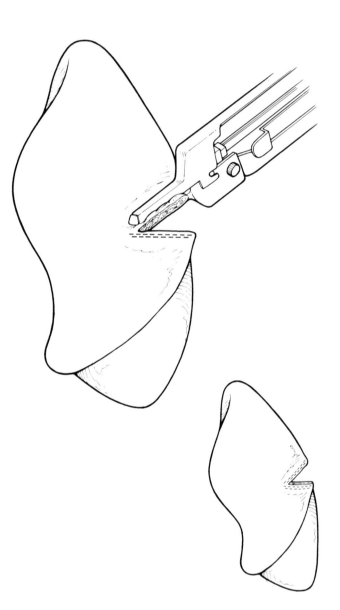

6

Mediastinal injuries (other than cardiac)

Diagnosis

If one suspects that a penetrating injury has traversed the mediastinum, several diagnostic steps are necessary. Mediastinal air may mean oesophageal or tracheal injury, but most often it results from injury to the lung itself. All patients with penetrating chest trauma should have a nasogastric tube placed, if for no other reason than to empty the stomach in preparation for a general anaesthetic. If blood is obtained, a barium swallow is performed as soon as the patient can cooperate sufficiently.

Endoscopy is done as an alternative, but has not been as accurate in detecting a leak. Tracheal injury is suspected by haemoptysis, mediastinal air and usually an active air leak into the pleura. Bronchoscopy should be diagnostic. Aortic injuries should be suspected on the basis of proximity alone, and though an aortogram may confirm the injury (particularly if the great vessels are involved), a normal aortogram never excludes a penetrating injury.

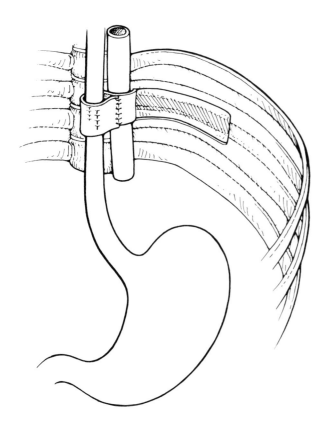

7

Wound closure

Oesophageal wounds are closed in two layers with interrupted sutures, preferably 3/0 or 4/0 non-absorbable monofilament material. If there is any delay in repair or if the closure is suspect due to contused tissues, a pleural flap is wrapped around the repair. Tracheal wounds are closed with a single layer of interrupted polyglycolic acid suture, usually 3/0, and this avoids late suture granulomas that occur with permanent suture. Aortic wounds are controlled by one's finger or with a partial-occlusion clamp and closed with felt-buttressed horizontal mattress sutures of 2/0 or 3/0 Dacron. A haematoma has usually temporarily controlled the wound or the patient would have exsanguinated, so that one has time to place proximal and distal tapes for control if necessary.

Cardiac wounds

Cardiac injury is likely to have occurred if a wound is over the precordium or if a projectile traverses the mediastinum. Eighty per cent of cardiac injuries never reach the hospital alive, yet occasionally when patients with cardiac wounds are admitted they may appear remarkably stable, only to deteriorate rapidly if observed. An aggressive approach should be taken towards such wounds, even if the weapon is as small as an ice pick. Most patients who reach the hospital will have signs of cardiac tamponade, with hypotension, elevated neck veins and CVP, and decreased heart sounds. If the patient is moribund, the only chance may be an immediate and expeditious left anterior thoracotomy in the emergency room, but ideally one should go through the same resuscitative measures noted earlier, transfusing crystalloid while type-specific blood is set up for the operating room.

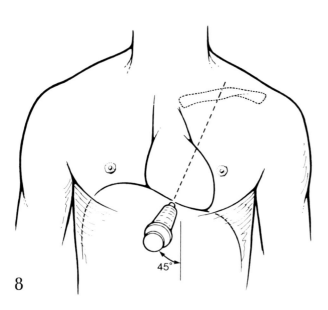

8

8

Pericardiocentesis

Pericardiocentesis is never used as definitive care in cardiac wounds, but may be very effective as a temporary measure while blood is crossmatched. Relief of tamponade also makes anaesthetic induction much safer, as otherwise these patients are very vulnerable to cardiac arrest during induction and intubation. Although pericardiocentesis is valuable, in inexperienced hands it is dangerous and may lead to additional penetrating cardiac wounds.

A needle with syringe attached is introduced to the left of the xyphoid, at 45° to the abdominal wall and aiming toward the left midclavicular line. Usually non-clotting blood is aspirated, but the important feature of a 'positive' tap is lowering of the CVP and elevation of the blood pressure. Improvement can be expected with removal of only 10–20 ml of blood and a guide wire is introduced (soft tipped or J-wire) and then a plastic catheter is threaded over the wire so that repeated aspiration can be done as required.

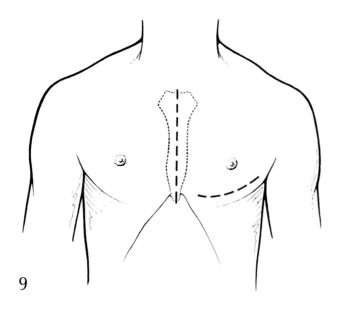

9

9

Choice of approach

In the operating room, a decision must be made regarding the operative approach. A left anterior thoracotomy is usually preferred, but it gives poor exposure to the right atrium and great vessels. Thus, a median sternotomy is selected if (1) penetration was from the right chest, so that injury of right atrium is likely; (2) the missile traversed the mediastinum, again potentially injuring the right atrium; (3) a previous left thoracotomy was done; or (4) the penetration is above the fourth interspace, making great-vessel injury more likely.

10

Left anterior thoracotomy

The illustration shows exposure of the heart and left hilum through a left anterior thoracotomy, fifth interspace, with the patient's left side elevated 30–45°. The pericardium is opened anteriorly (1 cm) and parallel to the phrenic nerve, and the anterior half is bisected as far forward as necessary; the two anterior halves are then distracted and anchored with a stay suture (or haemostat to save time if they are actively bleeding), forming a pericardial well. Gentle traction as shown will easily expose the entire surface of the right ventricle, which represents 55 per cent of the anterior cardiac surface and is thus the most common site for penetrating injuries. The posterior left ventricle is also easily exposed by retracting the heart anteriorly; this is often awkward through a sternotomy with a beating heart. Also shown is the relatively poor exposure of the right atrium and great vessels; this can be improved by extending the incision across the sternum, but the advantage of rapid exposure with a thoracotomy is thus lost. Again, if either right atrial or great vessel injury is suspected, a sternotomy should be performed. One should always prepare the left groin when exploring these patients through an anterior thoracotomy for that rare trauma case that requires cardiopulmonary bypass, and this also gives access to the saphenous vein if needed.

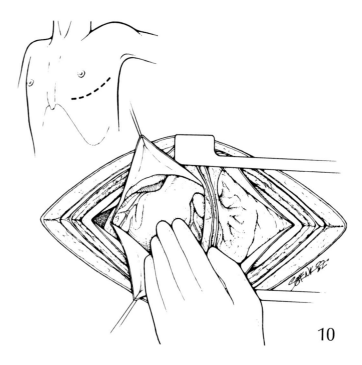

10

11

Wounds of right ventricle

Wounds of the right ventricle are often not actively bleeding at the time of exploration, but placement of sutures often causes renewed bleeding. For stab wounds, especially those less than 1 cm in length, it is sufficient to use one or two interrupted horizontal mattress sutures, with finger control while the sutures are placed. Stab wounds of the right ventricle can be closed with 2/0 or 3/0 Dacron sutures without felt buttressing, but left ventricular stab wounds and right and left ventricular gunshot wounds should be closed with felt buttressing, for there is a definite risk of subsequent false aneurysm if the sutures pull through the contused myocardium.

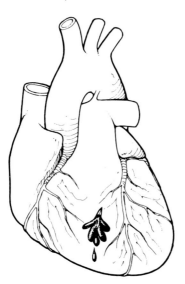

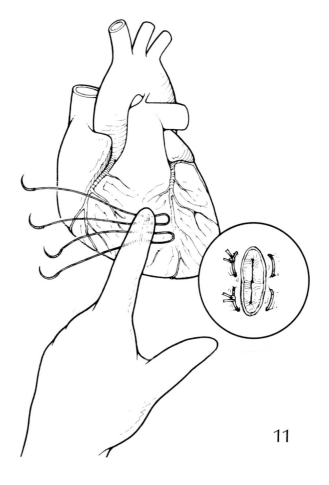

11

12

Special techniques

Junction of inferior vena cava and right atrium

Most right atrial injuries can be easily controlled with a partial occlusion clamp and then electively oversewn. An awkward area is at the junction of the inferior vena cava (IVC) and right atrium, as a clamp cannot usually be applied. If the laceration is not too large, a Foley balloon may occlude the bleeding site and allow elective placement of a running suture superficially to avoid rupturing the Foley balloon; then the Foley is removed and a deeper suture line placed. Larger lacerations in this area (IVC) require cardiopulmonary bypass for control.

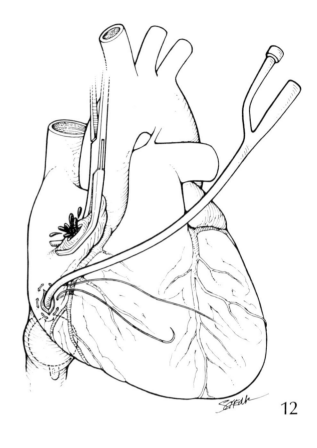

12

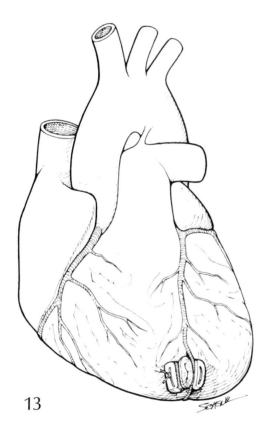

13

13

Injuries near a coronary artery

The technique illustrated is used to control injuries that are within a few millimeters of a coronary artery. The suture is passed beneath the artery so that the artery now passes within the buttressed suture. Obviously some septal branches (in the case of the left anterior descending artery) are compromised, but this does not seem to cause a clinical problem. If the artery itself is lacerated, it is simply ligated when the injury is in the distal half of the vessel, but more proximal injuries should be repaired with coronary artery bypass grafting on cardiopulmonary bypass.

Acute traumatic ventricular septal defect

Occasionally a penetrating wound will result in an acute traumatic ventricular septal defect (VSD). This is usually not noted initially, but instead a murmur is heard several days after the external cardiac wound is repaired. Although a rare case is described that requires immediate surgery, in most cases the VSD is haemodynamically trivial, and perhaps the majority actually close spontaneously.

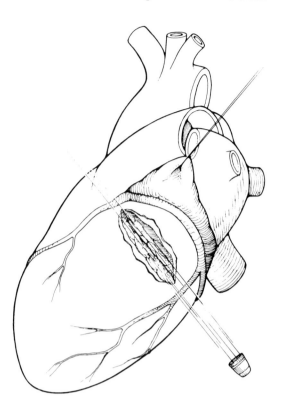

14

Extensive wounds not requiring cardiopulmonary bypass

A wound may be extensive and yet be reparable without using cardiopulmonary bypass. The illustration shows that occasionally a missile, instead of going through-and-through the myocardium, will 'crease' or split the myocardium as shown. Such wounds are invariably lethal if the trough created extends into the ventricular cavity, but the bleeding encountered in the case shown is from the open edges, rather than the ventricular cavity. Attempts to control the bleeding locally, including directly coapting the cut edges, will fail. A proper approach is to 'ring' the edges with felt-bolstered mattress sutures, using a finger to control bleeding and taking care to avoid coronary branches when possible. These sutures are then placed through the edge of a suitably shaped woven patch which is securely tied in place.

Personal results

Our experience at Parkland Hospital in Dallas, Texas illustrates the value of the management guidelines and technical principles discussed here. We have treated 156 cardiac wounds in the past 5 years; this includes all patients with cardiac wounds in whom a resuscitative attempt was made, and almost half the patients were gunshot victims. Fifteen patients died, for a mortality rate of 9.6 per cent. These results can only be achieved by having surgical residents available around the clock in the emergency room.

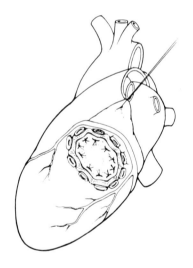

14

Tumours of the chest wall including neurofibromata

J. E. Dussek FRCS
Consultant Thoracic Surgeon, Guy's Hospital and The Brook Hospital, London, UK

Introduction

Tumours of the chest wall are relatively uncommon and the indication for resection will depend on symptoms, histology and their sensitivity to other forms of therapy. Usually primary tumours whether benign or malignant, require excision, but secondary deposits are normally only resected if they are insensitive to other forms of therapy and are causing symptoms. The aim of the operation is to excise completely all tumour bearing tissue with a generous margin, but with the minimum functional or cosmetic disturbance.

The decision whether to use a prosthesis to patch the defect following resection of a chest wall tumour will depend on the size and site of the resection. In general, if two or more ribs are to be excised and the defect is not covered by the scapula, a prosthesis is likely to be required. Similarly, excision of the sternum, either in part or entirety will require prosthetic replacement. Marlex mesh is suitable for small defects, but, where the area to be replaced is large, curved or stress-bearing, a Marlex methylmethacrylate sandwich may be used. As a general principle it is better to patch than not to patch.

Neurofibromas and Schwannomas present a particular challenge if they extend through the intervertebral foramen. These require close collaboration between thoracic surgeon and neurosurgeon. If it is suspected either clinically or radiologically that a neurofibroma extends through the intervertebral foramen, myelography, with or without computer-assisted tomography (CAT), is essential. If an intraspinal extension to the tumour is confirmed, that portion of the tumour should be excised first, and the thoracic portion of the tumour detached and allowed to retract into the thoracic cavity. This will usually be performed through a laminectomy approach and is ideally performed by a neurosurgeon. When the thoracic part of the operation is performed subsequently, there is no risk of traction on the spinal cord or nerve roots with the associated dangers.

Preoperative

Routine preoperative haematological, biochemical and appropriate radiological investigations should be performed. CAT scanning is particularly helpful in delineating the extent of chest wall lesions. Where intraspinal extension is suspected, myelography, with or without CAT examination, should be performed. Physiotherapy to clear secretions is obligatory. An iodine or similar skin prep is recommended and prophylactic antibiotics are advisable if prosthetic material is to be inserted. If it is anticipated that skin flaps will be required to close the ensuing defect it is beneficial to liaise with a plastic surgeon before the operation.

The operation

RESECTION OF CHEST WALL TUMOURS

1

The position of the patient will depend on the operation site, but for simplicity the excision of only three ribs will be shown here. A standard thoracotomy incision may be used for tumours in ribs alone, but the incision will need to be individually tailored for lesions involving sternum, costal margin or clavicles.

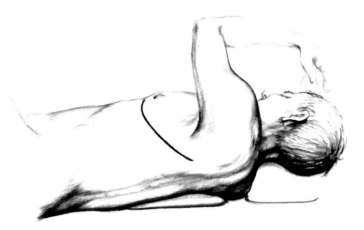

1

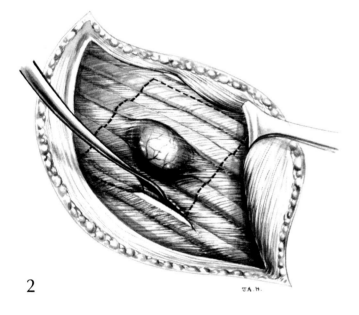

2

2

The incision is deepened down to the tumour. If it is malignant the dissection should stop short of the lesion itself. The periosteum of the upper and lower ribs to be resected is elevated using a Tudor Edwards periosteal elevator. This is most easily accomplished by first incising the periosteum with a diathermy point and then scraping the periosteum off the rib towards the rib edge. The elevator is inserted between bone and elevated periosteum, keeping close onto the bone itself, and then smartly moved laterally along the rib, keeping the curve of the instrument well under the rib.

3

The ribs are most easily divided using a Price Thomas costotome. It is advisable to raise a small length of periosteum at the site of division so the rib can be encircled without damage to the neurovascular bundle, which will probably need to be ligated. The intercostal muscles may be divided between the ribs using diathermy.

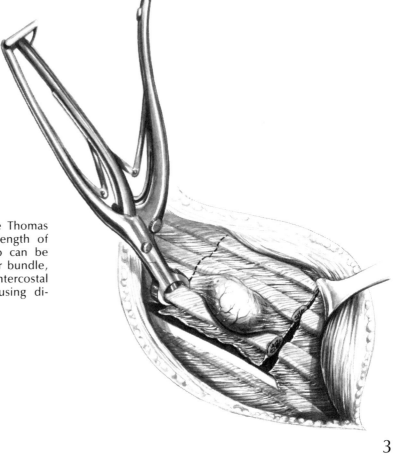

3

4

When two or more ribs are excised and the defect is not covered by the scapula, it is often advisable to fill the defect. A Marlex patch will often suffice, but, where rigidity or a curved shape are required, a Marlex methylmethacrylate 'sandwich' is recommended.

The affected portion of chest wall is removed and a chest drain inserted. The bony edges of the defect may be drilled now to accept the sutures required to hold the prosthesis. A spoon may be used to protect underlying structures.

4

5

A stainless steel gauze mesh may be used as a former and should be bent to the desired shape. A piece of Marlex mesh is then marked to the size of the defect to be filled. The methylmethacrylate is now mixed and applied to the Marlex inside the marked out area. A second layer of Marlex is then pressed onto the methylmethacrylate before it is dry. Coarse haemostats are useful to hold the Marlex to the gauze former. When the cement dries it becomes hot and hard. The 'sandwich' may now be handled.

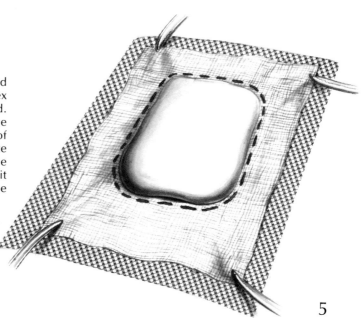

5

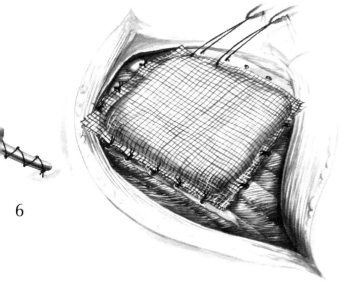

6

6

The prosthesis is sutured in place, preferably with an inert non-absorbable suture material, following which the wound is closed in an appropriate manner. It is preferable to cover the prosthesis with muscle and skin, although omentum may also be used, interposed between the prosthesis and skin.

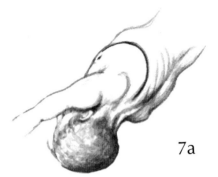

7a

RESECTION OF SCHWANNOMA OR NEUROFIBROMA

7a & b

Any intraspinal extension of the tumour should already have been resected. The patient is placed in an appropriate thoracotomy position to allow access to the tumour. Once the thoracic cavity is opened the tumour should be readily visible. It is usually covered by vascular pleura.

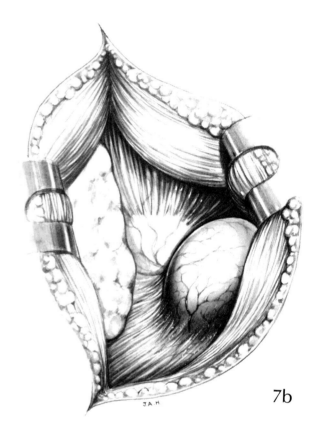

7b

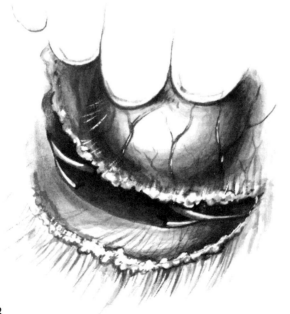

8

8

The pleura surrounding the tumour is incised all the way around the tumour just at the point where it reflects off the chest wall. This allows the tumour to be retracted. After a small amount of dissection the intercostal vessels are usually identified easily. It is advisable to ligate the artery and vein. The nerve leaving and entering the tumour should be identified and transected with a sharp knife several centimetres away from the tumour where possible. Where the tumour extends into the intervertebral foramen this is not possible.

9

At the end of the procedure the cut ends of the nerve should be clearly visible, and the bed in which the tumour has been lying will be completely clear.

If it is discovered that the tumour extends more medially than anticipated, it is advisable to resect as much of the intrathoracic component as possible. As little traction as possible should be exerted on the tumour itself, and especially the veins, in order to avoid intraspinal haemorrhage. Bleeding is controlled by local pressure or packing with absorbable foam. Excessive diathermy is absolutely contraindicated. Once the whole thoracic component is removed, the patient should be placed in the prone position and a laminectomy performed to give access to the intraspinal component. It is preferable to perform this under one anaesthetic.

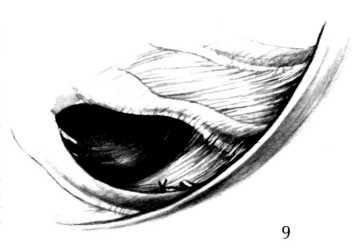

9

Postoperative management

Chest wall resection is often very painful and adequate postoperative analgesia is essential. Nerve blocks are very useful especially if performed with a cryoprobe, and thoracic epidural anaesthesia is of particular value.

Complications

Most problems relate to sputum retention and subsequent atelectasis or lobar collapse. This should be prevented by effective analgesia and physiotherapy, but may need treatment by bronchoscopy.

Problems with posture following laminectomy and thoracotomy require effective physiotherapy to prevent permanent deformity.

Illustrations by Peter Drury

Thymectomy

M. F. Sturridge MS, FRCS
Consultant Thoracic Surgeon, The Middlesex Hospital, London;
Consultant Surgeon, London Chest Hospital;
Honorary Consultant Thoracic Surgeon, The National Hospital for Nervous Diseases, London, UK

Introduction

Thymectomy is now indicated in the management of all cases of myasthenia gravis and is withheld only in the mildest cases and in very old patients. Myasthenia occurs when the gland is not clinically enlarged and is macroscopically normal but also in association with tumours of the thymus gland. Tumours of the thymus are detected early and are relatively small when they present with myasthenia whereas they are large and present late with signs of mediastinal compression when myasthenia is absent. The first section of this chapter will deal with thymectomy for myasthenia gravis and the second with the management of thymic tumours without myasthenia.

MYASTHENIA GRAVIS

Myasthenia gravis without tumour and myasthenia gravis with tumour appear to be different diseases. The former afflicts females twice as commonly as males. A wide age range is affected but the average age in a large series is around 30 years. About 70 per cent have demonstrable anti-acetylcholine receptor antibody in their serum and the prognosis following thymectomy is good. Myasthenia gravis associated with a thymic tumour is found equally in men and women and affects a population with an average age of 45 years. Antistriated muscle antibody is found in the serum typically and the prognosis is much less favourable from the myasthenic standpoint. The tumours are almost always benign and myasthenia is the prime indication for surgery in these cases.

The differential diagnosis of myasthenia can be difficult and is usually made by a neurologist. It is confirmed by the presence of antibodies or by intravenous injection of edrophonium 4 mg which produces a dramatic short-lived relief of symptoms and signs. All patients should have chest radiography with posteroanterior and lateral views to determine whether a tumour is present. Anterior mediastinal lateral tomograms and computerized axial tomography are useful adjuncts.

Preoperative preparation

The aim is to present the patient for the operation in an optimal state for a smooth uncomplicated recovery. If the symptoms are severe and particularly if they are 'bulbar', affecting swallowing and breathing, efforts should be made to bring the patient into remission by the use of steroids with or without immunosupressives. Plasmapheresis is another means of reducing the symptoms sufficiently to permit safer surgery in severe cases.

Attention is particularly directed to diaphragmatic breathing exercises to increase ventilation and reduce pain postoperatively. Repeated measurement of vital capacity using a Wright's respirometer encourages the patient and reassures the staff that therapy is optimal. The dose of anticholinesterase drugs should also be carefully assessed in relation to the patient's reduced activity in hospital but oral medication should be continued up to the time of operation.

The operation

Now that it is known that the disease is produced by degeneration at the acetylcholine receptor of nerve endings caused by an antibody produced in the thymus gland, though also in lymph nodes, only total extirpation of the thymus is acceptable as surgical treatment. This is only possible through a sternal approach.

1

The incision

The patient is placed horizontally in the supine position and the skin is prepared and towels placed as for cardiac surgery. A midline incision is made from the sternal notch to the lowermost point of the xiphisternum and is carried down to the periosteum of the sternum. The midline of the sternum is noted by palpation of the lateral margins between the costal cartilages and the sternum is divided longitudinally along all its length. Periosteal bleeding is controlled by diathermy and bleeding from the bone by plugging with bone wax.

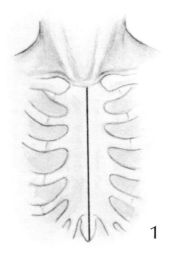

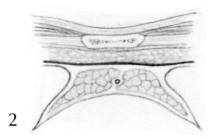

2

A sternal retractor is inserted and opened gradually to avoid fracture of the upper ribs which would cause postoperative pain below the clavicles. Fatty tissue behind the sternum is cleared laterally with a swab and the pretracheal fascia, extending down from the neck, deep to the sternothyroid muscles, is exposed. Inferiorly it is attached in an inverted horseshoe line to the anterior pericardium and laterally it blends with the extrapleural fascia. It forms the anterior capsule of the gland and is the key to the operation.

3

The thin fascia is incised in the midline and held on either side in a clamp for identification. By blunt dissection, the thymus is separated from its posterior surface and the fascia divided from its pericardial attachment to expose the lower poles of the gland on each side. The thymus differs from extrapleural fat in that it is larger and smoother in its lobulation, and pinker in colour. The lower pole can usually be easily mobilized and is held in a small tissue forceps. The gland can then be separated from the pericardium by blunt dissection and laterally from the pleura. Mobilization is continued upwards until the small arterial branch from the internal mammary artery is identified and divided between ligatures. The process is repeated on the contralateral side.

By retraction of the upper end of the wound the two upper poles of the gland are identified lying anterior to the left innominate vein and passing upwards into the neck. Blunt dissection and gentle traction will deliver these into the wound but a small arterial branch usually enters the uppermost end of them and this can be caught in a clamp and ligated before the upper poles are finally freed.

The gland is then separated from the innominate vein and its own venous drainage identified and ligated as it enters the inferior surface of that vein.

Haemostasis is not usually difficult. Special attention should be given to avoid undue clearance of extrapleural fat in the upper mediastinum as this may lead to damage to the phrenic nerves which enter the chest much more anteriorly than usually seen during thoracic surgery. Small accidental perforations of the thin parietal pleura do not require separate drainage since this thin pleura is relatively avascular and air can be expelled anteriorly before the chest is closed. The sternum is approximated securely with wire sutures and the wound closed in layers. A small suction drain (Redivac) may be left in the anterior mediastinum if there is doubt about the haemostasis.

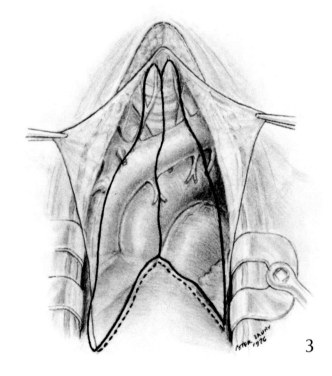

3

Postoperative care

The postoperative management of patients after thymectomy for myasthenia is best arranged in an intensive care area with full anaesthetic staffing since serious complications are most commonly associated with the patient's ability to breathe.

Ideally on leaving theatre a pernasal endotracheal tube should be present and artificial ventilation is continued probably for the first 24 hours. A nasogastric tube should also be present to enable the crushed anticholinesterase drugs to be given by the most effective route in a small quantity of water.

Anticholinesterases should not be restarted postoperatively until the patient's condition requires it. This can be assessed from time to time by intravenous injections of edrophonium 4 mg and observing whether this does or does not help the patient. Vital capacity is measured at intervals during the day using a Wright's respirometer or similar apparatus attached to the end of the endotracheal tube and artificial ventilation can usually be discontinued if the patient's airway remains uninfected and the vital capacity is greater than 1.5–2 litres. The endotracheal tube should be left *in situ* as long as there is doubt about the patient's safety without it – commonly for 3–4 days – and it is usually well tolerated. Intragastric feeds via the nasal tube can be started when bowel sounds return.

Complications

Haemothorax and pneumothorax are rare complications of thymectomy. A chest radiograph should be taken immediately after the patient's return from the operating theatre to demonstrate the presence of air or blood in the pleura. Small collections require no treatment but larger collections may require aspiration or water seal drainage of the affected pleura. Most complications are associated with the patient's myasthenia and include respiratory infection and weakness of the muscles of respiration and coughing. It seems best always to overcome these by respiratory assistance and tracheal aspiration rather than recourse to additional medical therapy in the first instance. Difficulty in swallowing may prevent administration of drugs and require replacement of the nasogastric tube.

THYMIC TUMOURS AND CYSTS

Thymic tumours and cysts are uncommon conditions. Benign tumours and cysts are usually detected during routine chest radiography or in the investigation of other diseases including myasthenia gravis. Malignant tumours are often large before they are discovered and then cause pain owing to invasion of bone and nerves of the anterior chest wall. Dermoids of the anterior mediastinum may become infected and cause symptoms of pulmonary or tracheobronchial disease.

In all of these the chest X-ray is usually the first and most useful pointer to the diagnosis if a shadow is found in the anterior mediastinum. Differentiation from cardiac abnormalities can be achieved by echocardiography or angiography in most cases. Pulmonary lesions are sometimes more difficult but computerized axial tomography is a new and impressive tool for this.

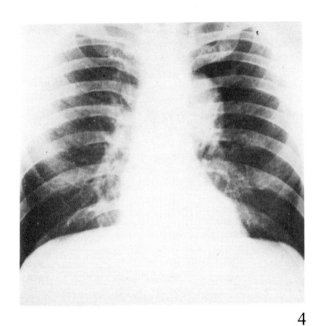

4

4

Having determined that the lesion is in the anterior mediastinum, the next factor is to decide whether it is likely to be benign or malignant. Small, well demarcated tumours are nearly always benign.

5

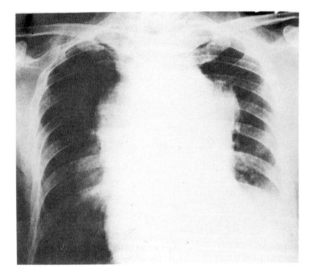

5

Malignant tumours tend to be large, have a flared outline and may demonstrate invasion by paralysis of the phrenic nerve which is not seen in even large benign tumours. If malignancy is suspected, needle biopsy should be employed to obtain the diagnosis with the minimum risk of tumour spread, and radiotherapy is then the treatment of choice.

If the tumour is considered benign it is best removed through an anterior sternotomy since this approach carries a much lower morbidity than a lateral transpleural one.

The operation is essentially similar to that above except that tumours tend to develop a false capsule of compressed tissues and cling to surrounding structures by inflammatory adhesions. Thus the tumour may be adherent to the pericardium and the pleura and may extend across the pleura to the lung, but it is essentially, macroscopically, non-invasive. It may engulf the phrenic nerve but not paralyse it. It may be possible to extricate the nerve intact but in large tumours it may be preferable to sacrifice the nerve to permit excision of the tumour *en bloc*. The whole thymus should always be removed.

Surgery of the thoracic duct and management of chylothorax

Sir Keith Ross MS, FRCS
Consultant Cardiac Surgeon, Wessex Cardiac and Thoracic Centre, Southampton General Hospital, Southampton, UK

History

The serious consequences of a thoracic duct fistula and chylothorax, which are fatal if persistent, have been appreciated for centuries. Lampson[1] in 1948 was the first to control a chylous leak successfully by ligating the duct low in its intrathoracic course, and since that time the lethality of the condition has been significantly reduced.

Surgical principles

The success and safety of thoracic duct ligation depends on the richness of collateral channels and lymphatico-venous connections between the thoracic duct system and the lumbar, azygos and intercostal veins.

Temporary rises in intraduct pressure and interruption of the transmission of thoracic duct contents to the venous system are made good within approximately 10 days of duct ligation[2].

Surgical injury to the duct may be anticipated, and therefore prevented, in planned procedures (e.g. coarctation resection) which are known to involve this risk.

For practical purposes, only 50 per cent of thoracic duct fistulae can be expected to close spontaneously, helped by restriction of fluid and food intake by mouth and continuous pleural drainage, whatever the cause.

In chylothorax complicating malignant disease, even when this is advanced, thoracic duct ligation, possibly combined with a favoured method for pleurodesis (e.g. iodized talc) may be the kindest and quickest way of ridding the patient of a most uncomfortable complication.

Preoperative

Recognition of chyle

Tables are available setting out the composition and characteristics of chyle[3] but there is seldom doubt about the nature of the pleural fluid when aspirated or when it appears in chest drainage tubes. The simplest test to confirm the diagnosis is to add ether to the fluid in a test tube; if the fat dissolves and the milky fluid becomes clear, the fluid is chyle.

Reduction of chyle flow and promotion of spontaneous fistula closure

For many reasons (e.g. multiple injury) it may be sensible to decide upon a period of conservative treatment for an established thoracic duct fistula. All oral feeding should be stopped and the patient's nutrition maintained intravenously. Observed chyle loss is replaced volume for volume with plasma. Alternatively, the patient may be given a strict fat-free diet and kept on restricted oral fluid intake, with intravenous fluid supplement to achieve the daily fluid requirements.

Although a chylous fistula may close spontaneously after a single pleural aspiration, its unpredictable nature demands that the pleural cavity be kept as empty as possible (and the lung fully expanded) by intercostal tube drainage and gentle suction (minus 3–5 mmHg).

A period of 7 days is all that should be allowed for a conservative regimen unless it is clear that the volume of chylous drainage is becoming progressively less or there are other strong contraindications to surgical closure of the fistula.

It is wise to challenge apparently successful spontaneous closure of the fistula by resuming full oral feeding before removing the chest drain(s).

The operation

Approach

The chest should always be opened on the side of the chylous effusion.

Postoperative chylothorax demands re-opening the chest on the previously operated side unless it follows median sternotomy when a lateral approach on the side of the effusion is indicated.

In bilateral chylothorax, a right-sided approach is best.

When a chylous leak complicates a previous surgical procedure a direct attack on the site of duct injury is usually possible, with ligation of the proximal and distal ends of the duct at the site where it was damaged.

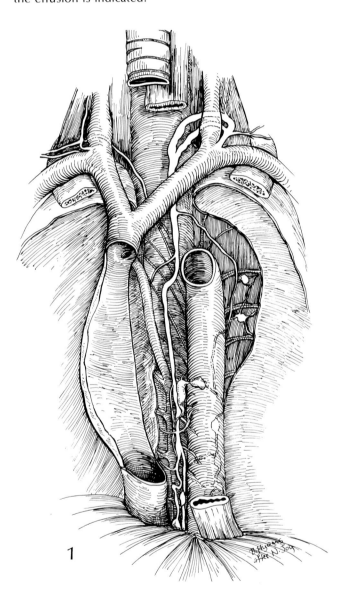

1

Elective duct ligation

1

When the course of the duct is 'normal' (found in only a little over half of individuals) the main duct is usually best approached by *right* thoracotomy, since it lies to the right of the aorta.

2

A standard posterolateral thoracotomy is made (see chapter on 'Surgical access in pulmonary operations', pp. 135–148) entering the chest along the upper or lower border of the unresected sixth rib, or a space lower if preferred.

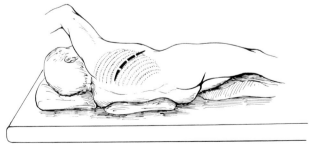

2

3

The pulmonary ligament is divided and the lung retracted forward.

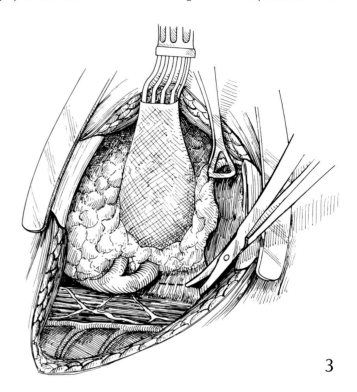

3

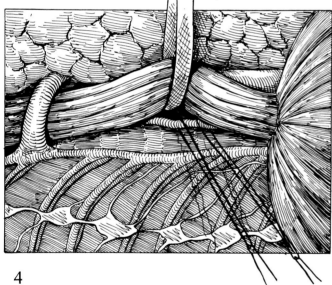

4

4

The oesophagus is retracted forwards and the thoracic duct (shown surrounded by two ligatures) is identified where it lies on the front of the vertebral column, a short distance above the diaphragm.

5 & 6

A left-sided approach to the main thoracic duct may be made by way of a standard left posterolateral thoracotomy to expose the aorta and its intercostal branches.

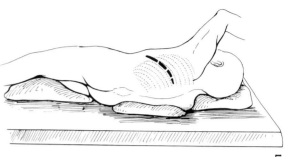

5

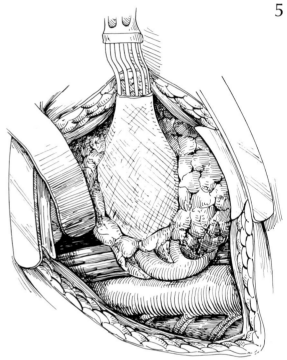

6

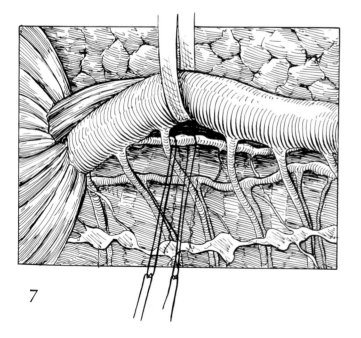

7

7

Following mobilization of the aorta, possibly with ligation of one or more intercostal arteries, the duct may be approached from in front of or behind (shown here) the retracted aorta.

Closure

After duct ligation the chest is closed in layers with a single basal pleural drain.

References

1. Lampson, R. S. Traumatic chylothorax: a review of the literature and report of a case treated by mediastinal ligation of the thoracic duct. Journal of Thoracic Surgery 1948; 17: 778–791

2. Ross, J. K. A review of the surgery of the thoracic duct. Thorax 1961; 16: 12–21

3. Ross, J. K. Surgical management of chylothorax. In: Rob, C. and Smith, R. eds. Operative Surgery: cardiothoracic surgery. 3rd edn. London: Butterworths, 1978, 349–354

Rigid and flexible bronchoscopy

D. K. C. Cooper   PhD, FRCS, FACC
Associate Professor, Department of Cardiothoracic Surgery, University of Cape Town Medical School and
Groote Schuur Hospital, Cape Town, South Africa

S. R. Benatar   FFA, FRCP
Professor and Head, Department of Medicine, University of Cape Town Medical School and
Groote Schuur Hospital, Cape Town, South Africa

Introduction

Attempts at visualizing the trachea and bronchi were made as early as the mid-nineteenth century, but it was not until the first half of the twentieth century that rigid endoscopy progressed rapidly under the influence of Chevalier Jackson[1]. Today, bronchoscopy plays an important role as a diagnostic procedure and, less commonly, as a therapeutic procedure in many chest diseases. The flexible fibreoptic bronchoscope developed by Ikeda[2] and introduced into clinical practice a little over a decade ago has extended the use of bronchoscopy from its previous sanctuary in thoracic surgery into the everyday practice of respiratory physicians. The use of bronchoscopy has been further extended into the investigation of diffuse lung disease by the development of broncho-alveolar lavage through the fibreoptic bronchoscope. Studies using this technique have contributed to rapid advances in understanding the pathogenesis of disorders such as sarcoidosis, extrinsic allergic alveolitis and idiopathic pulmonary fibrosis.

The proliferating use of fibreoptic bronchoscopy by respiratory physicians has meant that many bronchoscopists have never learnt to use the rigid instrument. Similarly, many thoracic surgeons, skilled in the use of the rigid bronchoscope, have neglected to acquire skill in the use of the newer flexible instrument. While it would be ideal for all operators to be skilled in the use of both instruments, this is not absolutely necessary in clinical practice; close co-operation between surgeons and physicians utilizing these procedures brings maximum benefit to the patient.

Training in bronchoscopy necessitates acquisition of extensive knowledge of chest diseases, practical skills in the use of the instrument, and visual training in bronchial anatomy, pathology and anatomico-radiological correlations. These attributes can best be acquired in training programmes in well established units under skilled operators available on a one-to-one basis; this training can be further enhanced by the use of practical and visual aids. Trainees need to perform in the region of 100 bronchoscopies to acquire an acceptable degree of skill.

Indications

Diagnostic

1. Observation
   (a) Mobility of vocal cords (recurrent laryngeal nerve injury or involvement by tumour); this is best shown in the awake, spontaneously breathing patient using the fibreoptic bronchoscope.
   (b) Patency and mobility of tracheobronchial tree.
   (c) State of mucosa.
   (d) Presence of tumours and foreign bodies.
   (e) Presence of secretions.
   (f) Origin of bleeding.
2. Aspiration of secretions for laboratory study (bacteriological, cytological).
3. Brushing of mucosa for cytological examination and examination for micro-organisms such as acid-fast bacilli and fungi.
4. Biopsy of tissue (bronchial wall and lung) for histological examination.
5. Assessment of pulmonary function by lobar sampling of gas.
6. Broncho-alveolar lavage to harvest alveolar cells and secretions.

Therapeutic

1. Removal of foreign bodies.
2. Aspiration of tracheobronchial secretions in debilitated patients who cannot adequately expectorate.
3. Aspiration of inhaled vomitus.
4. Aspiration of thick secretions causing postoperative collapse of a lobe or lung.
5. Treatment of haemoptysis (spontaneous or following biopsy).
6. Endobronchial resection of granulation tissue or endobronchial amyloidosis.
7. Restoration of a satisfactory airway by endobronchial resection of obstructing tumour or glands.

Choice of technique

Bronchoscopy may be performed with a rigid or flexible instrument. The major advantages of each are outlined in *Table 1*. The choice depends on the indications, the site of the lesion, the availability of the various instruments, and on the skill and preference of the operator. Conventionally, thoracic surgeons prefer the rigid instrument with the flexible bronchoscope as an accessory, whereas most respiratory physicians use the latter instrument alone.

Table 1 Advantages of different bronchoscopic systems

Rigid	*Flexible*
1. Aspiration of copious secretions.	1. Penetrates further into bronchial tree. Allows (a) biopsy and brushing of peripheral lesions with aid of fluoroscopy; (b) removal of small peripheral foreign bodies; and (c) early detection of bronchial carcinoma in patients with normal chest X-ray but positive sputum cytology.
2. Removal of foreign bodies and broncholiths.	
3. Assessment of mobility of tracheobronchial tree.	
4. Allows better evaluation of tracheal stenosis.	
5. Allows better control of haemoptysis. Safer biopsy of tumours such as adenoma which may bleed profusely.	2. Wider range of vision, especially within the upper lobe.
6. Requires less time.	3. Can be performed under local anaesthesia without discomfort.
7. Cost of instrument low.	4. Can be performed through a tracheostomy tube or endotracheal tube, and therefore can be used in patients on artificial ventilation.
8. Sizes of available instruments allow bronchoscopy in children.	
9. Better photographic records can be obtained.	5. Can be used in patients with rigidity of the vertebral column, e.g. ankylosing spondylitis, in whom extension of the head and neck is impossible.
	6. Allows examination of nasopharynx.

1

The flexible bronchoscope can be passed further distally to lobar, segmental and even subsegmental bronchi, which the rigid bronchoscope cannot reach, and can enter upper lobe and apical lower lobe segmental orifices which may not be adequately viewed with a rigid scope. The rigid instrument, however, allows for collection of large quantities of aspirate and much larger tissue biopsies.

In general, rigid bronchoscopy under general anaesthesia is a quicker procedure than flexible bronchoscopy under local anaesthesia, and therefore, although the extent of examination is more limited, a greater number of examinations can be performed in a limited time. This advantage is to some extent outweighed by the additional resources needed for rigid bronchoscopy, such as general anaesthesia and recovery room facilities.

Rigid bronchoscopy is probably preferred for most therapeutic procedures as it allows the passage of large forceps and large-bore suckers for the removal of inhaled foreign bodies, aspiration of thick secretions and of blood. Secretions can often be adequately aspirated through the flexible fibreoptic bronchoscope and this may be the method of choice where general anaesthesia is contra-indicated or where foreign bodies are located in the distal bronchial tree beyond the range of vision of the rigid instrument.

Diagram of normal bronchial tree, showing extent of vision by rigid and flexible bronchoscopy

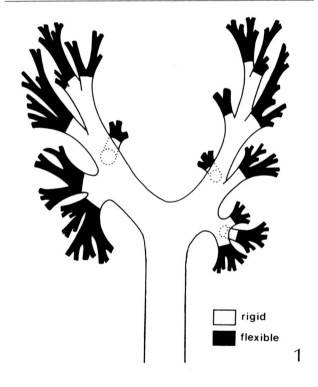

□ rigid
■ flexible

1

Relationship of mediastinoscopy to bronchoscopy

Before bronchoscopy is undertaken the indications for mediastinoscopy should be considered. In certain conditions, for example when lymphoma is strongly suspected, mediastinoscopy is accepted as a diagnostic procedure at the time of bronchoscopy. The role of mediastinoscopy in the assessment of operability in patients with bronchial carcinoma remains controversial, especially with the advent of such investigative techniques as computerized axial tomography (CAT) which may reveal the presence of enlarged hilar and mediastinal lymph nodes. If mediastinoscopy is to be carried out at the time of bronchoscopy, then general anaesthesia is usually preferred. Bronchoscopy should precede mediastinoscopy if a suspected bronchial carcinoma is likely to prove inoperable on bronchoscopic grounds, for example, if it lies close to the carina; mediastinoscopy would then prove unnecessary.

If it is the surgeon's policy to perform mediastinoscopy in all other cases or when mediastinal lymph node involvement is suspected, then it should usually precede bronchoscopy; this avoids the risk of bleeding from the site of bronchial biopsy while the patient remains anaesthetized for subsequent mediastinoscopy. If lymph nodes are encountered which are clearly pathological, biopsy or excision should be performed; bronchoscopy may then prove unnecessary.

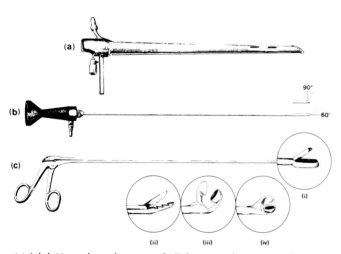

(a) Adult Negus bronchoscope. (b) Telescope, direct vision (inset – right angled vision). (c) Biopsy forceps: (i) Brian Taylor's; (ii) foreign body forceps (Chevalier Jackson's); (iii) Brock's angled; (iv) Brock's straight

If mediastinoscopy has not been performed, and it is decided to explore the mediastinum only after a bronchoscopically operable lesion has been seen, no biopsy should be taken at bronchoscopy. The scope should be withdrawn, mediastinoscopy performed, bronchoscopy repeated, and only then should a biopsy be taken, immediately before the patient is allowed to wake up and the cough reflex has returned.

With experience in the assessment of patients in whom bronchoscopy is indicated, the role and timing of mediastinoscopy become clarified.

Instruments

2

Rigid bronchoscope

The Negus instrument is a widely used standard bronchoscope, which comes in a range of sizes suitable for use in all age groups. In infants and children under the age of 6 or 7 years it is essential to choose a bronchoscope which will easily pass through the larynx; no attempt should be made to force an instrument which is just slightly too large. Post-bronchoscopy laryngeal oedema can be a major problem in such cases.

The basic design of the rigid bronchoscope has not changed over the years but there have been major improvements in optical systems and biopsy accessories. The bronchoscope requires a light source connected both to a light transmitter or carrier in the bronchoscope itself and to the various telescopes which can be passed down the lumen of the instrument. Three main telescopes are in common use, one allowing a 60° field of vision directly ahead, the others allowing a similar visual field but at 30° and 90° to the axis of the telescope. The right-angled instrument is essential for examination of the upper lobe bronchi and lower lobe apical bronchi.

A small range of biopsy and foreign body grasping forceps is available. Straight metal suckers, long enough to pass through the bronchoscope deep into the bronchial tree and wide enough (6 mm external and 4 mm internal diameter) not to become easily occluded by viscid aspirate, must be available, together with an adequate suction system. For the collection of tracheobronchial aspirate for bacteriological and cytological examination, sterile disposable sputum traps can be connected to the sucker.

Some form of 'bronchus blocker' should always be readily available to enable the operator to isolate the bronchial tree of one lung from the other in the event of profuse bleeding following tissue biopsy. Specific bronchus blockers are available, but a suitably sized catheter with distensible balloon tip (e.g. Fogarty) is equally satisfactory.

The bronchoscope and all accessory instruments to be passed into the bronchial tree should be clean. Some rigid bronchoscopes can be sterilized by autoclaving; all flexible equipment and telescopes for the rigid bronchoscope should be cleaned with 0.5 per cent hibitane in 70 per cent spirit before use and should *never* be autoclaved.

3

Flexible bronchoscope

A large variety of flexible fibreoptic bronchoscopes is available. They are delicate and expensive instruments, and should only be handled and used by trained personnel. They have a basic design, but many sophisticated accessories can be incorporated. A light source is again required. The operating head has an adjustable eyepiece, a finger-or-thumb-controlled lever or knob to manipulate the distal end of the instrument, and orifices for biopsy instruments and suction. The 5–6 mm diameter insertion tube contains the fibreoptic bundles, viewing lens system and a single operating channel, 1.8–2.6 mm in diameter. A variety of instruments, including forceps, brushes, balloon catheters and foreign body extraction devices, can be inserted through the channel and it can also be used for suction.

The field of view, which is about 105°, is considerably greater than that provided by the rigid bronchoscope. The tip of the bronchoscope can be angled to up to 180°, allowing manipulation into all lobar, segmental and even sub-segmental bronchi. Aspirate sampling units are available as attachments which allow tracheobronchial secretions to be sampled without contamination by oral and other airway micro-organisms. The use of a secondary attachment makes the flexible bronchoscope ideal for teaching purposes. Photography systems are available for still and moving films as well as video. Although a view of sub-segmental bronchi can be obtained in adults using the flexible system, progress of the scope down the bronchial tree is naturally limited by the diameter of the bronchus. In children, it may not be possible to see beyond the major bronchi.

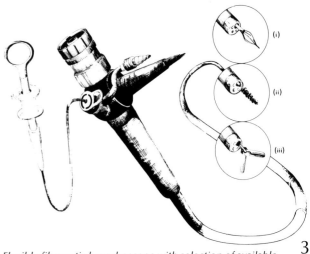

3

Flexible fibreoptic bronchoscope with selection of available accessories: (i) Basket; (ii) brush; (iii) biopsy forceps

To remove adherent material after use the instrument must be carefully cleaned externally with 70 per cent alcohol, and the operating channel must be brushed and flushed. The instrument is subsequently flushed and immersed in a 2 per cent glutaraldehyde solution (Cidex) for 20 minutes, though the control head should *never* be immersed in any solution. In addition, ethylene oxide sterilization can be performed intermittently if this facility is available.

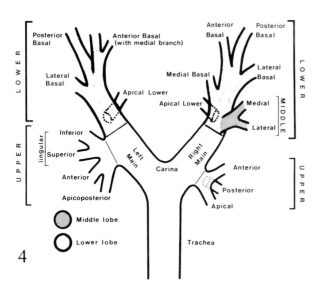

4

Bronchial anatomy

4

A good theoretical knowledge of bronchial anatomy is essential before bronchoscopy is undertaken. The bronchoscopic appearances of the normal tracheo-bronchial tree and of many of the pathological conditions which can affect it have been superbly described and illustrated by Stradling[3].

Preoperative

Preoperative preparation

When general or local anaesthesia is to be administered, the patient should have fasted for at least 6 hours before bronchoscopy. Patients undergoing rigid bronchoscopy prefer general anaesthesia. Many of these patients do not require premedication, but intravenous atropine 0.6 mg can be given if significant bradycardia occurs during the procedure.

Patients undergoing flexible bronchoscopy with local anaesthesia should receive premedication consisting of atropine 0.6 mg intravenously via an indwelling needle a few minutes prior to bronchoscopy. Very few patients require sedative drugs, but, if necessary, diazepam can be given intravenously. Anxious patients do well with atropine 0.6 mg and morphine 10 mg given intramuscularly 1 hour before the procedure.

Anaesthesia

General

Before general anaesthesia is induced for rigid broncho- scopy, the operator should check that the bronchoscopic lighting and suction systems are in working order, and that a 'bronchus blocker' which can easily be passed down the lumen of the bronchoscope is available. No muscle relaxant should be given until the operator is fully prepared.

For most diagnostic bronchoscopies in adults, anaes- thesia is induced with intravenous thiopentone, with subsequent muscle relaxation provided by a short-acting depolarizing drug such as succinylcholine, both of which may need to be repeated if the examination is prolonged. The pharynx and vocal cords may be sprayed with 2–4 per cent lignocaine. Oxygen is given by the Sanders technique[3] in which intermittent jets of oxygen blown down the bronchoscope inflate the lungs, keeping the patient satisfactorily oxygenated.

In infants and children inhalation anaesthesia without the use of muscle relaxants is preferable; some consider the Sanders technique dangerous to use in children when a foreign body, biopsy sample, or papilloma is present, as these may be blown distally by an ill-timed blast.

The flexible bronchoscope can be used in association with the rigid bronchoscope or endotracheal tube under general anaesthesia. When an endotracheal tube is inserted or when flexible bronchoscopy is performed through a tracheostomy tube, the fibrescope partially obstructs the airway and oxygen inflation is therefore essential. For this reason patients on mechanical ventila- tion require special care.

Local

Both types of bronchoscope can be passed under local anaesthesia, although this is not recommended with the rigid scope if an alternative is available, as it can be an uncomfortable experience for the patient.

For fibreoptic bronchoscopy, which is most commonly performed transnasally without an endotracheal tube, the most patent nasal passage is anaesthetized with 4 per cent lignocaine delivered from a MacIntosh nebulizer. The pharynx and vocal cords are anaesthetized by nebulizing 2 per cent lignocaine towards the back of the throat after instructing the patient to protrude the tongue as far as possible and then take a series of rapid shallow breaths. This procedure is repeated several times until adequate analgesia of the pharynx and upper larynx is obtained. A small cannula, introduced into the nasopharynx through the opposite nasal passage, is used to deliver oxygen at a flow rate of 5 litres per minute. Two per cent lignocaine jelly is applied to the anterior nares and to the distal 15–20 cm of the bronchoscope. Local anaesthetic is subsequently applied to the trachea and bronchi through the advancing bronchoscope (see below). To minimize the risk of inhalation, no patient who has received local anaesthesia to the pharynx and larynx should eat or drink for at least 2 hours after the procedure; clear fluids should be the first drink taken subsequently.

Position of patient

Rigid bronchoscopy

The distressed patient with a bronchial tree filled with secretions is best bronchoscoped while sitting upright in bed supported by pillows. The operator stands behind, leaning over the head of the patient. If a bronchopleural fistula or large lung abscess is suspected this position should also be used to avoid the possibility of aspiration into the other lung.

In all other cases it is usual for the patient to lie supine on the operating table with the head moderately extended and raised approximately 7.5 cm by a firm pillow so that the neck is flexed slightly. A mechanism for tilting the head of the table down in relation to the rest of the body greatly facilitates passage of the bronchoscope. A facility for tilting the whole table to bring the head down and feet up is essential in case of vomiting or of significant haemorrhage following biopsy.

In infants and children passage of the scope is greatly facilitated if an assistant's hand supports the upper thoracic spine, thus extending the neck.

A towel is wrapped around the head of the patient to protect the eyes, and the upper teeth and gums are covered by gauze swabs to prevent injury. The teeth must not be used as a fulcrum for the bronchoscope.

Flexible bronchoscopy

If the flexible bronchoscope is to be passed through a rigid bronchoscope or endotracheal tube under general anaesthesia, the position of the patient will be as described above. If the transnasal route is to be used the patient may be lying down or seated in a dental chair. The operator sits or stands behind or in front of the patient.

The operations

RIGID BRONCHOSCOPY

(The technique of passage of the bronchoscope will be described assuming the operator to be right-handed).

Introduction into oropharynx

The instrument is lightly lubricated with a suitable water-soluble jelly.

5

The position of the head of the patient is controlled by gripping the maxilla with the middle and ring fingers of the left hand, thus allowing the thumb and index finger to control the instrument.

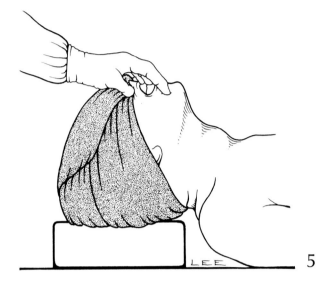

5

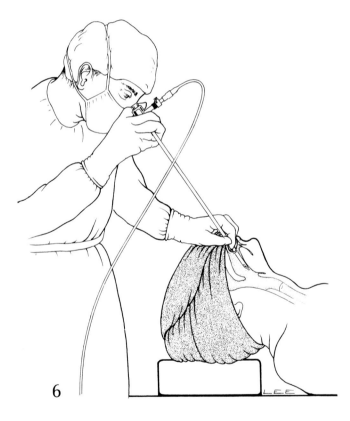

6

6

The operator stands behind the patient and holds the proximal end of the bronchoscope between the thumb and index fingers of the right hand, rather as he would hold a pen; the distal lip (or beak) of the scope is anterior.

Force must never be applied to the scope, nor the teeth or gums used as the fulcrum while the instrument lifts the tongue. The instrument should not be gripped with a fist as this gives very poor control and may result in the use of too much force.

7

The scope is then advanced in the midline gently past the uvula into the pharynx; from then on all further progress of the instrument is carried out under direct vision down the lumen of the scope.

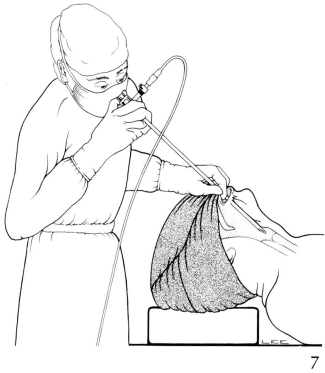

7

8

Identification of epiglottis

The distal end of the scope is lifted forward, mainly by the use of the operator's left thumb, which must also protect the patient's upper teeth and maxilla, and by slowly bringing the proximal end of the scope towards the horizontal plane; the root of the tongue is displaced anteriorly, bringing the epiglottis into view. Care must be taken to prevent the tongue and lips from being traumatized between the scope and teeth.

Occasional difficulty is experienced in visualizing the larynx, usually in patients with prominent teeth; exposure of the cords with a laryngoscope may facilitate the procedure.

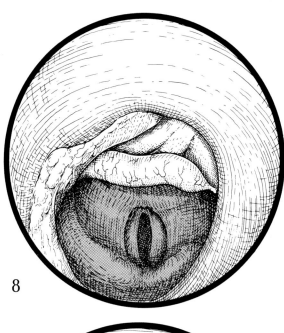

8

9

Visualization of vocal cords

The anterior lip of the scope is passed posterior to the epiglottis, which is then lifted forwards by bringing the scope further into the horizontal plane. This exposes the vocal cords, which are carefully inspected. Again care is needed not to use the upper teeth or gums as a fulcrum; the left thumb must continue to protect these structures. The scope is then rotated 90° to the right until its distal lip or beak lies in the same axis as the laryngeal inlet. The left vocal cord fills the centre of the operator's visual field. The scope is then passed gently onwards into the trachea.

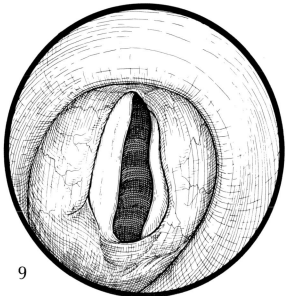

9

Advancing to the carina

Once the scope is in the trachea the head and neck are extended further by lowering the head of the table or removing the foam pillow. The instrument is rotated so that the beak is again anterior and is advanced to the carina. The wall of the trachea is inspected, any deviation of its course noted, and any loss of normal elastic mobility is transmitted through the scope to the operator's right hand. The proximal end of the bronchoscope tends to lie most easily towards the right corner of the mouth.

Inspection of bronchial tree

10

It is essential to examine the bronchial tree on both sides. The presumed normal side is inspected first. The scope can usually be passed easily into the right main bronchus, with slight extension and rotation of the head of the patient to the left. To enter the left main bronchus considerable rotation of the patient's head to the opposite side may be required.

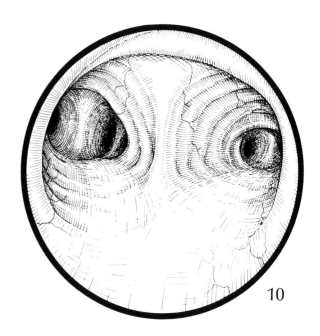

10

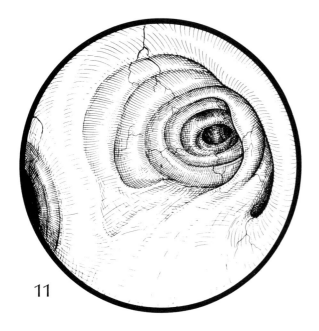

11

11

Right bronchial tree: upper lobe orifice

The orifice of the right upper lobe bronchus is situated close to the origin of the right main bronchus itself and can easily be missed if the scope is passed too far into the bronchus. Use of an angled illuminated telescope is necessary to obtain a good view of the right upper lobe bronchus and its segmental divisions.

12

Right bronchial tree: middle and lower lobe orifices

Right middle and lower lobe bronchi, with the exception of the apical lower segmental bronchus, can be viewed clearly by direct vision or with the straight telescope if a magnified view is required. An angled telescope is necessary for a clear view of the apical lower bronchus.

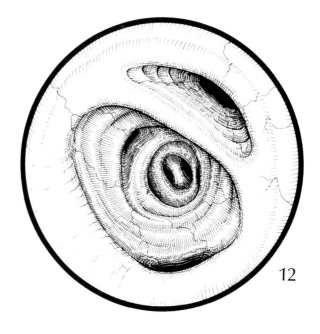

13

Left bronchial tree

A direct view of the origin of the left upper lobe bronchus and lingula division is frequently possible. An angled telescope is necessary to see into upper lobe segmental bronchi and the apical lower lobe bronchus. The basal segments of the lower lobe can be seen clearly with a straight telescope.

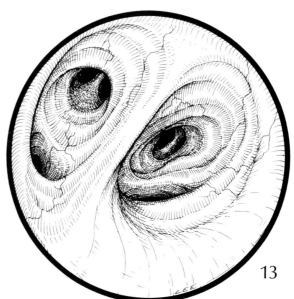

Taking a specimen of aspirate

Obtaining specimens from the bronchial tree during endoscopy is usually a vital part of the diagnosis. Secretion is removed, using a sucker and sputum trap. The sputum trap is kept upright to prevent losing the specimen. A small quantity of saline is then passed through the sucker to draw all removed material into the trap and ensure patency for immediate further use. This procedure is usually performed by the assisting nurse. Secretions may overlie tumours or other bronchial lesions which may bleed immediately if subjected to suction; aspiration must, therefore, at all times be performed gently and under direct vision.

Biopsy of tumours

Tumours, or suspicious areas of mucosa, should ideally be brushed before they are biopsied, as the latter may lead to bleeding which will obscure the visual field. If no tumour can be seen, but there is some distortion of the normal bronchial anatomy, 'blind' brushings from the depth of the bronchus may provide a diagnosis. The passage of a flexible bronchoscope (through the rigid scope or at a subsequent examination) may facilitate visualization of the lesion which can then be brushed or biopsied under direct vision. Bleeding following biopsy or brushing should be stemmed by intermittent suction and/or application of small, adrenaline-soaked gauze swabs.

Removal of foreign bodies

Foreign bodies may be obscured by secretions. They are usually readily removed with grasping forceps or by suction. In children the foreign body usually occludes a major bronchus and it may not be possible to withdraw it through the lumen of the bronchoscope. In this case the forceps grasping the foreign body and the bronchoscope must be gently withdrawn together.

After removal of any foreign body it is essential to have another look with the bronchoscope:

1. to assess any mucosal damage, bleeding or ulceration;
2. to remove distal retained secretions and promote reinflation of collapsed lung;
3. to ensure complete removal of the foreign body. This is particularly important following inhalation of peanuts as usually more than one are inhaled and they frequently fragment.

(Occasionally it is necessary to rebronchoscope after 2–3 days).

In all cases the airway should be adequately maintained until the anaesthetist and operator are satisfied that the patient is breathing spontaneously and has a satisfactory cough reflex.

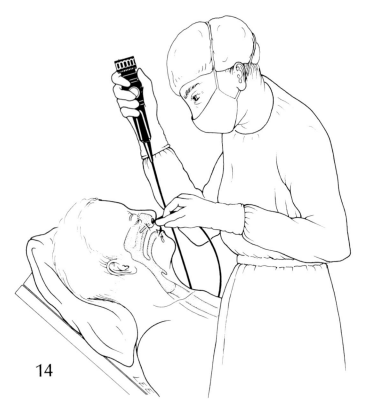

14

FLEXIBLE BRONCHOSCOPY

The advantages of transoral insertion of the fibreoptic bronchoscope through an endotracheal tube are that an airway is established and the bronchoscope can be removed and reinserted frequently and rapidly.

14

However, the transnasal route without an endotracheal tube is better tolerated by most patients and is preferred by the majority of operators. Once the larynx has been anaesthetized as described above, and inspected, the bronchoscope is advanced through the vocal cords, and the lower respiratory tract anaesthetized with successive 1–2 ml aliquots of 1 per cent lignocaine; 6 or 7 ml down each of the right and left main bronchi is usually sufficient. All lobar, segmental and subsegmental orifices on both sides should be examined routinely.

The major mucosal features of inflammation are mucopurulent exudates, mucosal erythema, longitudinal and transverse ridges, and dilated ducts of mucous glands. When these changes are localized rather than diffuse, carcinoma and other local lesions must be considered in the differential diagnosis. Additional mucosal features of bronchial carcinoma include loss of mucosal luminescence, increased mucosal granularity, thickening of bronchial spurs, and obvious endobronchial tumour which varies in appearance from polypoid masses to fungating lesions.

The use of fluoroscopy is of value in helping to direct the brush or biopsy forceps towards peripheral lesions not visible endoscopically. It is also useful in ensuring that the pleura is not penetrated during transbronchial lung biopsy. This procedure involves pushing an open 'crocodile' biopsy forceps through a distal bronchus into the lung parenchyma. Radiation time should be kept to a minimum, both to reduce patient and operator exposure and to prevent damage to the fibreoptic bundles. Protective lead aprons should be used by the operator, patient and assistant, and dosimeter badges worn by those involved in the procedure on a regular basis.

Patient co-operation, such as in taking deep breaths, can be helpful in directing the brush and forceps towards peripheral lesions and during transbronchial lung biopsy.

The 'wedge technique', which involves pushing the tip of the bronchoscope as far distally as possible to occlude the lumen of the bronchus, should always be used when transbronchial biopsy is performed as this permits better control of any complicating haemorrhage. Segmental broncho-alveolar lavage to harvest cells and secretions from the alveoli is also performed by 'wedging' the bronchoscope into a segmental bronchus and then alternately injecting and aspirating 30 ml aliquots of normal saline up to a total of 200–300 ml. This technique is used in the study and evaluation of a variety of interstitial lung disorders.

Postoperative care

Complications

Complications can be kept to a minimum by avoiding bronchoscopy whenever possible in high-risk situations, e.g. uncorrected bleeding diatheses, terminally ill fragile patients, patients with severe hypoxaemia and/or hypercapnia, and patients with unstable asthma.

Hypoxia

Prolonged examination in the apnoeic patient will give rise to hypoxia and may lead to cardiac arrest. Cardiac rate and rhythm should be monitored on an oscilloscope; the anaesthetist's duty to maintain the patient's oxygen saturation must take priority over the needs of the surgeon.

Bleeding

Some bleeding is almost inevitable after bronchial biopsy but is rarely a problem. The operator, however, should continue to observe the area biopsied until satisfied that the bleeding is negligible or has stopped. Occasionally a small gauze swab lightly soaked in adrenaline and held in a swab carrier needs to be pressed over the bleeding area for a few minutes to ensure clotting. With fibreoptic bronchoscopy, use of the wedging technique and the flushing of adrenaline solution (1:10 000) into the bleeding segment are of value in controlling bleeding and preventing aspiration of blood into more proximal airways.

Serious haemorrhage can follow blind biopsy or biopsy of a vascular tumour such as an adenoma. The patient is at immediate risk, not from blood loss but from hypoxia due to aspiration of blood into both lungs. In such cases the field of view of the operator may be rapidly and totally obscured. It is essential not to withdraw the bronchoscope. The patient should be tilted head down and turned on to the ipsilateral side to help prevent flooding of the opposite lung by blood. If the amount of bleeding cannot be readily controlled by suction or by the pressure of adrenaline-soaked swabs, then the site of bleeding should be isolated from the other lung by a bronchus blocker or Fogarty catheter. The catheter is passed until its tip lies in the offending bronchus and the balloon is dilated until it totally occludes the bronchus. Only then should the bronchoscope be gently removed, taking care not to dislodge the catheter.

A clean bronchoscope should immediately be passed carefully alongside the catheter down the trachea into the contralateral main bronchus and any blood in its lumen sucked out. Oxygenation of this lung should be continued for 5 minutes. The scope is then withdrawn and passed down again over the catheter, the balloon is deflated and the site of haemorrhage is inspected. In nearly all cases bleeding will have stopped; if not, the procedure should be repeated. Very rarely, thoracotomy is required to control the haemorrhage; the offending bronchus should be 'blocked' until this has been performed.

Pneumothorax

This is a potential complication of transbronchial lung biopsy. Its incidence can be kept to a minimum by careful biopsy under fluoroscopic control. Trans-bronchial biopsy should be limited to one lung to avoid the possibility of bilateral pneumothoraces. All patients should undergo fluoroscopic screening or chest radiography after transbronchial lung biopsy. Most pneumothoraces occur early though a few are only detected a few hours later. Only a small percentage require tube drainage.

Post-bronchoscopy laryngeal oedema in children

This may follow the passage of too large an instrument. Nursing in a steam tent may be the only treatment required in mild cases. Adrenaline nebulization administered by oxygen mask half-hourly or hourly controls the situation until the oedema resolves. Rarely, systemic steroids may be necessary.

Handling of specimens

Careful handling and labelling of all specimens obtained at bronchoscopy is necessary if maximum information is to be obtained. The interest and enthusiasm of skilled pathologists, cytologists and microbiologists greatly enhances the diagnostic yield. Bronchial and trans-bronchial biopsies should be placed in 10 per cent formalin for histology. Very small specimens obtained through the fibreoptic bronchoscope can be incorporated into a fibrin clot by adding a few drops of human plasma, rabbit brain thromboplastin and 0.02 M calcium chloride; this consolidated specimen is then placed in 10 per cent formalin. Brushings for cytology should be placed in 25 per cent alcohol, while brushings and biopsies for microbiological study should be submitted in saline. Specially designed, sterile, sleeve-protected brushes, which thus avoid contamination from proximal bronchial secretions, are available for accurate bacteriological sampling of distal lesions.

References

1. Jackson, C., Jackson, C. L. Bronchoesophagology. Philadelphia: W. B. Saunders, 1950

2. Ikeda, S. Flexible bronchofibrescope. Annals of Otology, Rhinology and Laryngology 1970; 79: 916–923

3. Stradling, P. Diagnostic bronchoscopy, 4th edn. Edinburgh: Churchill Livingstone, 1981

4. Sanders, D. R. Two ventilation attachments for bronchoscopes. Delaware Medical Journal 1967; 39: 170

Bronchography

John W. Jackson MCh, FRCS
Formerly Consultant Cardiothoracic Surgeon, Harefield Hospital, Harefield, Middlesex, UK

Introduction

This investigation in which a contrast medium is used to outline the bronchial tree is valuable in the assessment and diagnosis of certain pulmonary conditions. Modern diagnostic methods – tomography, angiography, and ventilation and perfusion studies – may provide much of the information that was formerly sought by bronchography but bronchography is still essential in determining the extent, distribution and severity of bronchiectasis particularly when there is a possibility of surgical excision. Knowledge of the exact distribution of the segments affected by bronchiectasis is also helpful to the physician and physiotherapist in the medical control of bronchiectasis. Fortunately, bronchiectasis in the United Kingdom is not the problem it was 30 years ago but it is still common in the developing countries. Surgery is indicated for localized disease particularly if it is confined to one lobe, e.g. middle lobe or lingula. Extensive bilateral disease might call for the excision of too much pulmonary tissue and in reaching a decision it is necessary to think not only of how extensively the bronchial tree is damaged but also, and equally important, of how well the remaining lung tissue will function after removal of the damaged segments. Bronchograms may be required in the investigation of bronchiectasis associated with Kartagener's syndrome, but surgery is not advisable in this condition where ciliary action is deficient owing to an ultrastructural abnormality in the cells of the respiratory tract. Nor is surgery advised where bronchiectasis is associated with IgA deficiency or cystic fibrosis. Bronchograms may be required whenever there is a troublesome productive cough, recurrent pneumonia and recurrent troublesome haemoptysis not explained by bronchoscopy. 'Dry' bronchiectasis may develop in an upper lobe as the result of collapse and scarring following tuberculosis; it is an occasional cause of recurrent haemoptysis.

Contrast media

Aqueous and oily suspensions of propyliodone (Dionosil) are available. The medium should be warmed to body temperature to reduce mucosal irritation and thoroughly mixed by shaking and repeated passage through a syringe and needle until a uniform suspension has been obtained. The oily suspension is less irritating to the bronchial tree, but being viscous will not pass through a fine needle; the tracheal catheter or needle must be of at least 1.5 mm internal diameter. Propyliodone is an organic iodide compound with little free iodine and as such does not provoke an iodide reaction; it is hydrolysed and absorbed from the bronchial tree in 2–3 days. The oily vector may take several weeks to clear, and surgery and repeat bronchography should be avoided for 4–6 weeks, although it is reasonable to proceed to outline the other lung after 5–7 days. With extensive or severe bronchiectasis the dye may linger for several weeks. For this reason it is best to outline the right bronchial tree first as residual oil in a left lung may make interpretation of the right lateral film, which is the most important diagnostic view of this lung, difficult. Because of the obliquity of the bronchial tree on the left the key diagnostic view for this side is taken in the right anterior oblique position and this is not obscured by the right lung. Simultaneous bilateral bronchograms are best avoided.

Method

In children bronchograms are best carried out under general anaesthesia, the contrast medium being introduced through a catheter passed down the endotracheal tube into the lung under investigation.

Preliminary bronchoscopy and bronchial toilet to clear secretions may be necessary where these are copious.

The investigation must be undertaken in the X-ray department under screening control, and successive small volumes of contrast medium introduced as the position is altered and each segment is outlined. It is important to avoid pooling and flooding of the bronchial tree and the amount of contrast medium used should be kept to a minimum. Ideally each lung should be investigated on a separate occasion. It is a mistake to think that having obtained good pictures of one lung it is safe to proceed to do the other during the same session. Usually these pictures will be inadequate and disappointing, making it necessary to repeat the investigation, and if there is any reaction it may be excessively severe.

Bronchograms should never be undertaken for the 'control of bronchiectasis', i.e. to see if it is progressing. Repeated bronchograms should be avoided and the investigation should only be carried out when a decision has to be made about surgery and the child is old enough to cooperate and participate in postoperative physiotherapy.

1, 2 & 3

In adults and teenagers the oil may be introduced into the bronchial tree down a plastic catheter passed through the larynx via the mouth or nose or, alternatively, by cricothyroid or cricotracheal puncture using a needle or fine catheter on an introducing needle (Angiocath).

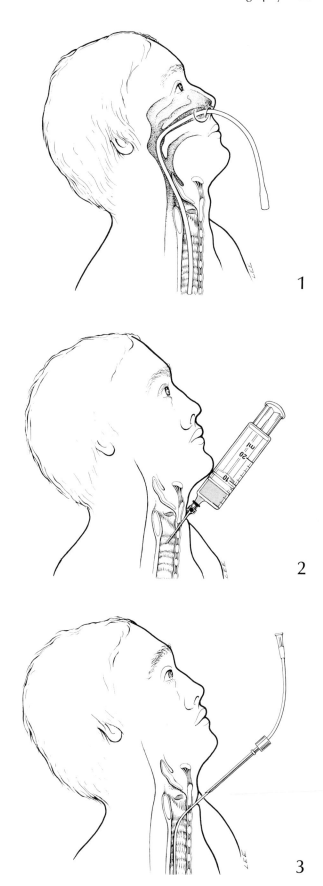

1

2

3

Preparation

The examination should be carried out during a period of remission from infection. Instruction in postural drainage and physiotherapy is advisable and if the sputum is infected a short course of an appropriate antibiotic should be administered. The interval should be used to instil confidence, secure cooperation and familiarize the patient with the various positions that he will be asked to assume during the examination. Mild sedation – diazepam 5–10 mg given orally 1 hour before the examination – is helpful in some cases. No attempt should be made to dry up secretions with an atropine preparation. It is essential to maintain the patient's full cooperation throughout the examination, which must be conducted in peace and quiet without distraction or disturbance. Talking, laughing, coughing and crying must be avoided. Lacrimation is often accompanied by a secretomotor disturbance of the upper respiratory tract and bronchorrhoea; the author prefers the apparently more barbaric method of cricothyroid (or cricotracheal) puncture to the transoral or transnasal routes as it causes less mucosal stimulation.

Anaesthesia

Nasopharyngeal intubation

Lignocaine (Xylocaine) 4 per cent is used for surface anaesthesia. One of the nasal passages and the oropharynx are sprayed and later the laryngopharynx and vocal cords are sprayed under direct vision but if this is not possible 2 ml of 4 per cent lignocaine may be introduced by cricothyroid puncture. It is important not to exceed 4 ml of 4 per cent lignocaine or its equivalent. The patient is allowed to rest while the catheter and contrast medium are prepared. The catheter is introduced into the larynx under direct vision or by viewing it on the X-ray screen, and positioned in the trachea; this may be facilitated by filling the catheter with contrast.

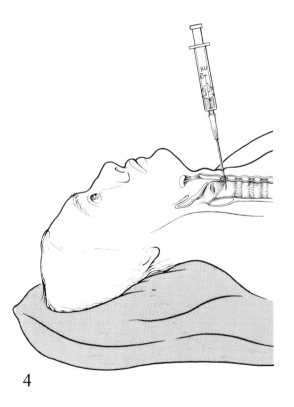

4

4

Tracheal puncture

For the cricothyroid (or cricotracheal) method the skin and superficial tissues of the neck are anaesthetized with up to 5 ml of 0.5 per cent lignocaine. Lignocaine (2 ml of 4 per cent) is introduced into the trachea using a short stout needle (19 gauge). It is easy to feel when the needle has entered the trachea. The piston is drawn back to ensure that the needle is not blocked by cartilage or lying submucosally. If air is obtained the patient is instructed to stop breathing in full expiration. The injection is then made and the needle removed immediately. A deep inspiration must follow and will distribute the anaesthetic throughout the bronchial tree. Some coughing results and lignocaine may appear in the sputum, thus anaesthetizing the larynx and pharynx. After a minute or two a second injection (2 ml of 4 per cent lignocaine) should be made in the same way. It is unusual for this to provoke further coughing. The patient is allowed to rest while the contrast medium is mixed and drawn up; 15–20 ml is all that should be required.

The patient is now instructed in and taken through the various positions he will be asked to assume before making any injection of contrast. To avoid bilateral filling the patient must remain inclined towards the side being examined and the operator stands on this side. Not more than 2 ml of contrast is introduced in any one position.

Positions for injection

5a & b

Position A

1.5–2 ml; Allow 30 seconds. Resting on the point of the elbow. Fills the apical segment of the lower lobe. Rest back to allow complete distribution.

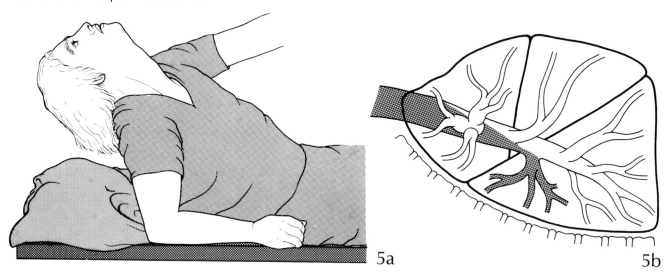

5a

5b

6a & b

Position B

1.5–2 ml. Sitting up but inclined backwards. Fills the posterior basal segments.

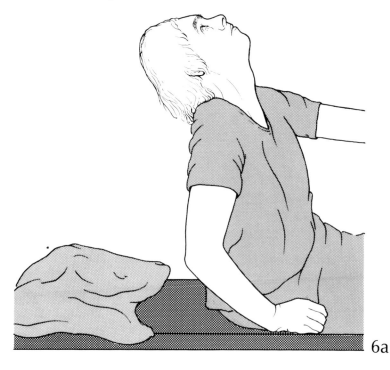

6a

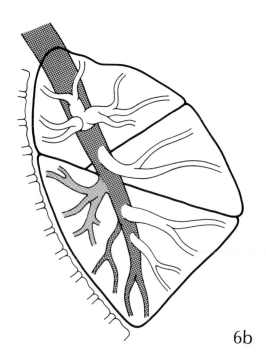

6b

7a & b

Position C

1.5–2 ml. Sitting straight up but still inclined to the side of the examination. Fills the lateral basal segment.

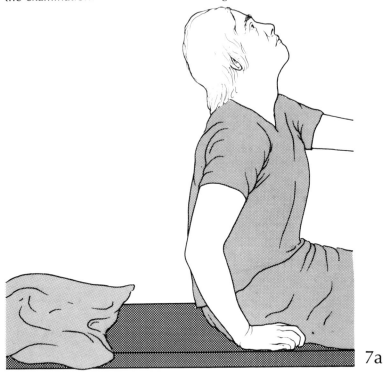

7a

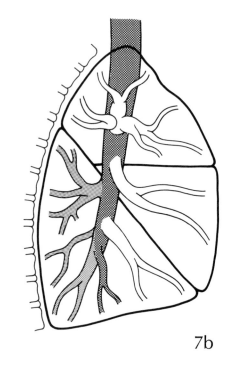

7b

8a & b

Position D

1.5–2 ml. Sitting up and leaning forward. Fills the anterior basal segment.

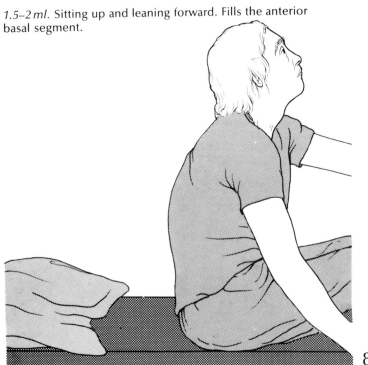

8a

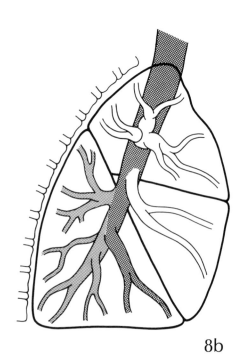

8b

9a & b

Position E

1.5–2 ml. Leaning further forward and arm hanging down.
Fills the middle lobe (or lingula).

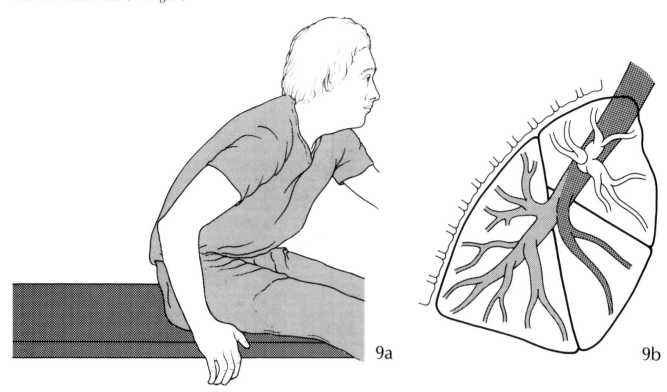

9a

9b

10a & b

Position F

4–5 ml. Lying on point of shoulder, head off the pillow.
Allows dye to enter upper lobe. Use 4–5 ml and remove
the needle.

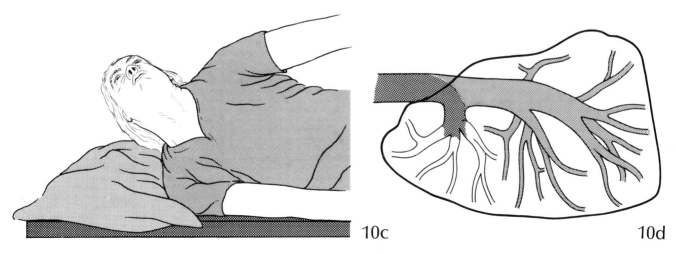

10c

10d

11a & b

Position G

Rest flat on table examination side down. Fills the posterior segment of upper lobe.

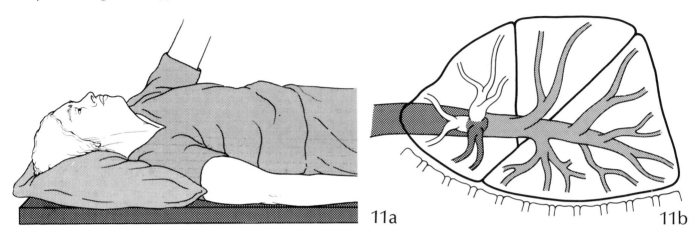

11a

11b

12a & b

Position H

Turn on face. Fills the anterior segment of upper lobe.

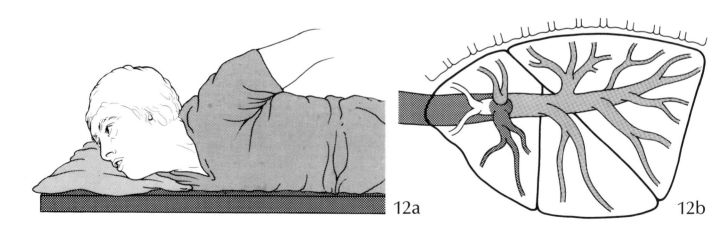

12a

12b

13a & b

Position I

Kneel up, shoulder on pillow. Fills the apical segment of upper lobe.

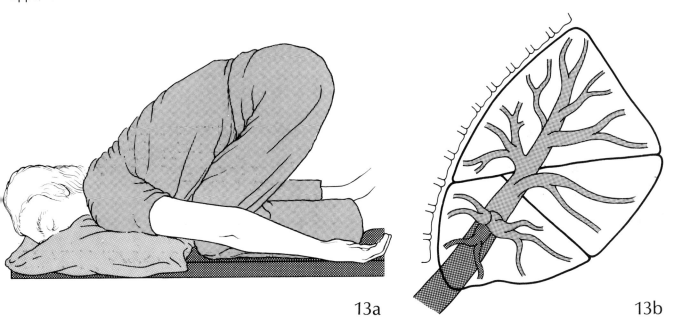

13a   13b

Technique of injection

Each injection must be made slowly, checking from time to time that the needle (or catheter) is correctly positioned. Quiet breathing, slightly deeper than normal, helps to distribute the dye. Prolonged deep inspiration and quiet expiration (rather like inhaling a cigarette) prevents coughing. Injection should be stopped if moist sounds are heard in the trachea or bronchi. Slow deep breathing is encouraged until the airway clears, and injection resumed in the next position using smaller quantities. Occasionally it will be necessary for the patient to 'clear the throat' but coughing should be avoided and prevented as this will result in alveolar filling. If medium reaches the mouth the patient should sit up immediately and the mouth should be wiped with a paper tissue. One should avoid getting contrast medium on the skin or clothing. The surgeon should wear a gown to protect his own clothes.

Postero-anterior and lateral radiographs are taken in the recumbent and/or erect positions and on the left side a postero-anterior radiograph is taken in the right anterior oblique position. Other views may be requested by the radiologist. If filling of one segment is incomplete a further injection of contrast in the appropriate position may be made.

After the radiographs have been judged satisfactory the patient is allowed to talk and cough and return to the ward where he should be postured by the physiotherapist and encouraged to cough up as much as possible of the medium. Where the dye has been introduced by cricothyroid puncture a small firm dressing should be applied and the patient should be instructed to press on this when coughing. Because of the effect of the local anaesthetic on the pharynx and larynx the patient should not be allowed to eat or drink for 4 hours.

If there is no undue reaction bronchography is performed on the other side in 5–7 days.

Further reading

Wardman, A. G., Willey, R. F., Cook, N. J., Crompton, G. K., Grant, I. W. B. Unusual pulmonary reactions to oily propyliodone (Dionosil) in bronchography. British Journal of Diseases of the Chest 1983; 77: 98–103

Aspiration of the chest

Rex De L. Stanbridge MRCP, FRCS
Consultant Cardiothoracic Surgeon, St Mary's Hospital, and Hammersmith Hospital, London, UK

Preoperative

Indications

Aspiration of the pleural cavity is indicated for diagnostic and therapeutic reasons.

Diagnostic tap is indicated to answer the questions 'What type of fluid is it?', i.e. serous, purulent, blood or chyle, and 'Is it infected or malignant?'.

Therapeutic reasons include drainage of a large volume of fluid which is causing respiratory embarrassment or of a small volume which may be causing fever. There is no limit to the volume of fluid which may be withdrawn from a pleural cavity at one sitting. Risks of pulmonary oedema are grossly exaggerated. As a general rule as much fluid as possible should be removed unless aspiration is undertaken for diagnosis only.

Anaesthesia

The procedure is performed under local anaesthesia of the chest wall with lignocaine hydrochloride in 0.5 or 1 per cent solution. This is 5 or 10 mg/ml. The maximum dose is 200 mg; thus up to 20 ml can be used. Usually, however, only 5–10 ml are needed.

A small intradermal weal is raised with a fine needle at the chosen site. The needle is then changed to a long fine one and this is advanced through the muscles of the chest wall and into the intercostal space, as the local anaesthetic is introduced.

It is necessary to assess the distance of the pleural cavity from the skin for two reasons:

1. To prevent unnecessary and deep movement of the aspirating needle into the thoracic cavity with probable injury of the lung or other organs.
2. To assess the thickness of the chest wall so that if a chest drain is inserted later the minimum distance necessary to ensure that the side holes are fully within the thoracic cavity can be measured (*see* chapter on 'Intercostal drainage', pp. 110–117). To do this it is useful to aim just at the upper border of a rib, actually to touch that rib and then to step the needle over the top of the rib. The distance between the muscle and the pleura is fairly constant; it is a matter of only 0.5 cm unless there is a heavy thickening of the pleura, as in chronic infected effusion. This method also avoids injury of the neurovascular bundle which lies immediately underneath the rib in the subcostal groove. It also allows accurate placement of the anaesthetic in the region immediately outside the pleura, thereby ensuring anaesthesia of the pleura, which is a very sensitive structure.

Between 5 and 10 ml of local anaesthetic are required to anaesthetize the track of the needle and the subpleural space. It is advisable to enter the pleural cavity with the needle to ensure that the right location for aspiration has been chosen. Thereafter this needle and syringe are not used for further administration of local anaesthetic. If it is known that multiple sites of aspiration are likely then it may be wise to anaesthetize these sites at this stage with clean apparatus.

The operation

1

Equipment

Disposable plastic needles, syringes and taps should be used, as these are airtight when fitted snugly. Glass syringes tend to leak over many years of use and are no longer ideal. The size of the equipment required depends on whether a large amount of effusion is to be aspirated or only a small amount for diagnostic purposes. A large-bore needle is required for large effusions and for purulent or thick effusions. The largest-bore needle you can find is the most suitable; a No. 15 blade will be required to make a nick in the skin to allow the insertion of such a needle. A secure three-way plastic tap, a 20 or 50 ml syringe, a simple dressing pack with gauze swab and gallipot for cleansing widely the skin area, and a standard urine drainage bag are all that are needed. Vygon and Pleuraset closed-system drainage-sets are recommended.

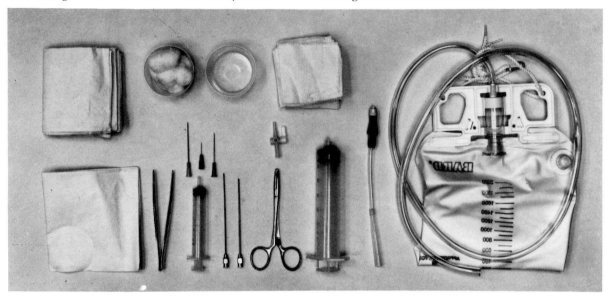

1

2

Position

If the patient can get out of bed he should be seated comfortably astride a chair by the bed with his head resting on his forearms, which are themselves resting on the bed. Pillows may be added according to the height of the patient. This is a stable position.

If the patient is confined to bed but can sit upright he should be leant well forward over a bed table and pillows so that his weight tends to hold him forward.

Site

The site of aspiration to be aimed at should be one fingerwidth below the fluid level as seen on the chest radiograph. The best way to determine this point is to mark the fluid level in relation to the anterior costal cartilages on the chest radiograph and then to identify the costal cartilage concerned on the patient and draw a horizontal line laterally around the chest to the site of aspiration. If the operator tries to go too low below a fluid level he will not know where the diaphragm lies and may easily penetrate the diaphragm, peritoneum, liver or spleen.

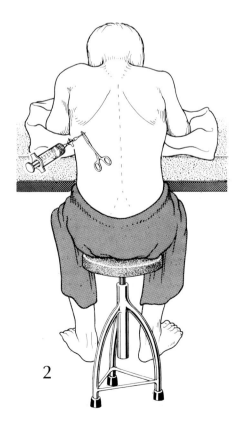

2

3a, b & c

Aspiration

A large-bore needle is inserted into the chest in the same manner as for the anaesthetic needle, finding the rib space and stepping over the lower rib with care, thereby preventing damage to underlying structures. Slight suction applied to the syringe, which is connected to the needle via the three way tap, helps to provide early confirmation of the effusion.

Fluid should be withdrawn slowly and steadily. A Spencer Wells or similar forceps attached to the needle at the skin level helps to prevent excessively deep movement of the needle into the thorax. The fluid is aspirated to fill the syringe (a). The three-way tap is then turned to connect the syringe with the drainage bag and the fluid is expelled into the bag (b).

Specimens should be taken for microbiology, cytology and chemistry at this stage.

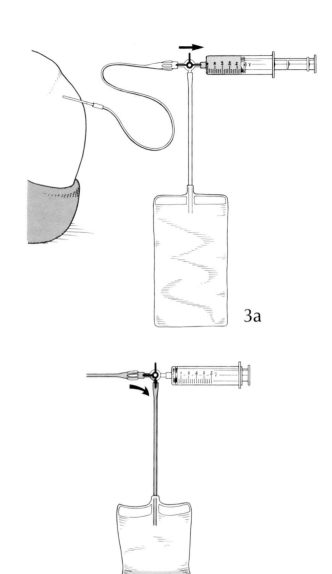

3a

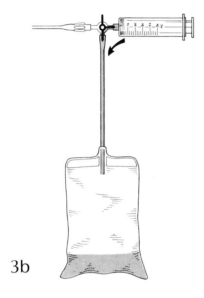

3b

3c

Syphon method If this method is to be adopted the three-way tap is now turned on again between the syringe and the patient, a further aspiration carried out and the three-way tap turned again to expel fluid into the drainage bag, which should be placed well below the level of the patient's chest. Care should be taken not to over-empty the syringe and to ensure that no air enters the drainage tube or the bag during this procedure. There should now be sufficient fluid to occupy the whole of the tube leading into the bag, and the three-way tap may be turned to connect the bag with the aspirating needle so that fluid syphons itself off into the bag (c). This technique is particularly useful for large effusions and has the advantage that it does not require frequent manipulation of the three-way tap, leaving the needle absolutely static during the procedure without any risk of damaging underlying structures. Transfer of fluid into the bag can be seen by the bag filling at the bottom and by the movement of tiny bubbles in the chest tube.

Termination of aspiration

As fluid is removed the lung expands and this often causes the patient to cough. This has sometimes been confused with pulmonary oedema, but it is due to alteration of the surfactant layer on the lung. When the patient starts coughing repeatedly this indicates that the volume of fluid remaining in the chest is now very small and aspiration should cease if injury of the lung is to be prevented. Also, towards the end of repeated aspiration it is often found that fluid enters the syringe in a jerky fashion, coming more easily on expiration. This too is a sign that the amount of fluid remaining is small. The needle is withdrawn and the puncture site is covered with a swab with collodion or a piece of Micropore tape applied, pinching the skin edges together without dressing.

Illustrations by Patrick M. Elliott

Biopsy of pleura and lung (including thoracoscopy)

Werner Maassen MD
Professor and Head, Ruhrlandklinic for Pneumonology and Thoracic Surgery, Essen, Federal Republic of Germany

Pleural biopsy

Indications and contraindications

A pleural biopsy to define the cause of a pleural effusion is always indicated, unless it is obvious clinically (pleurisy due to a pulmonary infarction, tuberculosis) or if an exploratory aspiration shows a purulent effusion, whether tuberculous or non-tuberculous. It is possible to aspirate most of the effusion during pleural biopsy, and this often facilitates further radiographic diagnosis and improves the patient's respiratory function at the same time. Circumscribed lesions of the pleura (pleural plaques, tumours) also require biopsy or endoscopic clarification. In cases of tuberculous pleurisy, the excised tissue can be examined both histologically and bacteriologically so that non-specific bacteria or tubercle bacilli can be identified and their resistance to antibiotic or antituberculous therapy can be determined.

An X-ray of the thorax in the decubitus or the head-down position often facilitates the diagnosis of pleural disease. This allows better localization for the pleural biopsy, especially needle biopsy, and leads to optimal results. In cases where limited lesions of the pleura are difficult to localize, the puncture point must be marked under fluoroscopic control with the patient's arm placed in the same position as for the examination. Occasionally, ultrasonic control can assist in more accurate direction of the instrument.

Anaesthesia

As a rule all pleural biopsies and thoracoscopy can be performed with local anaesthesia. For needle biopsy, usually not more than 10 ml of a 1 per cent lignocaine (lidocaine) solution is necessary. A maximum of 40 ml of 1 per cent lignocaine or its equivalent can be used in a patient of average size. For better pain alleviation, not only the soft tissue and the pleura should be infiltrated, but a small amount should also be placed at the upper margin of the lower rib of the chosen intercostal space. Should a need to cough occur on infiltration of the pleura, this shows that the lung is adherent to the chest wall at this point and that a needle biopsy of the pleura is not possible. For a pleural biopsy with the Abrams' needle only, the chosen location can still be used when pleural thickening is clearly identifiable on the X-ray and there is no effusion. If an effusion is present, an examination must be carried out in this area.

NEEDLE BIOPSY OF THE PLEURA

Instrumentation and technique

Three different types of needle are available for needle biopsy of the pleura: Silverman's, Abrams and Copes.

Silverman's splaying needle (See Illustration 11)

This can only be safely used where the pleura is clearly thickened and areas of the lung may be adherent. The splaying needle is encased in a cannula which is equipped with a stylet. The distance between the skin and the pleura is measured during infiltration of the anaesthetic (into the soft tissue and pleura) and then marked on the splaying needle by placing a clamp. Following a small skin incision, the instrument is inserted as far as the pleura. The stylet is withdrawn and the splaying needle is then pushed into the suspected centre of the pleural lesion. Tissue is caught by pushing the cannula forward and the needle is then withdrawn. Some authors advocate rotation of the needle through 360° several times to obtain better results.

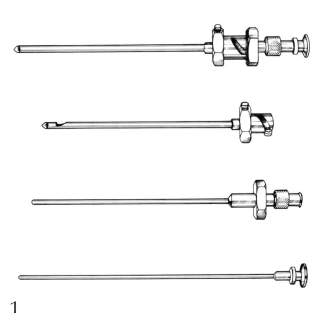

1

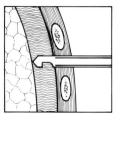

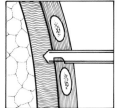

2

The Abrams' biopsy instrument

1

This consists of a short needle with a conical, and therefore relatively blunt, tip with a side notch for effusion aspiration and biopsy, and a sharp-edged inner hollow needle for severing and enclosing the tissue. A stylet for the inner cylinder completes the instrument.

2

Tissue is obtained by pushing the needle in until effusion is harvested. The examiner must then retract the needle until no more effusion is collected. At this point, the needle lies directly at the parietal pleura. Pleural tissue is drawn into the needle by sharp suction using a 20 ml syringe or, preferably, an aspirator; the inner cylinder is then pushed forward, thereby severing and enclosing the biopsy.

This procedure can be repeated several times. It is important here, as in all other puncture biopsies of the pleura, that the opening of the retractor needle faces downwards towards the upper margin of the lower rib of the chosen intercostal space, in order to avoid damage to the nerves and vessels at the lower margin of the upper rib.

Cope's biopsy instrument

3

This consists of an outer cylinder with a cutting edge at its tip, an oblique-cut stylet and a dull-edged hooked hollow needle for biopsy.

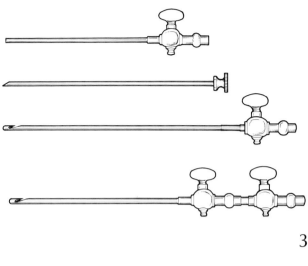

3

4

A skin incision is made through which the outer cylinder with stylet is introduced into the pleural space; the stylet is then withdrawn while the needle aperture is closed to prevent air from entering the cavity. The hooked trocar is then introduced into the needle – again with its cutting edge facing downwards. Using this needle it is possible to obtain pleural tissue from the inner surface of the lower rib and its upper margin, the tissue being enclosed by pushing the outer cannula forward. This procedure can be repeated several times without significant discomfort to the patient, until enough material has been collected.

After concluding the pleural biopsy, the outer cannula with stylet can be reintroduced into the effusion; after removal of the stylet an aspirator can be fitted and the effusion almost completely aspirated. Injury to the lung seldom occurs during this procedure as the outer cylinder is non-traumatic.

We prefer the *Ramel modification* of this instrument, for its outer cylinder is completely round and dull without a cutting edge. The cutting function is performed by the stylet which protrudes beyond the outer cannula. The method of taking the biopsy is the same. Drainage of pleural exudate is more easily accomplished using this needle because the tip of the cylinder causes less trauma than that of Cope.

Most hospitals provide a sterile thoracentesis tray which contains the following items.

50 ml Luer-lock syringe
16 gauge short-bevel needle
Three-way stopcock
Drainage tube
5 or 10 ml syringe
25 and 20 or 22 gauge needles
Towel
Fenestrated drape
Swab sticks and gallipots for antiseptic
Gauze squares and/or cotton balls

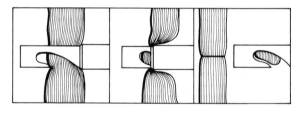

4

In addition to these items, the following should be assembled before the procedure is begun.

Sterile surgical gloves
Antiseptic solutions for skin preparation
Vial of 1 or 2 per cent lignocaine
Heparin, 1000 units/ml
Containers to collect fluid for laboratory examination
Aerobic, anaerobic, mycobacterial culture tubes
Vials containing anticoagulant for cell counts and various biochemical determinations
Glass syringe and cap for pH measurement
Empty 500 ml screw-top bottle for pleural fluid cytology
Empty 1 litre bottle or plastic bag for remainder of fluid to be removed
Adhesive tape to secure fenestrated drape
Plasters (Band-Aids) to cover puncture sites

Examination of the pleural effusion

Sufficient pleural effusion (30–50 ml) should have been obtained prior to the biopsy manipulation – if possible using the anaesthetic needle – in order to exclude any changes in pleural effusion caused by the biopsy procedure. The examiner should note the colour, transparency and viscosity of the fluid, as well as its milky appearance in cases of chylothorax. A leucocyte count is only important when empyema is present. In principle, however, a case of pleural empyema should not be subjected to pleural biopsy. An erythrocyte count of more than 100 000/ml constitutes a sanguinous exudate which usually indicates a tumour, although the same appearance is possible following pulmonary infarction or thoracic trauma.

A preponderance of polymorphonuclear leucocytes indicates an acute inflammatory disease such as pneumonia with parapneumonic effusion, pulmonary infarction, early tuberculous effusion or other inflammatory diseases. When lymphocytes form the majority of the leucocytes, tuberculosis or, less often, a tumour must be considered. Whether the effusion is exudate or transudate can be established by measuring the protein content. In the rare cases of rheumatic pleurisy, the glucose concentration is greatly reduced. A higher concentration of amylase in the pleural effusion than in the blood is characteristic of a pleural effusion which emanates from the pancreas. An increase in hyaluronic acid is typical for a pleural mesothelioma (Table 1).

Complications

Complications from needle biopsy of the pleura are rare. An air embolus occurs only in cases of inappropriate examination at the lower margin of the upper rib of the intercostal space or in cases of greatly thickened pleura with inadequate contractility of the vessels. Unequivocal injuries to the intercostal vessels with bleeding into the pleura can, in rare cases, necessitate a blood transfusion.

Radiological control after the puncture is very important in order to recognize a pneumothorax caused by the puncture. If such a pneumothorax is very large, drainage may be advisable and this must be undertaken immediately in cases where tension pneumothorax occurs.

Implantation of tumour cells is rare, but occasional instances of this have been reported[3]. From personal experience, this risk is greatest in cases of biopsy for mesothelioma.

Table 1 Typical findings in representative causes of pleural effusion (from Ball[1])

Condition	Appearance	Protein	WBC	Differential	Glucose	Amylase	pH	Cytology
Heart failure	Pale, hazy	Low	<1000	Mostly lymphs	N*	N	>7.35	Negative
Tuberculosis	Serous	High, often >5.0	2000–10 000	Mostly small lymphs	Usually N	N	7.20–7.40	Very few mesothelial cells
Malignant tumour	Often bloody	High	2000–10 000	Mostly small lymphs	Usually N	Sometimes slightly increased	occ. <7.30	Often positive
Pneumonia	Serous	High	Often >10 000	Mostly polys	N	N	>7.30	Negative
Empyema	Purulent	High	Often >30 000	Mostly polys	Very low	N	<7.20	Negative
Pulmonary infarct	Often bloody	High	Variable	Mostly polys	N	N	>7.35	Negative
Rheumatoid arthritis	Often greenish	High	2000–10 000	Mostly mononuclears	<20 mg/100 ml	N	>7.35	Negative
Pancreatitis	Serous, occasionally bloody	High	Often >10 000	Mostly polys	N	Very high	>7.35	Negative
Mesothelioma	Often viscid, often bloody	High	2000–10 000	Mostly mononuclears	N	N	>7.35	Negative
Asbestosis	Serous	High	Variable	Mostly mononuclears	N	N	>7.35	Negative
Chylothorax	Chylous	Low	<1000	Mostly mononuclears	N	N	>7.35	Fat droplets

* N = Normal

5

SURGICAL PLEURAL BIOPSY USING SUTLIFF'S METHOD

Using this method a small section of rib can be removed subperiosteally under local anaesthesia, the parietal pleura beneath it exposed and a biopsy taken for histological examination.

Parietal pleura can also be obtained after incising the intercostal musculature, but this method is not widely used.

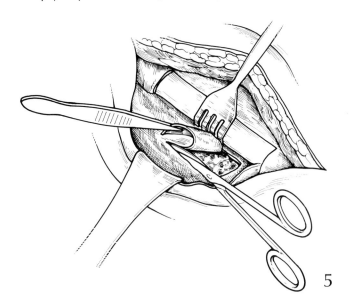

5

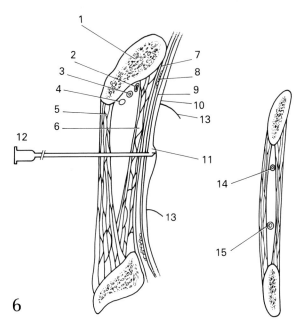

6

1. Rib; 2. Intercostal vein; 3. Intercostal artery; 4. Intercostal nerve; 5. External intercostal muscle; 6. Internal intercostal muscle; 7. Fascia intercostalis; 8. Fascia endothoracica; 9. Pavietal pleura; 10. Visceral pleura; 11. Pleural space; 12. Pneumothorax needle; 13. Pleura interlobaris; 14. Ramus cranialis of intercostal artery; 15. Ramus candalis of intercostal artery.

THORACOSCOPY

Instrumentation and technique

6

Thoracoscopy takes a mid-position between needle biopsy of the pleura and surgical pleural biopsy. A prerequisite is extensive pleural effusion which can be drained and replaced by air or, when no pleural effusion is present, a free pleural space allowing for the creation of a pneumothorax. The pneumothorax should be filled with carbon dioxide in order to avoid air embolism. A pneumothoracic apparatus and a pneumothorax needle with a side notch are necessary. In the lateral position, the pneumothorax is created between the third and fifth intercostal space in the anterior midaxillary line; in the supine position, it is made in the second or third intercostal space in the midclavicular line; and with the patient in the face-down position, the sixth to seventh intercostal space medial to the scapula should be chosen.

7 & 8

A trocar with stylet is necessary for thoracoscopy, whereby the stylet can be withdrawn and the thoracoscope introduced into the pleural cavity.

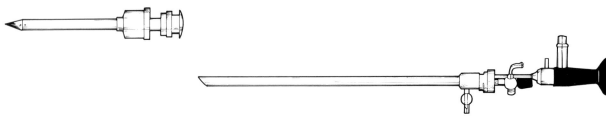

7

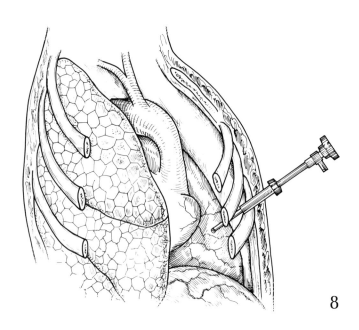

8

9

Optical equipment with various viewing angles allows an endoscopy of the pleural cavity and, in conjunction with forceps, tissue biopsy. A thoracoscope with a laterally placed eyepiece allows for puncture of the lung or mediastinum as well as coagulation and biopsy with larger forceps under visual control*.

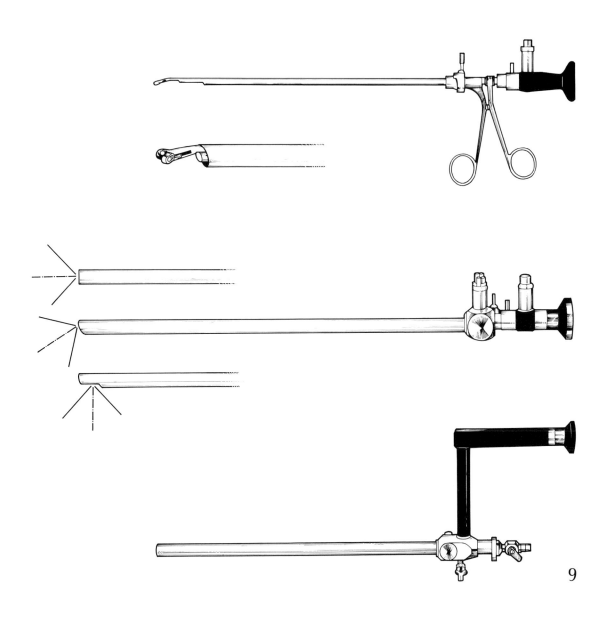

9

* K. Storz, Tuttlingen, Federal Republic of Germany

10

As a rule, thoracoscopy is used only for clarification of pleural processes. Some examiners also employ it for fine needle aspiration of diseased areas of the lung as, for example, tuberculosis, infarction pleurisy or isolated pulmonary tumours, and for lung biopsy of diffuse pulmonary diseases. We avoid biopsy in cases of peripheral pulmonary tumours as the surgical removal of these is necessary in any case. Pulmonary biopsy should only be undertaken by experienced examiners. Pleural biopsy in the region of the parietal pleura and, when great care is taken, in the visceral pleura, is normally without risk.

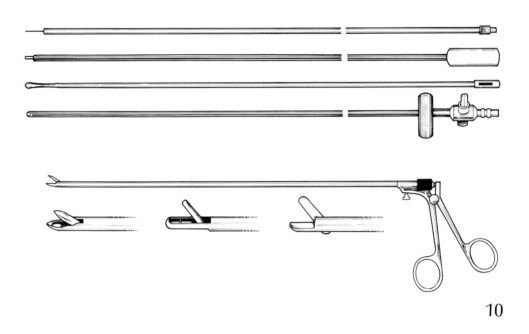

10

Postoperative care

Pneumothorax, either caused at or developing after thoracoscopy, must be sucked out as quickly as possible. This is achieved using a suction drainage tube introduced through the trocar. The suction system is the same as for a thoracotomy. Following a simple pleural biopsy, 24 hours is usually sufficient for complete drainage of the exudate and expansion of the lung. With pulmonary biopsies, a small fistula of the pulmonary parenchyma always results which, as a rule, necessitates suction drainage for several days until the lung is safely expanded and the biopsy site closed.

Complications

Haemorrhage is very rare and can usually be controlled by coagulation. A blood transfusion is necessary in 1 per cent of cases. Fatalities are practically unknown; a lethal outcome could be imagined only as a result of severe respiratory insufficiency.

Results

Positive results from a needle biopsy of the pleura can be expected in 50 per cent of cases. Repetition of the procedure produces a higher percentage. The diagnosis of tuberculous pleurisy can be made in about 80 per cent of cases when the results of the biopsy and bacteriological tests are combined. In the literature[3], 60 per cent of surgical pleural biopsies yielded positive results; in our experience the aetiology was clarified in 82 per cent of patients examined using this procedure. Non-specific pleurisy and resolving pleurisy may yield negative biopsies; these can be of value in terms of diagnostic exclusion.

Thoracoscopy naturally provides more diagnostic information than needle biopsy of the pleura: the yield is 80–90 per cent, depending on the experience of the examiner. The rigid thoracoscope gives better results than the fibreoptic bronchoscope.

Lung biopsy (without transbronchial biopsy)

Indications

Biopsy of the pulmonary parenchyma can be used for diagnosis of peripheral round foci. Fine needle biopsy is best suited for this but we seldom use it because, even when the results of the examination are negative, the pulmonary coin lesion, as long as it is isolated, should always be extirpated because of the high rate of malignancy. Fine needle biopsy to prove a neoplasm is malignant only seems justified in cases of high operational risk or when radiotherapeutic and/or chemotherapeutic support is to be provided. The danger of seeding tumour cells within the lung and especially in the region of the chest wall must not be ignored. Needle biopsy is more justified in cases of multiple circular foci in that the patient is thereby spared more complicated examinations and, furthermore, surgical extirpation is usually not feasible.

Diagnosis of diffuse pulmonary disease is important, but normally, needle biopsy does not provide sufficient representative tissue, especially for additional investigations such as radiographic microanalysis, ash-analysis, or immunofluorescent examinations in patients with immunological diseases. Surgical procedures would take priority in these cases. Transbronchial lung biopsy provides reliable evidence only for sarcoidosis, tuberculosis and carcinomatous lymphangiosis. Tissue obtained by surgery allows for more exact diagnosis in other pulmonary diseases with diffuse changes. It is also easier to see whether, in cases of extrinsic allergic alveolitis and other interstitial pulmonary diseases, the processes may be reversible if treated with corticosteroids.

A single fine needle aspiration can, in cases of disseminated malignant lung affection, provide cytological evidence of a tumour. In the same way, demonstration of the pathogenic agent with its sensitivities is possible in cases of inflammatory pulmonary changes which occur during immunosuppressive therapy.

When choosing the methods of investigation for pulmonary affections with dispersed foci, the diseases which lead to corresponding changes in the mediastinal lymph nodes must be borne in mind. In these cases a mediastinoscopy is indicated rather than a surgical lung biopsy. This applies to sarcoidosis at all stages, lymphogranulomatosis and silicosis.

Anaesthesia

For needle aspiration in the area of the lung, anaesthetic infiltration of the soft tissue and pleura similar to that for pleural biopsy is sufficient. General anaesthesia is usually necessary for surgical lung biopsy.

FINE NEEDLE ASPIRATION BIOPSY

Technique

Following local infiltration anaesthesia, a fine aspirating needle which is attached to a suction system with a drainage bottle can be introduced into the focus under fluoroscopic control.

Choice of the site of puncture is made according to the location of the round lesion. If the latter lies in the anterior pulmonary segment, the puncture is made ventrally in the appropriate intercostal space; if in the posterior pulmonary segment, it should be dorsally.

A very fine aspiration needle should be used so that the procedure can be repeated several times, especially if it is not certain that the focus has been reached. The needle must be completely retracted before being reintroduced so that repeated insertion, will cause only insignificant lesions in the lung and visceral pleura and the development of a pneumothorax following the procedure is normally prevented. If the needle is not completely retracted, but several attempts at reaching the focus are made from the original point, the lung is more severely traumatized and subsequent pneumothorax more likely.

11 & 12

Nordenstrom[2] has developed a special aspiration needle with a simple mechanism which allows not only an exact puncture of the focus but also, by turning the needle, a better biopsy specimen.

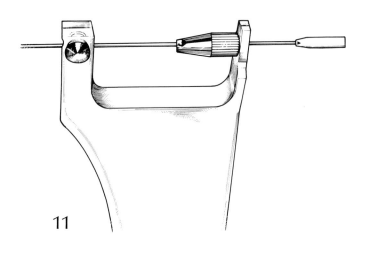

11

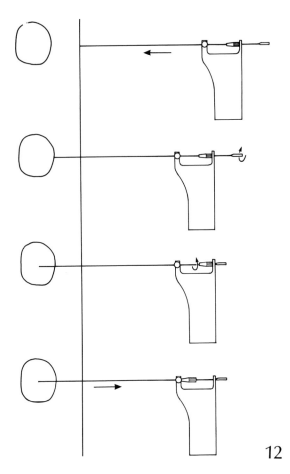

12

Postoperative care

Following examination, pneumothorax should be looked for using fluoroscopy and again, later, by means of a radiograph of the thorax in expiration. As a rule, a small pneumothorax will be resorbed. Drainage is only necessary in cases of large pneumothorax or tension pneumothorax. Intrapulmonary haemorrhage is rare with fine needle aspiration and usually only appears as haemoptysis; equally uncommon is bleeding in the area of the chest wall.

Complications

In an accumulated study by Otte, Schiessle and Könn[3] of 1953 biopsies with histological work-up, subsequent pneumothorax occurred in 12 per cent, with fatal outcome in 0.2 per cent and there were 3 implantation metastases. In 2301 cases of biopsy with cytological analyses, a similar complication rate of 13 per cent pneumothorax development with 0.3 per cent fatality was reported[3]. In other studies with smaller patient populations the rates of subsequent pneumothorax lie between 10 per cent and 39 per cent, even with experienced examiners[3].

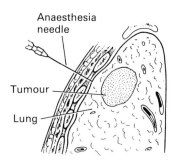

13a

BIOPSY WITH A SPLAYING NEEDLE AND OTHER PROCEDURES

Technique

13a–d

The Silverman needle is the most commonly used. Following infiltration anaesthesia (a), the needle, which is closed by a stylet, is introduced into the tumour under fluoroscopic control (b). After the stylet has been withdrawn, the splaying needle is introduced and advanced through the cylinder into the tumour of diseased pulmonary tissue (c). The needle can now be repeatedly rotated 360°. Finally the cylinder is pushed forward, thus protecting the tissue obtained (d).

Some examiners use the Menghini needle, designed for blind liver biopsy, for biopsy of peripheral pulmonary foci; however, this procedure cannot be recommended as the danger of pulmonary traumatization and cell implantation is greater.

A drill core trephine biopsy is also not recommended as the complication rate is higher and the results not significantly better.

Postoperative care

Radiographic examination for pneumothorax is necessary, and the patient should be observed for 24 hours. Not all biopsy procedures can be undertaken on an outpatient basis.

Complications

Complications from retractor needle biopsies are the same, but somewhat more frequent, than from fine needle aspiration. They should be treated as mentioned above.

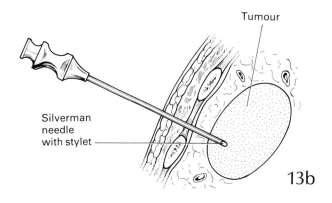

13b

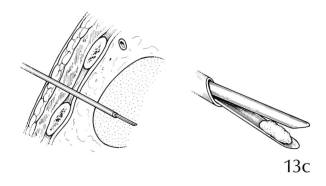

13c

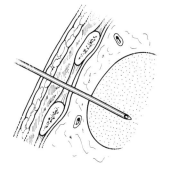

13d

OPEN LUNG BIOPSY

Klassen[4], in 1949, pioneered a method of open or surgical lung biopsy for differential diagnostic clarification of diffuse pulmonary diseases.

Anaesthesia

Endotracheal anaesthesia is usually sufficient. The use of a double lumen tube is only recommended for special techniques.

Technique

14

Under general anaesthesia, the pleura is opened through a small intercostal incision, and the lung is either pulled out or inflated by the anaesthetist so that it herniates through the intercostal space.

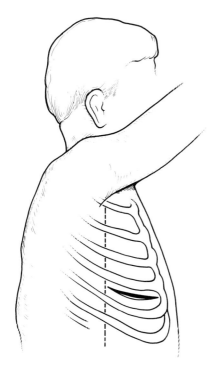

14

15

A wedge-shaped excision between two clamps is taken from the lung.

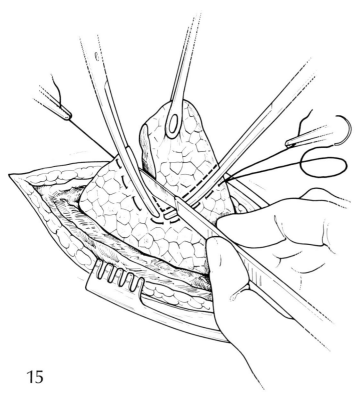

15

16 & 17

The pulmonary parenchyma is then closed using mattress sutures and a second row of stitches is oversewn for safety. A stapling device can be used (*see* chapter on 'Use of stapler in lung surgery', pp. 000–000).

The thoracic wall is closed by the usual technique.

The amount of pulmonary tissue harvested by this method allows for histological, mineralogical and biochemical analyses. As a rule, thoracic drainage attached to a suction system is used for at least 24 hours, as after a thoracotomy.

The examination involves only a minor operation and can be undertaken in both children and geriatric patients. Care is advised in cases of severe global respiratory insufficiency and badly scarred diseased pulmonary tissue, as for instance with longstanding pulmonary fibrosis.

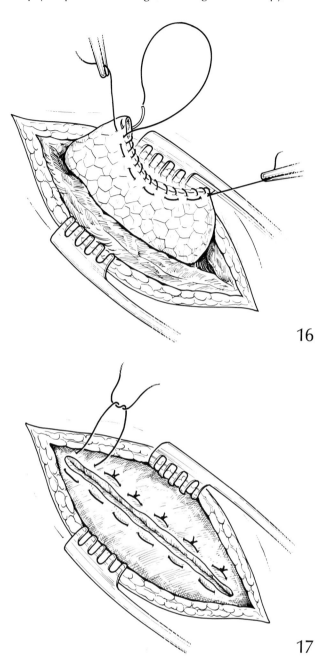

16

17

Postoperative care

The patient must be observed for 24 hours, after which time the drain can be removed as long as there is no further pleural exudation. With a normal course, the patient can be discharged from hospital on the third day after the procedure at the latest, provided a postoperative radiograph shows no significant abnormality.

Complications

Previously, the postoperative mortality rate for this procedure was 1.5 per cent. Today, with appropriate technique and attention to contraindications, postoperative fatalities are extremely unusual. Occasionally haemothorax results, or pleural empyema with a bronchopleural fistula in rare instances. However, with current experience and technique, these complications are practically negligible. Reactive changes of the pleura with restriction of mobility of the diaphragm are more frequent following this procedure than after thoracoscopy or that described in the next section. This procedure should, therefore, not be used bilaterally and its repetition is generally contraindicated.

RESULTS OF THE DIFFERENT PROCEDURES

A survey of 1953 fine needle biopsies of the lung with histological work-up showed positive results in 70 per cent[3]; 2301 biopsies with cytological investigations also clarified the aetiology in 70 per cent of cases.

In our clinic, by combining the two procedures, 80 per cent of fine needle aspiration biopsies are positive. Needle biopsy of the lung is mainly used for diagnosis of peripheral pulmonary coin lesions. Unilateral or bilateral pulmonary diseases with diffuse foci are diagnosed by lung biopsy.

By these means an unequivocal diagnosis can be made in 90 per cent of the cases examined. At this point, a word of warning in relation to the so-called lingula biopsy is necessary, as changes in the lingula are not always representative of processes in other pulmonary segments. We prefer open lung biopsy from the anterior basal segment in cases of left-sided pulmonary pathology and from the same segment or the anterior segment of the upper lobe in right-sided disease. Palpation is necessary to verify whether tissue representative of the disease has been harvested.

Open pleural and lung biopsy using author's technique[5, 6]

Indications

This technique is used to diagnose the same diseases for which surgical pleural and lung biopsy are used. It can be employed for diagnosis of purely pleural processes, as well as for identification of diffuse pulmonary diseases and lesions of both the pleura and the lung. It is not suitable for diagnosis of larger multiple pulmonary round foci, although smaller disseminated foci can be diagnosed.

Technique

The procedure is unique in its combination of endotracheal anaesthesia with a double lumen tube and the use of a mediastinoscope for entering the pleural cavity. Following a small intercostal incision in the midaxillary line in the fifth or sixth intercostal space, the muscle layers are bluntly separated with the scissors. Two small retractors allow a view of the intercostal musculature which is then divided with scissors to a width of about 2 cm. The parietal pleura is visible and incised to provide a point of entry.

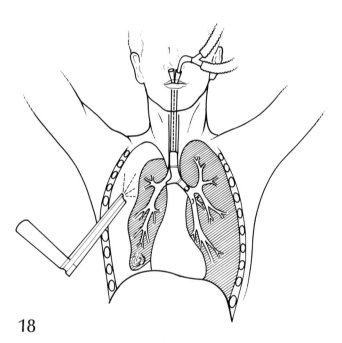

18

With one-sided contralateral artificial respiration, the lung collapses following opening of the parietal pleura. The mediastinoscope is introduced and allows inspection of the pleural cavity and lung with both the naked eye and the optical equipment necessary for thoracoscopy. Under observation, more pleural tissue can be harvested, especially in the region of identifiable lesions, which are more pronounced dorsally than ventrally. This form of examination is sufficient for the diagnosis of isolated pleurisy.

18

19a, b & c

Should a pulmonary disease with disseminated foci be present, the pulmonary tissue is grasped with forceps and pulled through the thoracic incision along with the mediastinoscope. The pulmonary tissue can usually be harvested by means of a single ligature above which the biopsy can be resected using a diathermy needle.

The method of resection between two clamps with appropriate subsequent suturing as outlined by Klassen[4] is also satisfactory.

Following completion of the procedure, a drain is placed in the pleural cavity and connected to a suction apparatus with 50–100 cm H_2O negative pressure. At the same time, the anaesthetist inflates the lung, having first reconnected both sides of the lung. The musculature, with the exception of the intercostal muscles, is closed with two or three interrupted sutures. The thoracic drain can be removed immediately while the lung is momentarily inflated. The procedure is completed by closing the skin with interrupted sutures.

Postoperative care

A radiograph of the thorax in expiration is taken 3–4 hours after the intervention in order to exclude a pneumothorax. Postoperative observation is necessary for only a few hours and the patient can be mobilized immediately. Usually he has recovered fully by the evening of the operation day.

Complications

Fewer complications occur with this method than when using Klassen's technique. Out of 2000 cases examined using this procedure, there were only 3 fatalities. The patients involved were all suffering from end-stage pulmonary fibrosis with preoperative respiratory insufficiency. We have had no bleeding, empyema or other serious complications. The total number of complications as a result of postoperative pneumothorax and seeded metastases, even in cases of pleural mesothelioma, is below 1 per cent.

Results

This method has the advantage of being less extensive than Klassen's open lung biopsy. There are practically no reactive changes in the pleura. In particular, the mobility of the diaphragm is not compromised. The procedure is so well tolerated that we undertake examination of patients from other hospitals on an outpatient basis. These cases constitute 45 per cent of our open pleural and pulmonary biopsies. Pleural drainage is left in place for one or two days in exceptional cases only – those with larger pleural effusions or with severely fibrotic lesions of the lung.

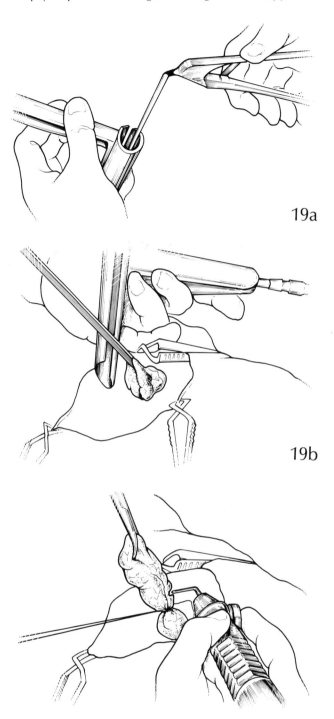

19a

19b

19c

A positive histological result was obtained in 82 per cent of cases of isolated pleurisy, and the same percentage in cases of unilateral combined diseases of the lung and pleura.

A positive diagnosis was made in 92 per cent of the cases of bilateral diffuse pulmonary disease, and this corresponds to the results of the more complicated lung biopsy method of Klassen.

DIAGNOSTIC THORACOTOMY

If all the above procedures do not clarify the aetiology, a classical diagnostic thoracotomy cannot be avoided (see chapter on 'Resection of lung', pp. 149–177.

References

1. Ball, W. C. Thoracentesis and pleural biopsy. In: Sackner, M. A., ed. Diagnostic techniques in pulmonary disease. Part II. New York, Basel: Marcel Decker, 1981: 541–566

2. Nordenström, B. E. W. Needle biopsy of pulmonary lesions. In: Sackner, M. A., ed. Diagnostic techniques in pulmonary disease. Part II. New York, Basel: Marcel Decker, Inc. 1981: 623–654

3. Otte, W., Schiessle, W., Könn, G. Bioptische Diagnostik endothorakaler Erkrankungen. Stuttgart: Thieme Verlag, 1971

4. Klassen, K. P., Anlyan, A. J., Curtis, G. M. Biopsy of diffuse pulmonary lesions. Archives of Surgery 1949; 59: 694–704

5. Maassen, W. Direkte Thorakoskopie ohne vorherige oder mogliche Pneúmothorax anlage. Endoscopy 1972; 4: 95–98

6. Maassen, W. Thorascopie et biopsie pulmonaire sans Pneúmothorax initial. Ponmon et Coeur 1981; 37: 317–320

Further reading

Sackner, M. A. (ed.). Diagnostic techniques in pulmonary disease. Part II. New York, Basel: Marcel Decker Inc., 1981

Scalene node biopsy

Rex De L. Stanbridge MRCP, FRCS
Consultant Cardiothoracic Surgeon, St Mary's Hospital, and Hammersmith Hospital, London, UK

Definition

The scalene node fat pad lies in the scalene triangle whose borders are the internal jugular vein medially, the subclavian vein inferiorly, and the omohyoid muscle superiorly. The scalenus anterior muscle forms the floor. Nodes deep in this triangle are beyond the reach of the palpating finger on clinical examination. The supraclavicular lymph glands occupy a more superior, lateral and superficial position.

Preoperative

Indications

The operation is indicated to establish diagnosis or to define malignant metastatic spread in a variety of lung and mediastinal conditions. It has also been used to assess spread from intra-abdominal and testicular tumours.

Positive biopsies are obtained in 70–80 per cent of cases of sarcoidosis[1,2] and in 20–25 per cent of cases of carcinoma of the bronchus without palpable neck glands[1]. The percentage yield is improved if dissection is made farther into the upper mediastinum[3] and with the experience of the surgeon[2]. Palpable glands give positive biopsies in 83–93 per cent of cases[1]. Oat cell cancer and bronchial adenocarcinoma more frequently metastasize to scalene nodes than squamous cell carcinoma[1,4]. A positive biopsy in lung cancer indicates inoperability. Mediastinoscopy is now often preferred to scalene node biopsy in the assessment of non-palpable glands.

Which side?

When no palpable gland is present, the choice of side follows the usual lymphatic drainage of the lung. The right side is preferred for lesions of the right lung and left lower lobe, and for hilar and bilateral lesions. The left is preferred for left upper lobe neoplasms and neoplastic lesions below the diaphragm. There are variations in lymphatic drainage such that bilateral exploration is often advisable[1,5]. When there are palpable glands present, they should be submitted to biopsy.

Anaesthesia

The operation can be performed under local anaesthesia using a direct local infiltration of 0.5 per cent lignocaine. Even under local anaesthesia, the incidence of vascular complications is low[2]. For added safety and improved exposure, general anaesthesia with endotracheal intubation is recommended.

The operation

1

The incision

The patient lies supine with a sandbag beneath the scapulae, the head turned to the opposite side and the arms alongside the body. The incision starts at the anterior border of the clavicular head of the sternomastoid muscle, 2 cm above the clavicle, and is extended parallel to the clavicle for at least 5 cm. It therefore centres on the lateral border of the sternomastoid muscle.

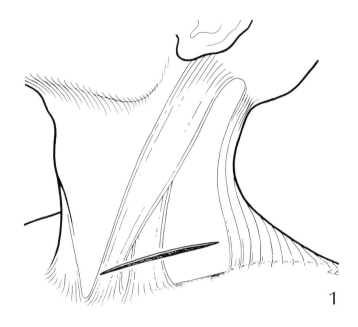

2

Superficial dissection

The skin, platysma and fascia deep to the platysma are divided, revealing the prescalene fat area between the sternomastoid muscle and external jugular vein. The supraclavicular nerves should be preserved in the lateral part of the incision. The external jugular vein may be retracted laterally. If it is engorged, ligation and division is advised.

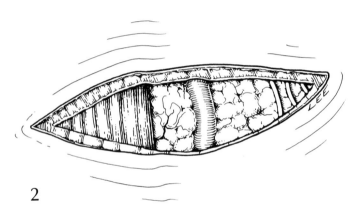

3

Exposure of internal jugular vein

The sternomastoid is retracted medially and the omohyoid superiorly. Superolateral retraction of the scalene fat pad exposes its medial border with the internal jugular vein. The fat pad is gently and easily dissected away from the vein using scissors.

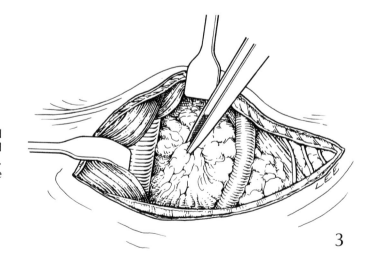

4

Inferior exposure

The inferior border of the incision is retracted downwards and dissection of the medial border of the fat pad is continued inferiorly until the junction of the internal jugular vein with the subclavian vein is encountered. A large lymph node (the thoracic duct node) invariably occupies this junction and should be removed. The scalenus anterior muscle is visible along the floor and the subclavian artery is defined inferiorly. The scalene fat pad is mobilized superiorly, fully exposing the floor of the scalene triangle. Particular attention should be given at this stage for any possible leakage of chyle.

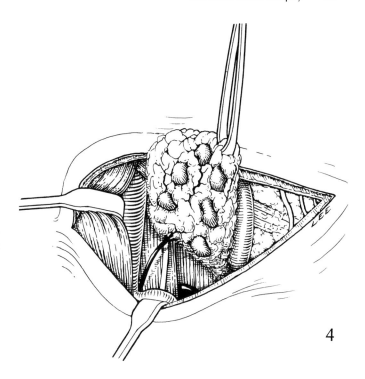

4

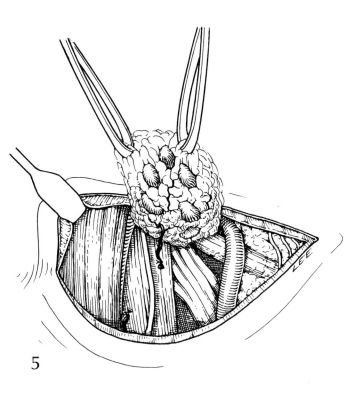

5

5

The posterior floor

The fascia overlying the scalenus anterior muscle also envelops the phrenic nerve. Mobilization of the scalene fat pad is easily accomplished by lifting the fat pad off the fascia, leaving the nerve intact. The superficial cervical artery (transverse cervical) crosses the triangle and enters the scalene fat pad. Although the artery can be dissected free, it is often easier to divide it. In the lateral border of the floor lie the cords of the brachial plexus.

Completion

Dissection is completed when the scalene fat pad is mobilized up to the level of the omohyoid muscle. If required, further lateral dissection under the supra-clavicular nerves may be carried out. The specimen should contain at least five lymph nodes. Digital palpation of the mediastinum along the border of the internal jugular vein, lateral to the trachea, may give an impression of deeper mediastinal gland involvement. The platysma and skin are closed separately. Drainage is not necessary.

Complications

These are uncommon. The chances of an air embolus will be increased if the patient is in the head-up position when a great vein is injured. Using a wet swab which should be immediately available limits the quantity of embolism, as does asking the awake patient to cough. Postoperative chyle leaks can be managed by pressure dressings and needle aspiration. Reports of damage to each of the nerves encountered in the operation have been described. Nerve blocking due to local anaesthesia may affect the brachial plexus, sympathetic chain, phrenic or recurrent laryngeal nerves. Pneumothorax may also be caused during administration of the local anaesthetic[1].

References

1. Brantigan, J. W., Brantigan, C. O., Brantigan, O. C. Biopsy of nonpalpable scalene lymph nodes in carcinoma of the lung. American Review of Respiratory Diseases 1973; 107: 962–974

2. Stjernberg, N., Truedson, H., Björnstad-Peterson, H. Scalene node biopsy in sarcoidosis. Acta Medica Scandinavica 1980; 207: 111–113

3. Harken, D. E., Black. H., Clauss, R., Farrand, R. E. A simple cervico-mediastinal exploration for tissue diagnosis of intrathoracic disease. New England Journal of Medicine 1954; 251: 1041–1044

4. Brousseau, J. D., Reinecke, M. E., Banerjee, T. K., Magin, G. E., Lawton, B. R., Ray, J. F. III. The continuing importance of scalene node biopsy in lung cancer patients. Wisconsin Medical Journal 1977; 76: 97–99

5. Yee, J., Llewellyn, G. A., Williams, P. A., May, I. A., Dugan, D. J. Scalene lymph node dissection: a study of 354 consecutive dissections. American Journal of Surgery 1969; 118: 596–601

Illustrations by Margot B. Mackay

Mediastinoscopy

Joel D. Cooper   MD, FACS, FRCS(C)
Professor of Surgery and Head, Division of Thoracic Surgery,
University of Toronto, Toronto, Ontario, Canada

Preoperative

Indications and contraindications

In 1959, in an attempt to identify preoperatively patients with mediastinal involvement from carcinoma of the lung who would not benefit from surgical resection, Carlins proposed the use of cervical mediastinal exploration. This procedure continues to be used primarily for the assessment of patients with carcinoma of the lung, but is also used to establish the diagnosis of other intrathoracic conditions, especially sarcoidosis.

Thymic tumours and other anterior mediastinal tumours cannot be approached safely by this method as these tumours lie in front of the great vessels. Superior vena caval obstruction is not a contraindication *per se*. Once the bleeding from the skin incision has been stopped and the distended veins in the neck retracted laterally, there are no engorged veins in the pretracheal area and it is safe to take a biopsy.

There remains controversy regarding both the indication of preoperative mediastinoscopy in patients with lung cancer, and the significance and implications of the presence of positive mediastinal lymph nodes. There is general agreement that the presence of tumour metastases in superior mediastinal lymph nodes significantly alters prognosis and must be taken into consideration in deciding whether or not to proceed with surgical resection.

For more than 20 years we have routinely employed mediastinoscopy for the preoperative assessment of patients with lung cancer not already shown to be inoperable. We find that the information so obtained is critical for accurate preoperative staging, and for selecting the best treatment modality for each individual patient.

It has been proposed that non-invasive mediastinal imaging, using CT scan or magnetic resonance imaging, may replace routine preoperative mediastinoscopy. Clini-cal trials to date have demonstrated that the images obtained with these two methods cannot replace the precise information obtained by direct visualization and biopsy of superior mediastinal lymph nodes.

Equipment and preparation of patient

Cautery, insulated cautery forceps, small right angled retractors, mediastinoscope, cupped mediastinoscopy biopsy forceps, insulated suction (used for dissection and for cautery), long aspirating needle with attached syringe, and a long strip of wide gauze packing are required.

Mediastinoscopy is performed under general anaesthesia which is administered through a cuffed endotracheal tube. Whether or not it has been performed previously, bronchoscopy is usually carried out immediately prior to mediastinoscopy. If a small cell anaplastic tumour is found on quick section of a bronchoscopic biopsy, or if a tumour has extended up the airway to the point of unresectability, then mediastinoscopy would not be performed. Some surgeons are concerned that endoscopic biopsy prior to mediastinoscopy might resolve in troublesome bleeding into the airway during mediastinoscopy. Such has not been our experience, but we have no hesitancy in briefly interrupting the mediastinoscopy and inserting a flexible bronchoscope down the endotracheal tube to clear the airway of accumulated blood, if this should occur.

The endotracheal tube should be positioned at the left corner of the mouth, and the anaesthetic apparatus located to the left of the patient's head to permit easy visualization down the mediastinoscope from the head of the table.

1

The neck is extended and the shoulders are elevated with an inflatable balloon or a sandbag. The patient's head is stabilized with a doughnut ring under the occiput. The neck and anterior chest down to the xiphoid are prepared and draped. The table should be level or slightly tilted foot downwards to reduce venous congestion.

The anatomical relationships, critical to an understanding of this procedure, are difficult to convey merely by displaying the structures seen at any one time through the end of the mediastinoscope. For this reason, a series of anatomical dissections were performed and utilized to prepare some of the drawings used for illustration.

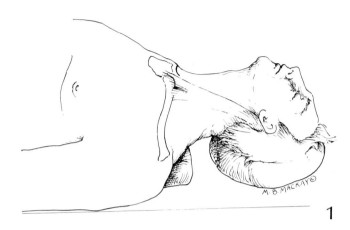

1

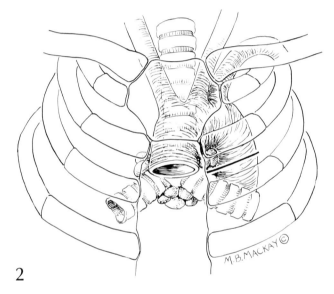

2

The operation

2

A 4 cm transverse incision is made just above the suprasternal notch. The pretracheal muscles are separated vertically in the midline to expose the anterior surface of the trachea.

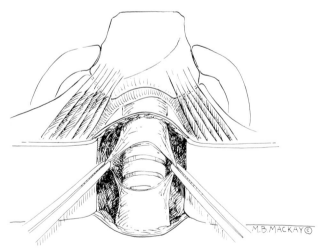

3

3

The thyroid isthmus is retracted superiorly and the tracheal surface is exposed just below the isthmus. The tendency to dissect downward into the mediastinum at this point should be avoided, and it is safer and simpler to expose the upper part of the trachea by incising the pretracheal fascia and then carry the dissection down along the anterior surface of the trachea.

4

The index finger is inserted into the pretracheal space, and blunt dissection carried out along the anterior surface of the trachea down to the carina. The aortic arch is readily palpated anterior to the left main bronchus, and the innominate artery is palpated anterior and to the right of the mid trachea. Further blunt dissection with the finger is performed to open a channel to the right and left of the trachea. At this point the finger breaks gently through the pretracheal fascia, as the superior tracheobronchial and paratracheal lymph nodes lie outside the fascial envelope.

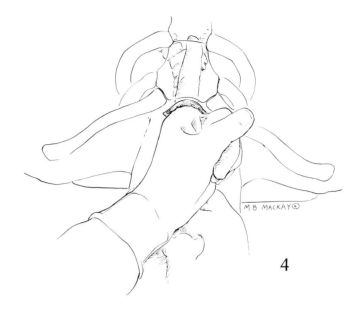

4

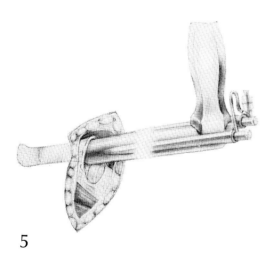

5

5

The finger is withdrawn and the mediastinoscope is then inserted. This may be facilitated by retracting upward on the lower flap of the pretracheal fascia with a small right angled retractor. The mediastinoscope is advanced down to the carina. The plane in front of the mediastinoscope is developed with the use of blunt dissection, using the sucker through the channel of the mediastinoscope. An insulated sucker is useful as it permits cautery to be applied to the tip of the sucker.

Cadaver dissections

6

The innominate artery as well as the innominate vein have been divided and retracted laterally to expose the distal trachea. The aortic arch has been retracted inferiorly. The paratracheal lymph nodes, the superior tracheobronchial nodes and those in the subcarinal (inferior tracheobronchial) region are accessible. The right pulmonary artery crosses just anterior to the carina and right main bronchus. The azygous vein is readily seen just proximal to the right tracheobronchial angle. Even to the experienced eye, vascular structures may be mistaken for lymph nodes and it is strongly recommended that even the most apparent lymph node be routinely aspirated with a long needle and syringe prior to biopsy.

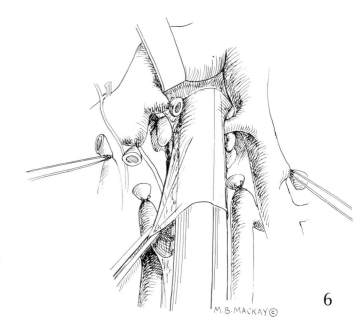

M.B.MACKAY©

6

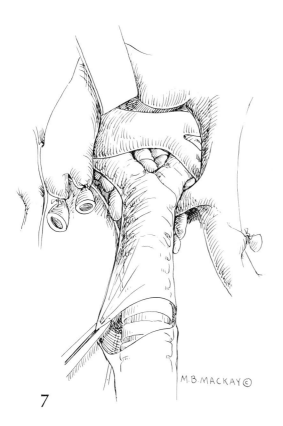

M.B.MACKAY©

7

7

The aortic arch is retracted to the left and the posterior pericardium has been incised further, exposing the right pulmonary artery and the subadjacent anterior subcarinal lymph nodes. Initial attention can be directed to any firm or enlarged nodes previously identified by palpation. Many positive mediastinal lymph nodes, however, are not grossly abnormal to palpation or inspection, and hence routine biopsy of subcarinal, paratracheal, and tracheobronchial angle lymph nodes should be undertaken.

The left recurrent laryngeal nerve lies approximately 1 cm lateral to the trachea and can usually be visualized in the mid tracheal plane. A lymph node is commonly found just above the left tracheobronchial angle node, immediately medial to the left recurrent laryngeal nerve. Biopsy of this lymph node should be done from the medial aspect of the node, as approach from its lateral aspect may cause injury to the recurrent nerve.

Potential hazards, therefore, include vascular injury to the azygous vein, the right pulmonary artery, the aorta, or the innominate artery. Dissection of the subcarinal lymph nodes may be associated with bleeding from bronchial arteries which on occasion may be significant. The long narrow gauze packing should always be immediately available. Most instances of haemorrhage should be dealt with by packing through the mediastinoscope and waiting for the bleeding to stop. Rarely, thoracotomy on the side of the haemorrhage proves necessary.

Closure

The pretracheal muscles may be approximated with a catgut suture, and a subcutaneous interrupted catgut suture will obliterate the dead space.

Anterior mediastinotomy

8

For patients with left upper lobe tumours, left anterior mediastinotomy is commonly performed if preliminary cervical mediastinoscopy is negative, as there is evidence that the lymphatic spread from that lobe is frequently to the anterior mediastinal group of nodes. This procedure gives access to any structures lying in the left anterior mediastinum, i.e. in front of the great vessels, which cannot be approached by mediastinoscopy. The cervical incision made for mediastinoscopy is left open, and a small transverse incision made in the second left interspace just lateral to the sternal border. Dissection is carried down to the intercostal membrane which is incised. Care should be taken to avoid injury to the internal mammary vessels at this point. The anterior mediastinal area is then explored with the surgeon's right index finger, best accomplished with the surgeon standing on the right side of the table. The left index finger should be inserted through the cervical mediastinoscopy incision, with the tip of the finger posterior to the aortic arch. This helps guide the palpating right index finger to the subaortic space. The anterior surface of the aortic arch and the anterior mediastinal lymph nodes should likewise be palpated. Following palpation through the second interspace incision, the mediastinoscope can be inserted to visualize, aspirate and biopsy any palpable lymph nodes.

If the pleural space has not been opened, it may be incised at this point for a more thorough examination of the left hilar area. If the pleural space has been opened, but the lung not biopsied or injured, a red rubber catheter is placed in the pleural space and withdrawn with the lungs inflated after wound closure. If biopsy or damage to the lung has produced an air leak, then an intercostal drainage tube should be inserted and connected to underwater seal.

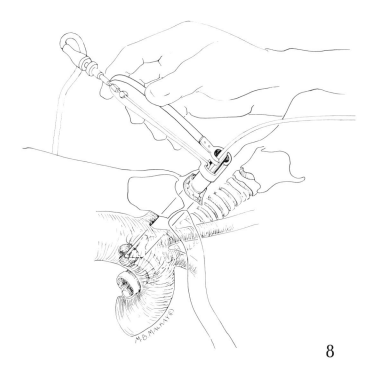

8

Results and complications

Utilizing routine mediastinoscopy for preoperative assessment of lung cancer, patients selected for thoracotomy have a resectability rate of 93 per cent, with 84 per cent having a complete, potentially curative, resection.

Of patients found to have positive mediastinal lymph nodes at preoperative mediastinoscopy, only a highly selected group, amounting to approximately 1 patient out of 5, is submitted to subsequent thoracotomy. Even with this highly selected, relatively favourable group of patients with positive mediastinoscopy, the overall 5 year actuarial survival is only approximately 9 per cent.

A recent review of 1000 consecutive mediastinoscopies at our hospital demonstrated no mortality, two cases of significant haemorrhage requiring thoracotomy, five wound infections, and six pneumothoraces. In this series there were no left recurrent laryngeal nerve palsies, though this complication did occur in our previous series.

Illustrations by Gillian Lee

Intercostal drainage

Rex De L. Stanbridge MRCP, FRCS
Consultant Cardiothoracic Surgeon, St Mary's Hospital, and Hammersmith Hospital, London, UK

Preoperative

Indications

Drainage is indicated whenever there is a large volume of air or fluid in the chest or when the volume of air or fluid is causing respiratory embarrassment.

Air

Drainage rather than aspiration is particularly indicated in cases of bilateral or tension pneumothorax. Shallow pneumothorax without surgical emphysema should be left alone; with surgical emphysema it should be drained.

Blood

Following chest injury haemothorax may respond to drainage alone and pneumothorax should be drained, even if small, if the patient is artificially ventilated or has surgical emphysema. Bilateral apical and basal drains may thus be required. Excessive drainage is defined as more than 500 ml of blood in 1 hour or sufficient air leak to embarrass the patient's respiration and indicate a need for thoracotomy.

Chyle

Intercostal tube drainage for chylothorax is not usually successful in allowing for spontaneous resolution. Surgical control is best (see chapter on 'Surgery of the thoracic duct and management of chylothorax', pp. 59–62).

Pus

Tube drainage may be required in the following circumstances:

1. In children.
2. When there is virulent infection that cannot be controlled by antibiotics.
3. When a lung abscess has ruptured into the pleura causing positive-pressure pyopneumothorax.
4. When an empyema ruptures into the lung and threatens to drown the patient.
5. When there is a postoperative bronchopleural fistula for which immediate surgery is not feasible.
6. When an acute empyema has not responded to daily aspiration and instillation of antibiotics together with enzymatic debridement agents.

Malignancy

In malignant pleural effusions intercostal tube drainage carries the risk of tumour implantation in the tube track and rarely helps the patient. Pleurodesis or local cytotoxic therapy is advised if symptoms warrant.

Surgical

At the onset of a bronchopleural fistula immediate drainage of the hydrothorax is required to prevent spill over into the other bronchus.

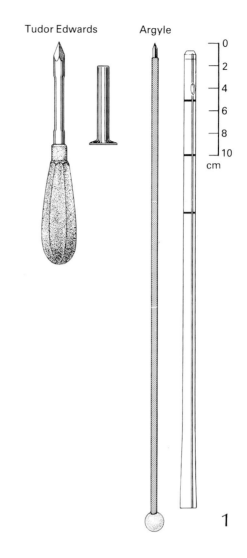

Tudor Edwards   Argyle

1

Equipment

1 & 2

The Tudor Edwards empyema trocar and cannula is preferred because it is sharp and short, ensuring easy and accurate entry to the thorax without danger of damage to underlying structures. The catheter runs freely through the cannula and can be positioned easily and correctly. Three sizes are available: *Small* ¼ inch (6 mm) accepts a 16 Fr catheter. *Medium* ⅓ inch (8 mm) accepts a 22 Fr catheter. *Large* ⅜ inch (9.5 mm) accepts a 28 Fr catheter.

The small size should be used in infants only; the medium size may be used in children and to release air in adults. The large size is best for both air and blood in adults as the chance of occlusion by fibrin, clot or debris is less the larger the bore of the tube.

The Argyle-type thoracic catheter contains a radio-opaque marker line interrupted at the most proximal side eye so that its position can be identified by X-rays. Non-radio-opaque transverse marker lines are present to facilitate the positioning of the tube in the chest. The tip of the Argyle catheter, however, is not sharp and considerable force is required to push it through the chest wall; it may plunge and penetrate lung or other vital structures. It is therefore best used through a Tudor Edwards cannula; if this is not available extensive dissection with artery forceps down to the intercostal muscles or pleura reduces the force required for insertion.

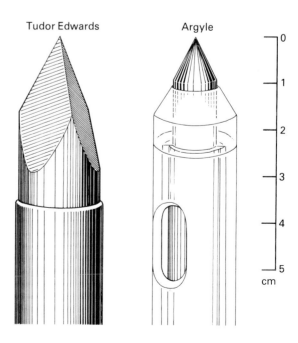

Tudor Edwards   Argyle

2

3

The Malecot or De Pezzer catheter on an introducer has advantages in that the mushroom head can be located near the chest wall.

A Foley-type catheter with an inflatable balloon is not suitable as its walls are too soft and the outer end will not pass through the cannula.

A Tinkler tube is a specialized type of Foley tube which works well within the chest. It is useful for long-term drainage but requires a special introducer for insertion.

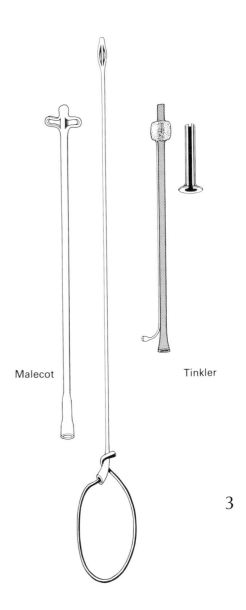

Malecot

Tinkler

3

Position of the patient

Positioning the patient correctly for drain insertion is important. The position required will be different for anterior or posterior insertions at the apex or at the base of the chest.

4

Basal effusions

If the patient can get out of bed he should be seated comfortably astride a chair by the bedside, with his head resting on his forearms, which are themselves resting on the bed. Pillows may be added according to the height of the patient. This is a stable position.

If the patient is confined to bed but can sit upright he should be leant well forward over a bed table and pillows, so that his weight tends to hold him forwards.

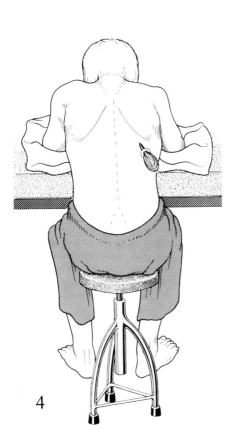

4

5

Apical insertion

For an anterior drain the patient is placed in a semi-recumbent position supported on many pillows.

For an apical posterior shoulder tube the patient should sit upright as for a basal tube but with the arm of that side fully extended downwards as if pulled by a heavy object. This pulls the scapula out of the way of drain insertion.

If the patient is unconscious, on a ventilator or shocked the affected side is placed uppermost.

Site of drainage

First check the side with reference to clinical signs and radiographic appearances.

For empyema and effusion select a site one space below the upper level of fluid. This guarantees that the fluid and not, for example, the diaphragm is entered. If contrast has delineated the lower level of the empyema the site one space above this is selected. A posterior site, 4 finger-breadths from the midline, is suitable for most effusions. This space is chosen by reference to the anterior rib markings on the radiograph rather than by counting ribs posteriorly, which is difficult.

For pneumothorax an apical-posterior shoulder site is optimal. This is comfortable and leaves a posterior scar. The site is 4 finger-breadths (8 cm) lateral to the vertebral bodies, in line with the upper border of the scapula and above the second rib posteriorly. The scapula is retracted laterally by downward displacement of the straightened arm.

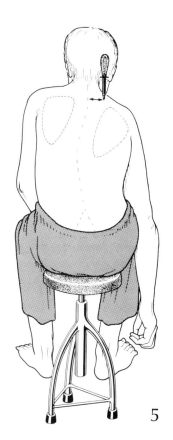

5

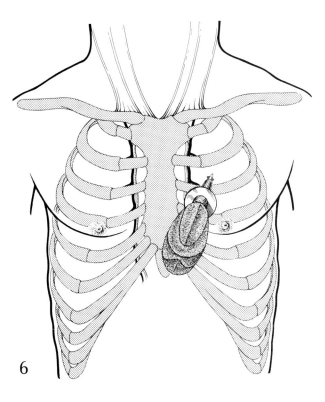

6

6

For tension pneumothorax and for pneumothorax in children the second intercostal space anteriorly, 5 cm from the sternal edge and with the patient in a semirecumbent position, is the quickest and easiest site.

Anaesthesia

Lignocaine 0.5% is used as described in the chapter on 'Aspiration of the chest', pp. 82–84. A few minutes are allowed for the anaesthetic to achieve its full effect. Instruments, cannula, catheter, sutures, connections and underwater-seal bottles are checked. The depth of the pleura is noted for assessment of minimum depth of insertion of the chest drain.

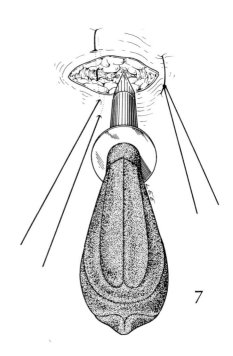

7

The operation

7

A horizontal incision, long enough to accept the Tudor Edwards trocar and cannula, is made, 1.5 cm long when a 28 Fr catheter is to be used. A vertical mattress suture is placed for closure when the drain is finally removed. A single suture of adequately strong material (e.g. 0 nylon, 90 mm needle) is placed posterior to the incision to fix the drain when inserted.

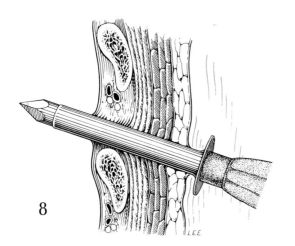

8

8

The trocar and cannula enter the pleural space under gentle pressure after lightly stepping over the upper border of the chosen rib.

9

The cannula is held and the trocar removed. The opening in the cannula is immediately sealed with the thumb to prevent air entering the thorax. However, in draining a pneumothorax it is useful to leave the cannula open to hear air passing into and out of the chest; this confirms that the cannula is correctly sited.

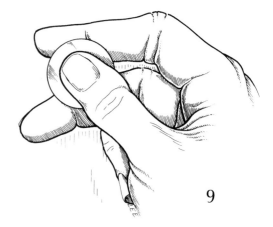

9

10

The catheter is inserted via the cannula to the required depth. Keeping the Argyle trocar in the catheter aids correct positioning. The black lines on the Argyle catheter are used for assessment of depth of insertion.

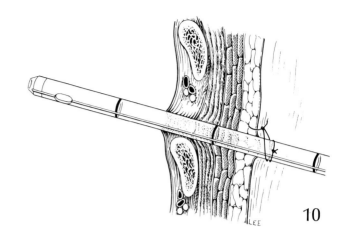

10

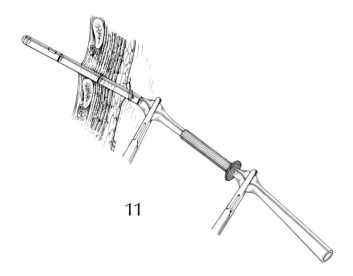

11

11

The Argyle trocar is removed and the drains clamped. The surrounding cannula is withdrawn, if necessary between clamps to prevent air entry. Removing the cannula over the wider flange end of the catheter can be difficult; lubrication and a very firm pull while steadying the proximal end of the catheter is helpful. The catheter is now tied firmly with the suture already placed.

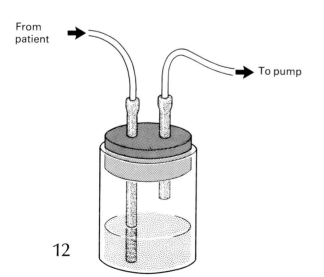

From patient

To pump

12

12

The catheter is connected to the underwater tube of the underwater-seal bottle and the other tube connected to a suction pump if required. Connection sites should be securely taped.

Postoperative care

Large clamps are kept at hand in case of accidental disconnection. Suction is recommended for all cases of pneumothorax and haemothorax. Slower drainage is advised for pleural effusions in excess of 1 litre. A suction pressure of 20 cmH₂O is usually adequate. A range of pressures used and their equivalents in different units of measurement are shown in the table.

The pump ought to be able to maintain a negative pressure throughout the respiratory cycle. If the air leak is bigger than the suction pump can overcome a stronger pump should be used. Drainage is improved with an increase in the height between patient and bottle, with absence of U loops, with low levels of fluid in the underwater-seal bottle or column and with suction.

A radiograph is taken to confirm the position of the tubes and to observe the immediate effects of drainage.

Table 1. Comparative pressures for suction pumps

	cmH_2O	$mmHg$	$cmHg$	$inchHg$	kPa
Normal range used	10	7.5	0.75	0.3	1
	20	15	1.5	0.6	2
	30	22	2	1	3
	40	30	3	1.2	4
Very high or excessive	70	50	5	2	6.5
	135	100	10	4	13
1 atmosphere	1030	760	76	30	100

Table 2. Comparison of volumes swept by suction pumps

Pump type	Suction rate (l/min)
Roberts	0.25
Tubbs Barrett	3
Vernon Thompson	30

13

Alternative drainage

A one-way (Heimlich) valve connected to a urine bag will allow the patient to walk about freely. In the double Heimlich valve the proximal chamber is compressible to allow continuing suction. A Uribag also contains a one-way valve and is useful for well established cases with only a small persistent leak.

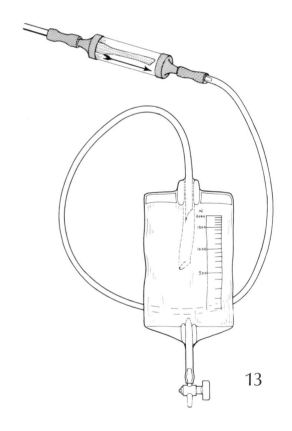

13

Removal

Air

Drains may be removed when the lung is fully expanded radiologically and when there has been no bubbling of air for 24 hours with the drains on suction and no bubbling on coughing with the drains off suction.

Fluid

Drains may be removed when the rate of fluid loss is less than 150 ml per day and there is no further requirement for a drain.

It is unnecessary to test-clamp the drains before removal if the above criteria have been adhered to.

A two-person technique is advised. One removes the drain, the other ties the mattress suture (see Illustration 7). Sedation or anaesthesia are not usually required. However, as the jerk of removal may cause pain with a sharp indrawing of breath the drains should be removed while the patient holds his breath in full inspiration. A gauze swab with collodion suspension is placed on the wound immediately after the purse-string suture has been tied.

After removal an immediate chest radiograph is traditionally advised. This is unnecessary if the proper technique has been applied and the patient is clinically well. It is more important to check the expansion of the lung with a chest radiograph before removal than after it. During removal of the drain it is quite acceptable and sometimes useful to keep the drain on suction without clamping.

Complications

After 10 days the risk of infection increases and there arises a small risk of haemorrhage from pressure erosion of an intercostal vessel. Decisions are made with regard to insertion of another chest drain, continuing drainage or decortication.

Illustrations by Gillian Lee

Management of spontaneous pneumothorax

R. E. Lea FRCS
Consultant Thoracic Surgeon, Southampton General Hospital, Southampton, UK

Introduction

Spontaneous pneumothorax occurs as a result of a leak of air from the lung. This may be due to rupture of a small bulla at the apex of the lung, but often no site for the leak can be identified. It can occur at any age but is commonest in previously fit young patients in their late teens and early twenties. It is also seen in elderly patients, usually with a history of lung disease. The leak of air results in a variable degree of collapse of the lung which is frequently associated with a sharp pain on the affected side. The aim of management is complete re-expansion of the lung. If the pneumothorax is small (less than 30 per cent of the lung volume on chest X-ray) conservative management may be sufficient, with no active treatment. If larger, the patient should be admitted to hospital and an intercostal drain inserted. For persistent or recurrent pneumothorax, or if the opposite side has been involved, pleurodesis by iodized talc poudrage, or a thoracotomy with pleurodesis or parietal pleurectomy is indicated.

THE OPERATION

INTERCOSTAL DRAIN INSERTION

Position of patient

1

The most comfortable position for the patient is semi-supine. The tube should be inserted either in the second intercostal space in the midclavicular line or the fifth intercostal space in the anterior axillary line, just posterior to pectoralis major. The latter is usually more comfortable.

Anaesthesia

After cleaning the skin with 1 per cent povidone iodine, lignocaine 1 per cent is infiltrated into the skin and underlying intercostal muscles.

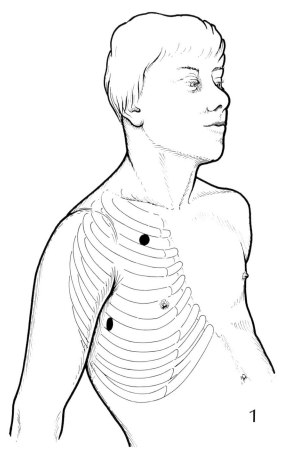

1

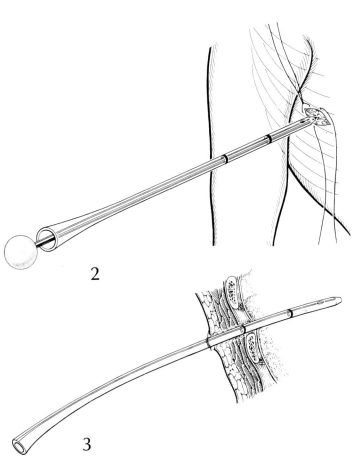

2

3

Insertion of drain

The most convenient type of drain to insert is the catheter supplied complete with an internal trocar (Argyle); the trocar is removed after insertion of the drain. Alternatively a trocar and cannula can be used, the catheter being inserted through the cannula after removal of the trocar. In an adult the minimum catheter size should be 24 Fr.

2 & 3

A 1 cm incision is made through the skin. Two sutures of zero nylon are inserted, one to fix the drain, the other – a vertical mattress suture – to close the wound when the drain is removed. The trocar is pushed into the pleural space. Care should be taken to avoid pushing the trocar too far; the lung or a mediastinal organ may be injured. (Alternatively, a tract is made through the underlying intercostal muscles by blunt dissection using a small pair of artery forceps or other suitable instrument. The dissection is continued until the pleural cavity has been entered. The catheter and indwelling trocar is then pushed gently down this tract into the pleural space – Editor). The trocar is withdrawn and the catheter is connected to a chest drainage bottle containing an underwater seal. A dressing is applied and the tube further anchored by adhesive strapping.

Subsequent management

Re-expansion of the lung is confirmed by chest X-ray. If not fully expanded, low pressure suction can be applied with a Roberts (or other suitable) pump. The drain is removed once the air leak has stopped and the lung is fully expanded.

(An alternative to the waterseal system is to connect the catheter directly to a simple one-way flutter valve contained in a plastic unit (Heimlich valve). With this system the patient can be ambulant – Editor.)

4

TALC PLEURODESIS

The aim is to promote adhesions between the lung and chest wall in patients with a persistent or recurrent pneumothorax. A trocar and cannula is inserted into the pneumothorax as described (*see Illustrations 2 and 3*) and 2 g of iodized talc are introduced with an insufflator. A catheter is then inserted and connected to a chest drainage bottle. If talc is not available, 50 ml of 50 per cent dextrose can be used; this can be instilled through the catheter. Iodized talc and 50% dextrose produce pleural irritation and adhesion formation.

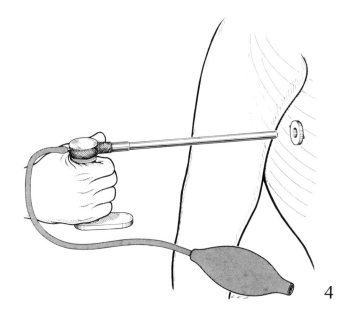

4

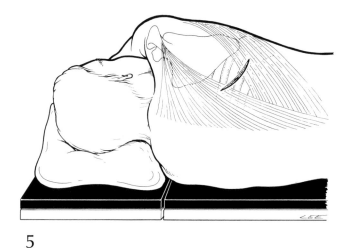

5

THORACOTOMY, OVERSEWING OF BULLAE, AND PLEURODESIS OR PLEURECTOMY

5

Position of patient

The patient is placed in the full lateral position, with the affected side uppermost, and securely fastened to the operating table.

Anaesthesia

The procedure is carried out under general anaesthesia, preferably with a double lumen endobronchial tube. High inflation pressures must be avoided.

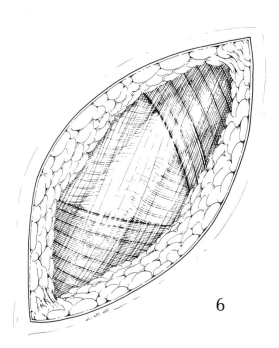

6

6 & 7

The incision

A 10–12 cm long incision is made over the auscultatory triangle. In this site, only little muscle has to be divided, at most 3 cm of the posterior edge of latissimus dorsi. After exposing the fifth rib, the periosteum is divided by diathermy. The pleural cavity is entered by using a rougine to separate the intercostal muscle from the upper border of the rib. To allow easier spreading of the ribs the costo-transverse joint is separated. A small retractor is inserted.

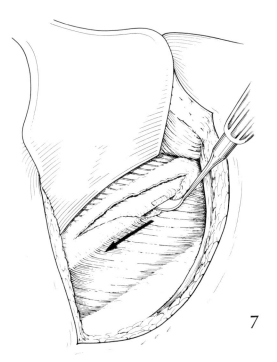

7

8

The lung is carefully examined for bullae, which are commonest at the apex. If small, they are best ligated or oversewn. Occasionally the base of a large bulla can be stapled and the redundant cyst excised.

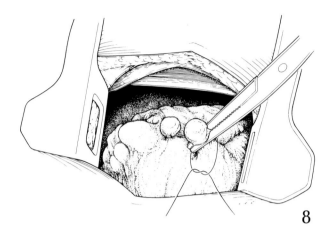

8

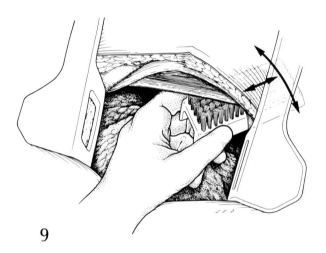

9

9

Pleurodesis

Both parietal and visceral pleural surfaces are firmly abraided with either a sterile bristle brush or numerous dry swabs, to encourage rapid adhesion between the lung and chest wall. Apical and basal drains are inserted and connected to underwater seals.

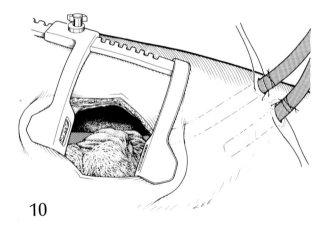

10

10

Apical parietal pleurectomy

Alternatively the parietal pleura is stripped and excised from the upper border of the wound to the apex of the chest. The remainder of the parietal and visceral pleura is firmly abraided (as above), and apical and basal drains inserted. (Personal experience would suggest that recurrence of pneumothorax is less likely after apical pleurectomy when compared with pleurodesis alone).

Closure

Intercostal and muscle layers are closed with absorbable synthetic sutures, and a subcuticular suture is used to close the skin.

Postoperative care

A minor air leak is not unusual. The drains are removed when no longer functioning.

Tracheostomy

Mary P. Shepherd MS, FRCS
Consultant Thoracic Surgeon, Harefield Hospital, Harefield, Middlesex, UK

Introduction

Wherever possible tracheostomy should always be carried out as a planned procedure under general anaesthesia, in an operating theatre, using aseptic technique with good lighting and assistance.

The indications for tracheostomy have diminished in recent years. With the development of sophisticated endo- and nasotracheal tubes with double and/or low-pressure cuffs, and the recently described 'mini' tracheostomy, formal tracheostomy may often be avoided. Provision of an airway in an emergency can be achieved by endotracheal intubation. In the very rare instance when this, or the passage of a rigid bronchoscope, is not possible, immediate laryngotomy or tracheotomy may be required.

An airway provided by endotracheal tube may be maintained safely for several days. This can often be achieved transnasally, a technique especially useful in infants. Should an artificial airway be needed for longer periods, formal tracheostomy may be necessary. The technique of fashioning a permanent tracheostomy will not be described here.

Preoperative

Indications

Tracheostomy may be indicated in the following circumstances.

1. When intermittent positive pressure ventilation (IPPV) with frequent aspiration of secretions may be required for a prolonged period of time.

   (a) After chest trauma which has resulted in an unstable, paradoxically moving segment of chest wall, respiratory embarrassment and possible damage to the underlying lung.
   (b) Where pulmonary infection results in respiratory embarrassment and copious pulmonary secretions.
   (c) In some infants or children in severe congestive cardiac failure.
   (d) In some postoperative cardiac surgical patients.
2. When separation of the pharynx and larynx is necessary.
   (a) Guillain-Barré syndrome.
   (b) Severe head injury.
   (c) Bulbar poliomyelitis.
3. When assisted removal of retained secretions is repeatedly required.
   (a) In patients who continue to be unable to clear retained secretions.
   (b) After lung resection despite bronchoscopic aspiration.

Equipment

Tracheostomy tubes

Tubes, varying in shape, are available in graded lengths and diameters. Silver tracheostomy sets (usually used for permanent tracheostomy) include inner and outer silver tubes with obturator and special forceps for insertion. Red rubber tubes irritate the trachea and cannot be recommended.

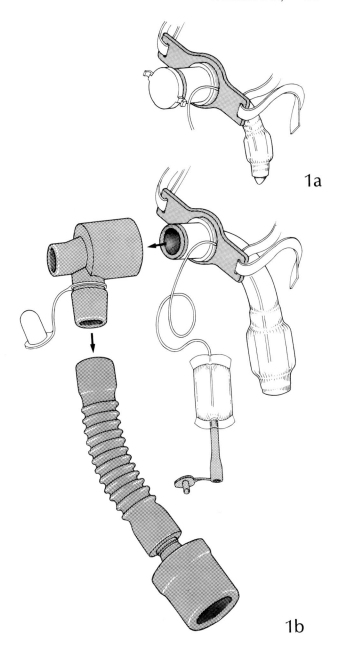

1a

1b

1a & b

Plastic tracheostomy tubes are the type of choice for infants and children (a) and adults (b). They are obtained with and without cuffs and with (a) and without (b) an obturator.

A selection of sterile and uncuffed plastic tracheostomy tubes must be available when a tracheostomy is performed. The largest tube which will pass easily through the surgical stoma in the trachea should be selected.

The appropriate sterile connections for maintenance of anaesthesia and oxygenation after insertion of the tracheostomy tube must be ready for immediate use. Diathermy should be available if possible, to ensure meticulous haemostasis throughout the procedure.

Anaesthesia and position of patient

After suitable premedication a general anaesthetic is given.

2

The intubated patient is placed supine on the operating table. Full extension of the neck is facilitated by placing a sandbag under the shoulders. The head may be stabilized by a padded ring under the occiput.

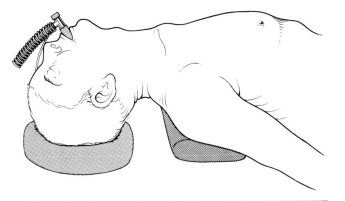

2

The operation

3

The incision

A transverse skin crease incision is made halfway between the sternal notch and the cricoid cartilage, 3–4 cm long in the adult and 1.5 cm long in the infant or child. This is deepened through the superficial fascia in the line of the incision.

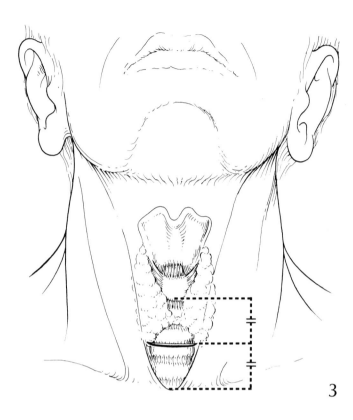

3

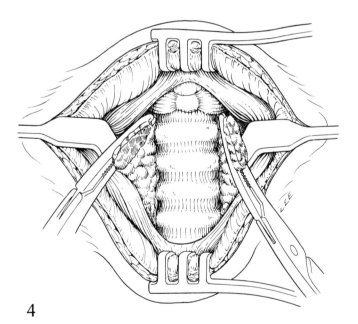

4

4

The deep fascia and strap muscles are separated in the midline. The thyroid isthmus is identified and may be retracted, or divided between ligatures, or clamped and sutured. The inferior veins may also require ligation and division. Exposure is facilitated by the use of a self-retaining retractor. The second and third tracheal rings are exposed by division of the pretracheal fascia.

In the adult

5

A transverse stitch is inserted into the anterior wall of the trachea immediately above the second tracheal ring and then brought through the subcutaneous tissues at the centre of the lower skin edge.

A plastic, cuffed tracheostomy tube with a diameter approximately two-thirds that of the trachea is selected and the cuff tested. A second tube one size larger than the selected one is also identified.

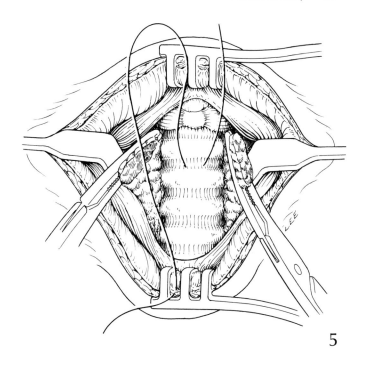

5

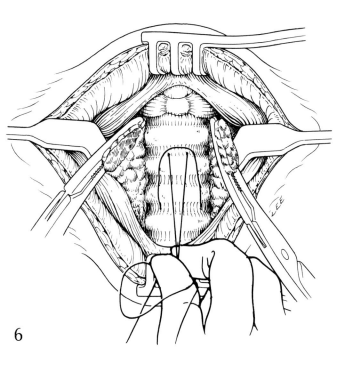

6

6

By gentle downward traction on the tracheal stitch, the trachea is stabilized. It is then incised with a scalpel horizontally above the stitch (but below and well clear of the first tracheal ring), dividing the central two-thirds of the trachea. Every effort must be made not to puncture the cuff of the endotracheal tube.

Both ends of this incision are then extended vertically downwards through the second and third tracheal rings. Scissors are often useful for this manoeuvre.

The free edge of the ∩-shaped flap (after Bjork[1]) of the anterior wall of the trachea is pulled gently forward by traction on the stitch to enable the tracheostomy tube to be inserted easily. The two ends of this stitch are tied to approximate the flap of anterior tracheal wall to the subcutaneous tissues of the lower edge of the incision. Thus a track is formed to facilitate subsequent tube changes.

In the infant or child

7a & b

The trachea is stabilized with a skin hook (a) or stay sutures (b) and is incised vertically, exactly in the midline, through the second, third and fourth tracheal rings. No cartilage is removed or displaced.

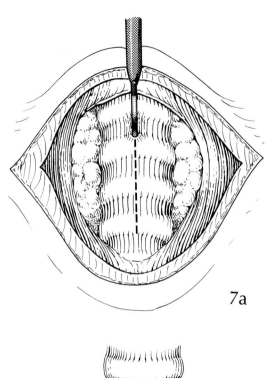

7a

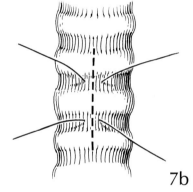

7b

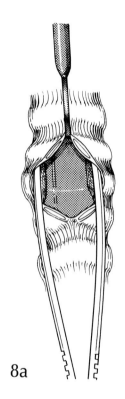

8a

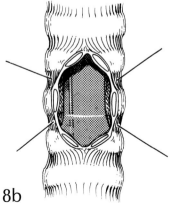

8b

8a & b

The edges of the tracheal incision are held apart by McIndoe's forceps (a) or the stay sutures (b) to allow insertion of the tube of a diameter about 1.5 mm less than that of the trachea.

Insertion of tube

9

The anaesthetist frees the endotracheal tube, deflates the cuff and slowly withdraws it. When the tip of the endotracheal tube reaches a point immediately above the tracheal stoma, the moistened tracheostomy tube with its obturator is slipped into the trachea. While the tracheostomy tube is held firmly in place by an assistant, the obturator is removed and the trachea is aspirated through the tube. The sterile anaesthetic connections are attached to restore the ventilatory system.

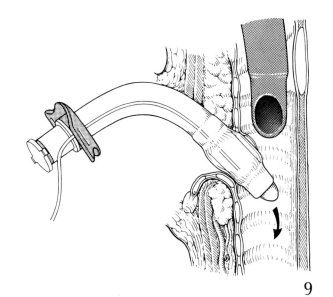

9

10

The tracheostomy cuff is inflated so that the trachea is just occluded around the tube. Note is taken of the volume of air required to achieve this.

The sandbag is removed from behind the patient's shoulders. Frequently no skin sutures are necessary, but if they are required the skin edges should only be loosely approximated around the tracheostomy tube.

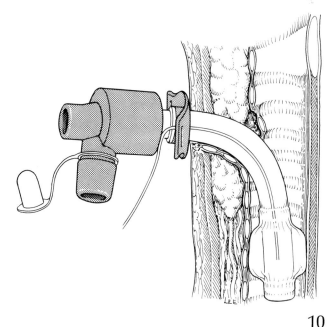

10

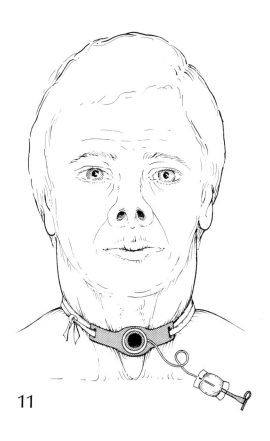

11

11

The tracheostomy tube is held securely in place using one piece of tape. This is threaded through one flange, both ends passed behind the neck, one end threaded through the other flange, and the ends tied, using a knot and not a bow.

Stay sutures, if used, are left in place to be removed on the third or fourth postoperative day.

Inflation of both lungs must be ascertained. In the infant or child it is possible for the tracheostomy tube to enter the right main bronchus. The tube can be withdrawn slightly be elevating it from the skin surface with a plastic foam pad.

Postoperative care

A patient with a tracheostomy should be nursed in an area allowing close observation. An infant or child must be attended by a special nurse at all times. Scissors, to release the tracheostomy tube in an emergency, and a sterile replacement tube of the same size and shape must always be available at the bedside. While a patient has a tracheostomy, frequent reassurance must be given that the loss of voice is only temporary. Pencil and paper should be provided.

The well-placed tracheostomy tube should be kept as still as possible to minimize the effects of movement and traction on the trachea. This applies particularly when IPPV is used.

Tracheal aspiration is carried out as often as necessary:

1. A mask is worn by the attending nurse and a sterile soft catheter used for each aspiration.
2. Using sterile disposable gloves, a catheter is inserted gently as far as it will readily go. This may be 12–18 cm. Following lung resection, however, the catheter should be introduced only to a point in the trachea just beyond the end of the tracheostomy tube, approximately 8–10 cm.
3. Suction is applied only when the catheter is in position and being withdrawn. A Y connection is useful in this respect.
4. The left main bronchus may be entered if the head is turned gently well to the right.
5. The aspiration procedure should only take 10–15 seconds, i.e. as long as a person can comfortably hold his or her breath.

Prophylactic antibiotics are not given. It is possible for sterile secretions to be kept so, if the aseptic techniques of management are strictly adhered to. Tracheal aspirate is cultured regularly and the appropriate antibiotic given systemically (and/or by direct instillation into the trachea if necessary).

Cuff management

The cuff of a tracheostomy tube should only be inflated if IPPV is required or if there is a risk of aspiration of secretions or food. The volume of air used to inflate the cuff should be the smallest which occludes the trachea around the tube. A small air leak is often acceptable; over-inflation must be avoided. The practice of intermittent cuff deflation is hazardous as it can lead to over-inflation, and this in turn can cause pressure necrosis of the trachea, tube collapse or cuff prolapse.

Changing the tracheostomy tube

It may not be necessary to change the tube for a week or more. Changing the tube is always preceded by pharyngeal aspiration and tracheal aspiration after deflation of the cuff. If difficulty is experienced in passing the suction catheter, or a rise in IPPV inflation pressure is noted, the tube must be changed and checked immediately. These observations may indicate a decrease in the lumen of the tube by crusting, kinking or cuff prolapse.

Extubation in the adult

A cuffed tracheostomy tube is replaced with an uncuffed plastic tube of the same size.

The practice of using a spiggot to obstruct the tracheostomy tube is not advocated, although it allows the return of speech. Airway obstruction of a degree relative to the size of the tube *in situ* is produced.

After 1–2 days the uncuffed tube is changed for one a size smaller.

This is repeated until an uncuffed tube of about 1 cm in diameter is reached (33 Fr approximately). Finally this tube is removed and a firm, sterile dressing is applied to the stoma in the neck. Speech is restored. Should tracheal aspiration be required, this is readily carried out through the stoma, employing the same aseptic technique.

The stoma will close spontaneously during the course of about a week. Formal closure, even after the Bjork flap type of tracheostomy, is seldom required.

Extubation in the infant and child

The tracheostomy tube is changed for one a size smaller. After 3–4 days the tube is again changed for one a size smaller. This is repeated until a tube size 3.5 mm approximately is reached. This tube is removed and a firm sterile dressing applied to the stoma in the neck. Immediately following extubation, bronchoscopy is advisable to confirm that the airway is clear.

Complications

Complications following tracheostomy include: infection of the tracheostomy and/or tracheobronchial tree; haemorrhage resulting from pressure effects or infection; and pneumothorax.

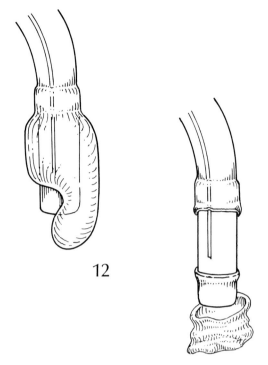

12

13

12, 13 & 14

Obstruction of the tracheostomy tube may be due to:

1. crusting with dried secretions;
2. collapse of the tracheostomy tube due to an over-inflated cuff;
3. herniation of an over-inflated cuff over the end of the tube (*Illustration 12*);
4. detachment of the cuff from the tube (*Illustration 13*);
5. displacement of the tube from the trachea into the tissues, also producing surgical emphysema (*Illustration 14*).

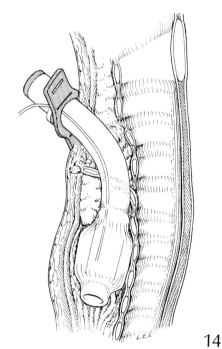

14

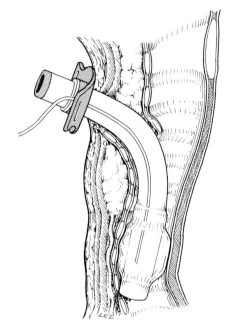

15

15 & 16

Trauma to the trachea may result from:

1. inappropriate type of suction catheter;
2. inappropriate technique of tracheal suction;
3. over-inflation of the tracheostomy tube cuff;
4. inadequate fixation or inappropriate shape of tracheostomy tube allowing:
   (a) pressure necrosis of the tracheal cartilage around the stoma or in the region of the cuff;
   (b) the tip of the tube to impinge on the anterior tracheal wall which can result in innominate artery erosion (*Illustration 15*);
   (c) the tip of the tube to impinge on the posterior tracheal wall which can result in tracheo-oesophageal fistula (*Illustration 16*).

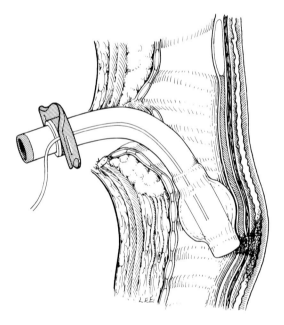

16

Tracheal stenosis

Subglottic stenosis can occur if the tracheostomy is too high, especially in the infant or child.

19 & 20

Stomal stenosis occurs more often in the infant or child and is due to:

1. removal of tracheal cartilage;
2. pressure necrosis and/or infection of tracheal cartilage;
3. granulomatous polyps (*Illustration 17*);
4. forward angulation of the trachea (*Illustration 18*) by inappropriate tension exerted by ill-positioned ventilator connections.

Infrastomal stenosis may be due to:

1. Mucosal ulceration and/or infection at the level of the tracheostomy tube cuff;
2. mucosal ulceration and/or infection in the region of the tip of the tracheostomy tube.

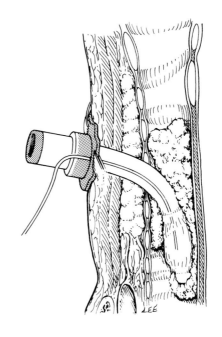

17

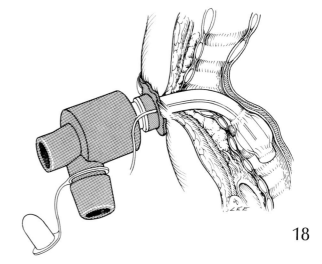

18

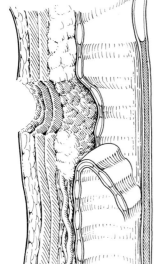

19

19

In adults, the flap of the anterior tracheal wall may fall back into the tracheal lumen if it becomes detached from the subcutaneous tissues when the tracheostomy tube is changed or removed.

Reference

1. Bjork, V. O. Partial resection of the only remaining lung with the aid of respirator treatment. Journal of Thoracic and Cardiovascular Surgery 1960; 39: 179–188

Further reading

Andrews, M. J., Pearson, F. G. Incidence and pathogenesis of tracheal injury following cuffed tube tracheostomy with assisted ventilation: analysis of a two-year prospective study. Annals of Surgery 1971; 173: 249–263

Burke, A. The advantages of stay sutures with tracheostomy. Annals of the Royal College of Surgeons 1981; 63: 426–428

Clarke, D. B. Tracheostomy in a thoracic surgical unit. Thorax 1965; 20: 87–92

D'Abreu, A. L., Abbey Smith, R. eds. D'Abreu's practice of cardiothoracic surgery. 4th ed. London: Edward Arnold, 1976

D'Abreu, A. L., Brian Taylor, A., Clarke, D. B. Intrathoracic crises. London: Butterworths, 1968

Feldman, S. A., Crawley, B. E. eds. Tracheostomy and artificial ventilation in the treatment of respiratory failure. 2nd ed. Baltimore: Williams & Wilkins, 1972

Harley, H. R. S. Laryngotracheal obstruction complicating tracheostomy or endotracheal intubation with assisted respiration: a critical review. Thorax 1971; 26: 493–533

Hewlett, A. B., Ranger, D. Tracheostomy. Post Graduate Medical Journal 1961; 37: 18–21

Johnson, D. G., Jones, R. Surgical aspects of airway management in infants and children. Surgical Clinics of North America 1976; 56: 263–279

Spalding, J. M. K., Lucas, B. G. B., Wilson, K. et al. Respiratory units: intermittent positive pressure respirator: tracheostomy. Proceedings of the Royal Society of Medicine 1966; 59: 29–36

Stell P. M. Tracheotomy and tracheostomy. In: Ransome, J., Holden, H., Bull, T. R. eds. Recent advances in otolaryngology. Edinburgh and London: Churchill Livingstone, 1973: 275–294

Stool, S. E., Campbell, J. R., Johnson, D. G. Tracheostomy in children: the use of plastic tubes. Journal of Paediatric Surgery 1968; 3: 402–407

Watts, J. McK. Tracheostomy in modern practice. British Journal of Surgery 1963; 50: 954–975

Warwick, R., Williams, P. K., eds. Gray's anatomy. 35th ed. Edinburgh: Longmans, 1973: 1183

Illustrations by Barbara Hyams

Surgical access in pulmonary operations

Peter Goldstraw FRCS, FRCS(Ed)
Consultant Thoracic Surgeon, Brompton Hospital, Middlesex Hospital and
University College Hospital, London, UK

Introduction

A wide spectrum of surgical pathology may affect the lungs and other organs of the chest. With a sound knowledge of anatomy and an appreciation of the exposure required the surgeon may tailor the site and extent of his incision. There is, therefore, no 'standard' thoracotomy incision. Commonly used incisions include the following.

Choice of incision

The lateral thoracotomy incision is shown in detail in *Illustrations 10–21*. The patient lies in the lateral position and the incision passes between two ribs, dividing all the attachments of one rib to the other. Depending on individual preference the patient may be inclined backwards and the incision carried further anteriorly (the anterolateral approach) or placed in the prone position

and the incision carried more posteriorly (the posterolateral approach). In either event the incision between the ribs is total and access is gained by the bucket-handle movement of the ribs above separating from those below. There is little justification now for the removal of the rib, particularly in children where such a manoeuvre encourages the later development of scoliosis.

The lateral thoracotomy incision provides excellent exposure of the whole of the ipsilateral lung and its hilum, the mediastinum and diaphragm. In the left chest this incision exposes the lower oesophagus and descending aorta, while on the right access is given to the whole of the intrathoracic oesophagus.

Median sternotomy has been greatly popularized by cardiac surgeons. It may be used to resect anterior mediastinal tumours and affords access to both pleural spaces, permitting bilateral pleurectomy or limited procedures on the lungs to remove bilateral bullae or metastases. A limited upper sternotomy is adequate for thymectomy and gives access to the trachea as far inferiorly as the carina. As an extension to a cervical incision this approach is occasionally necessary for the removal of a large retrosternal goitre.

MEDIAN STERNOTOMY

1

The patient is positioned supine, with a sandbag placed transversely beneath the shoulders to elevate the manubrium and hence render the sternum horizontal. A vertical skin incision is made from the suprasternal notch to the tip of the xiphoid.

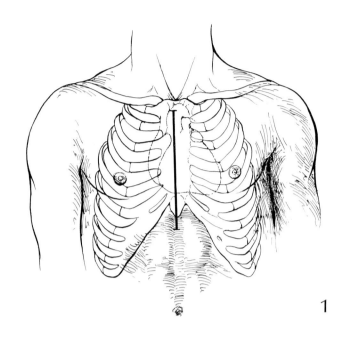

1

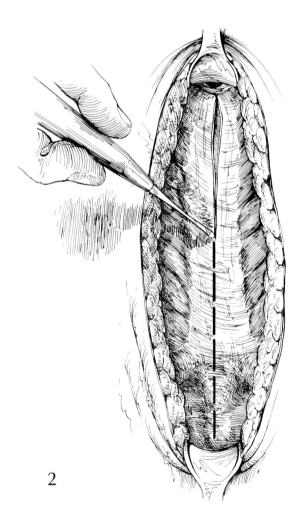

2

2

Diathermy is used to make a vertical incision in the periosteum of the sternum, taking care to remain in the midline. The transverse suprasternal ligament is divided and a finger insinuated into the superior mediastinum. At the lower margins of the incision the xiphoid process is divided vertically and a finger may then be insinuated into the retrosternal space. This finger may then strip the pleura to each side.

3

Using a vertical sternotome the sternum is divided longitudinally. If the anaesthetist allows the lungs to deflate during this manoeuvre, there is less chance that the pleura will be opened inadvertently.

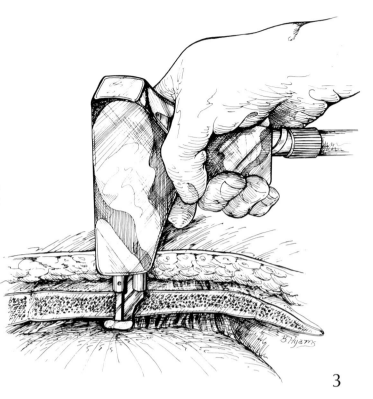

3

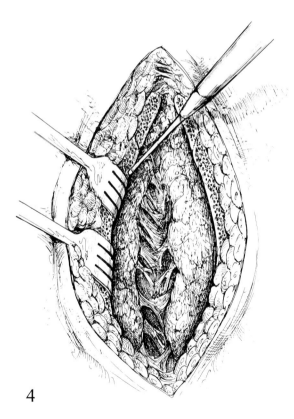

4

4

The sternal margins are elevated using retractors. Diathermy is used to control bleeding from the periosteal surfaces. Any bleeding from the cancellous bone may be controlled with small quantities of bone wax. This procedure is then repeated by the assistant for the opposite sternal margin. A parallel-sided, geared retractor can then be inserted to spread the sternal edges.

Closure

The sternal margins should be firmly approximated using interrupted wire sutures. The pectoralis muscles are approximated in the midline and skin closed.

The cosmetic appearance of this operation may be considerably improved if a transverse submammary skin incision is utilized. This approach has been popularized by Professor A. G. Brom of Leiden. It requires considerably more dissection to elevate the skin flaps to the sternal notch, but access is unhindered.

COMBINED THORACOLAPAROTOMY

Thoracic incisions may be continued into the abdomen, and this may be necessary to resect residual tumour in the lungs, mediastinum or abdomen.

The median sternotomy extended as a midline laparotomy allows limited access to both lungs and pleural spaces and the lymph node chain along the abdominal aorta and pelvic brim.

5 & 6

The left thoracolaparotomy incision, along the eighth or ninth rib, crosses the costal margin, divides the diaphragm circumferentially and may then pass obliquely to the linea alba or extend as a paramedian laparotomy. This incision gives good access to the lower oesophagus, stomach and spleen and in addition is used to resect tumour deposits in the left lung, mediastinum and abdomen. It affords good access to the nodes behind the crura of the diaphragm – a common site for lymph node metastases ascending from the abdomen and testes.

The right thoracolaparotomy incision mirrors that on the left. The liver is dislocated laterally with the hepatic veins. We have used this incision to resect residual tumour deposits in the right lung, main carinal nodes, liver and para-aortic chain.

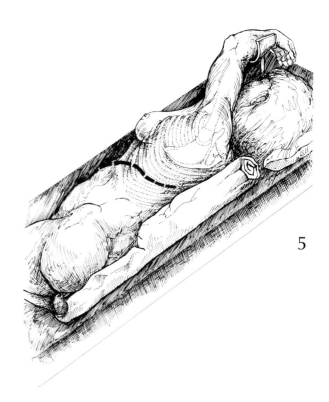

5

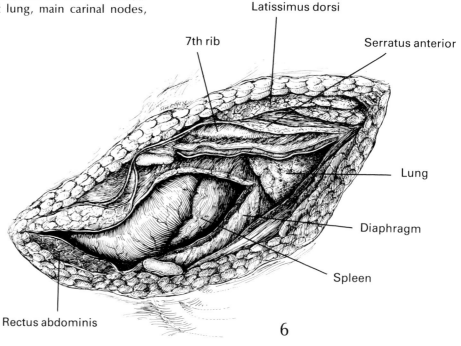

6

7 & 8

TRANSVERSE BILATERAL THORACOTOMY

This incision, once popular for cardiac operations, is now rarely used. It entails division of the serratus anterior and pectoralis muscles on each side, entering the pleural spaces through the fifth or sixth interspace, and completing the incision by transverse division of the sternum with sacrifice of both internal mammary arteries. It is a painful incision but allows more extensive exposure of the lungs, particularly the posterior aspect of the lower lobes.

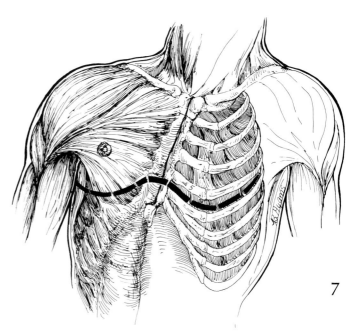

7

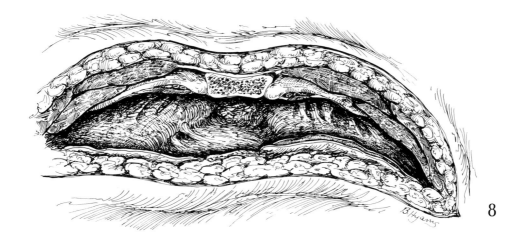

8

LIMITED INCISIONS

Short transverse intercostal incisions may be made anteriorly through the second interspace to biopsy anterior mediastinal masses. On the left this anterior mediastinotomy is a valuable staging procedure when assessing upper lobe tumours. Similar limited incisions anteriorly through the fifth interspace allow biopsy of the lung and pleura, and on the left also permit biopsy and fenestration of the pericardium.

Preoperative

Preoperative preparation

Intensive physiotherapy of a high order is essential following any operation on the lungs. All patients will therefore benefit from a short period in which to practise the manoeuvres their physiotherapists will be utilizing after surgery. Those patients producing large volumes of sputum can be considerably improved but will require several days of intensive physiotherapy aided by antibiotics and antispasmodics as appropriate. The length of preoperative preparation required depends not only upon the extent of the proposed resection but also upon the severity of the underlying lung disease. Those patients with severe chronic conditions producing large volumes of sputum may require prolonged treatment to create the optimum conditions even if only minor surgery is proposed.

In most hospitals the operative site is shaved the day before surgery. This allows time for the superficial abrasions to become colonized by bacteria and may predispose to wound sepsis. Depilatory creams are expensive and can cause irritation. We have found the best compromise to be shaving of the operative field in theatre after the induction of anaesthesia.

Anaesthesia

9a–d

After the induction of anaesthesia, bronchoscopy is recommended as a final check on the situation and to permit bronchial toilet. It will often provide useful information for the anaesthetist, aiding the positioning of the double-lumen tube. A double-lumen endobronchial tube greatly facilitates exposure within the chest, and avoids conflict between anaesthetist and surgeon. Correct positioning of a Robertshaw tube is shown in (a) and (d), while (b) and (c) show some common malpositions.

It will be appreciated that the right-sided tube is the more difficult to position, and hence its use is reserved for operations requiring division of the left bronchial tree. For all other operations a left-sided tube (d) is to be preferred irrespective of the side of the thoracotomy. An improperly positioned double-lumen tube does not protect the contralateral lung and may hamper exposure. The surgeon must thus be prepared to accept an endotracheal tube if his anaesthetist cannot confidently position the endobronchial tube. After intubation, monitoring lines and intravenous drips are inserted as necessary. For most major resections a peripheral drip and central venous catheter are desirable.

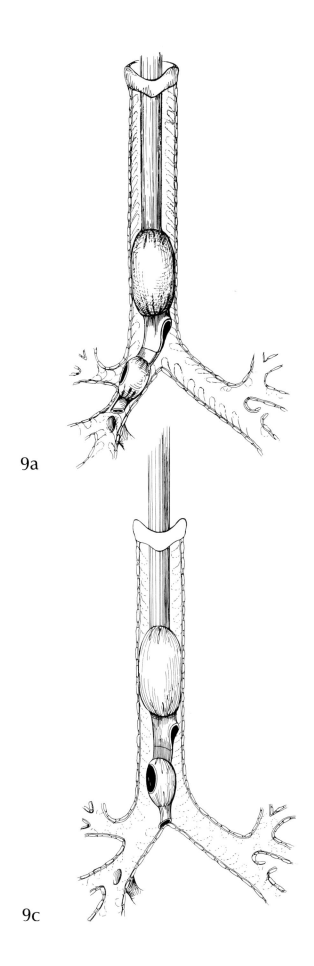

9a

9c

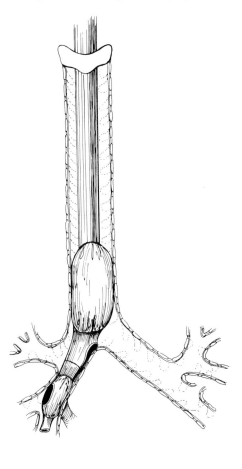

9b

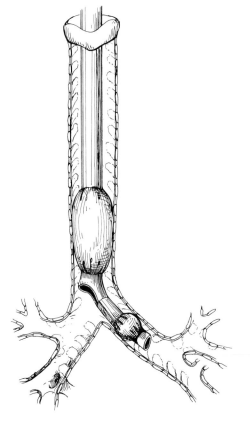

9d

Lateral thoracotomy

10

Position of patient

The patient is secured in the full lateral position. This may be achieved with a pillow and sandbags, but is facilitated by a support bag containing small polystyrene beads which becomes a firm mould when air is evacuated. The bottom leg is flexed and the uppermost knee supported on a pillow. The upper arm rests on a support.

It is at this stage that we undertake shaving of the operative site. The skin is then prepared with an alcohol-based antiseptic containing iodine or chlorhexidine. Care should be taken not to spill excessive spirit over the patient and diathermy plate. Conventional draping with sheets and a transparent adhesive incise drape is adequate. We prefer to spray the operative field and surrounding area with an adhesive aerosol, and to use a single large sheet of 150 gauge transparent polythene. This forms the incise drape and dispenses with the need for additional sheets. The diathermy quiver and sucker are held in place using thin adhesive strips. This simple method has the advantage of giving clear vision of all drips, catheters and anaesthetic tubes and is far cheaper than commercially available incise drapes.

The skin incision commences 3 cm beneath the nipple and extends in a gentle arc 2 cm below the angle of the scapula, to end midway between the spinous processes and the posterior border of the scapula. In the female the position of the breast must be noted and the mobile position of the nipple is misleading. The incision is inevitably made lower and is best started lateral to the breast.

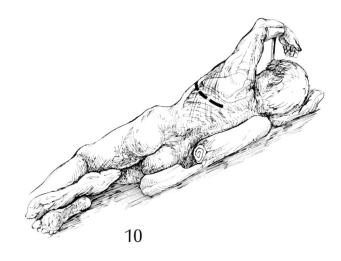

10

11

The incision is carried deeper using the diathermy spatula. Lattisimus dorsi is transected towards the lower margin of the incision since the lower segment is inevitably denervated. The fascia posterior to serratus anterior continues as a firm sheet onto the posterior border of the scapula. The incision through this fascia is carried inferiorly along the posterior edge of serratus anterior. This muscle is then divided towards the lower part of the incision from its posterior margin anteriorly until the belly arising from the desired rib is encountered. The ribs are counted from above, the highest palpable rib being the second. The first rib is obscured by scalenus posterior except over a short segment near the vertebrae.

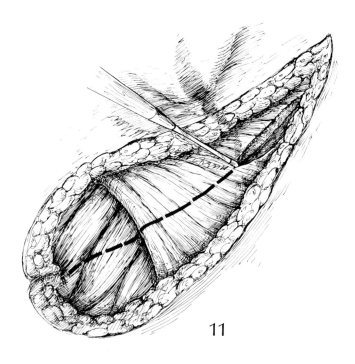

11

12

An incision through the bed of the fifth or sixth rib will give access to the pulmonary hilum; the fifth rib is used for upper lobectomy, the sixth for lower and middle lobectomy, and either may be used for pneumonectomy.

The belly of serratus anterior arising from the chosen rib is cut from the upper border of the rib and the diathermy is used to score the lateral aspect of the periosteum, extending posteriorly until the border of the erector spinae is encountered and notched.

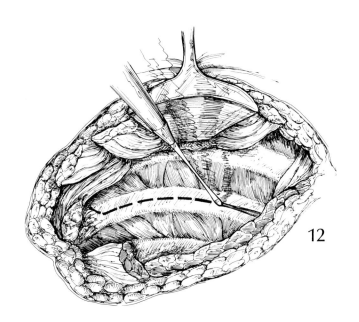

12

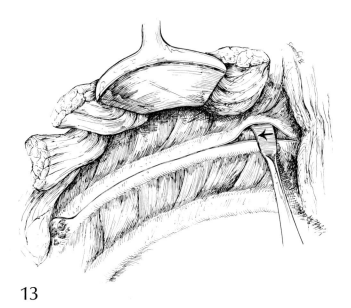

13

13

The edge of a raspatory is inserted into this notch and drawn along the upper surface of the rib. For this first stroke the handle of the raspatory is kept flat against the chest wall and the blade lifts the periosteum from the rib. A second stroke in the same direction, keeping the handle of the raspatory vertical, exposes the parietal pleura. The inferior border of the rib is then exposed at the posterior angle.

14

Using a costotome 1 cm of the posterior angle of the rib may be excised. This manoeuvre adds little to the exposure, but decreases tension on the posterior attachments of the rib, reducing the frequency of severe post-thoracotomy pain.

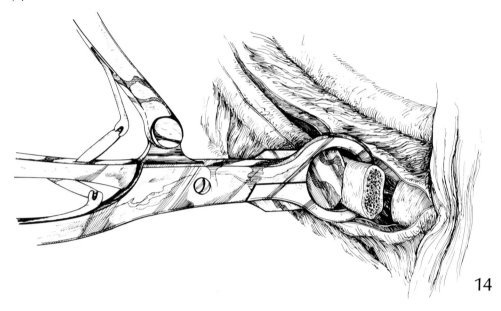

14

15

The pleura is incised where adhesions are least likely.

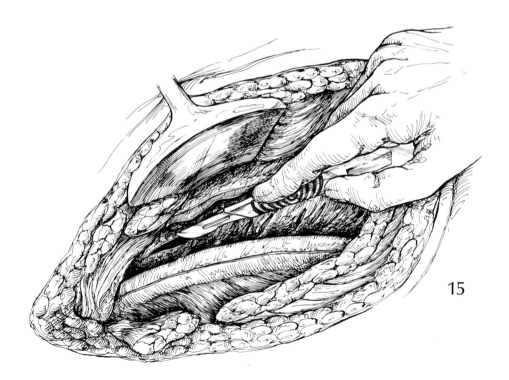

15

16

If the pleural space is free the pleura is split the length of the incision and two Price-Thomas retractors inserted. It is often helpful to have a deeper blade on the upper arm of each retractor to allow for the extra depth imposed by the scapula. Progressive steady retraction will then provide adequate exposure for the majority of intra-thoracic procedures. A headlight is a great asset in the dark recesses of the thoracic cavity.

17

If adhesions are encountered a Tudor-Edwards retractor is used to gently separate the rib margins and a Roberts forcep is used to evert the pleura. Sharp dissection is then undertaken to clear a sufficient area to allow safe introduction of the Price-Thomas retractors.

Should the tumour involve the pleura over the incision or dense inflammatory adhesions make access difficult an extrapleural mobilization aids access. This is a bloody plane and the pleural space should be re-entered once free of the troublesome area.

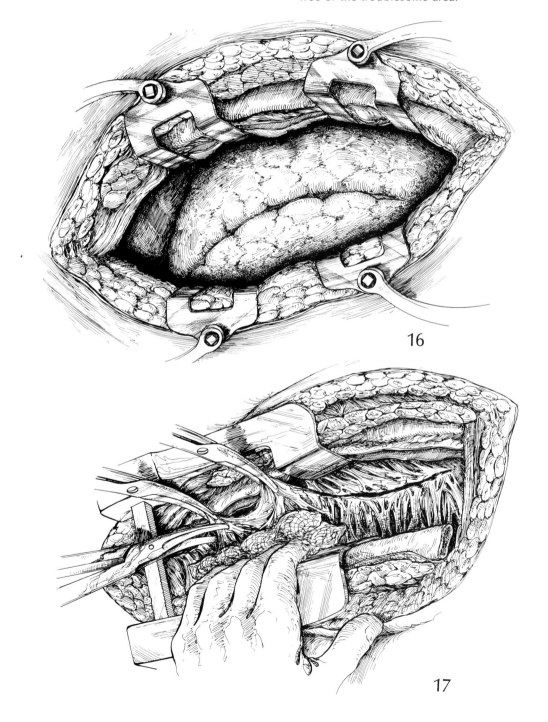

16

17

18

If it is necessary to resect a portion of chest wall over the upper lobe the incision can be extended posteriorly and superiorly midway between spinous processes and the posterior border of the scapula to the vertebra prominens.

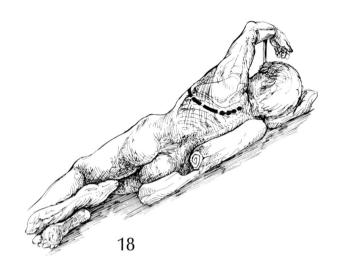

18

19

19

The underlying muscles – trapezius, the rhomboids and serratus posterior superior – are divided near their origins from the spine through their aponeuroses. This extension allows forward displacement of the scapula and gives access to the first rib. It may be necessary to divide the costal components of serratus anterior and scalenus posterior to expose the second, third and fourth ribs anteriorly.

To mobilize and deliver a large bulky tumour it may be necessary to divide one or two ribs above, below, or both above and below the incision. One centimetre of each rib is excised from the posterior angle to prevent painful clicking of the ribs postoperatively. The intervening intercostal bundles may have to be divided and both ends of the vessels transfixed.

20

If particular difficulty is encountered mobilizing over the apex or in the costodiaphragmatic recess a second thoracotomy may be performed utilizing the existing incision through skin and muscle. The muscles are retracted to expose a rib two or three places away from the original incision and the pleural space is entered as before.

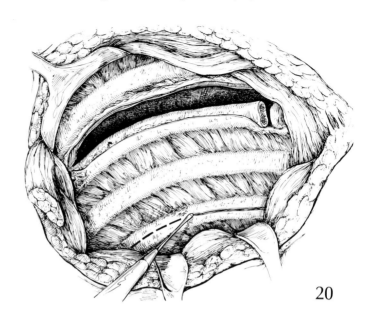

20

Chest drainage

After pneumonectomy a drain is unnecessary unless bleeding is expected. If a drain is omitted then air should be aspirated from the pneumonectomy space after chest closure, when the patient is supine and extubated. Aspiration continues until the mediastinum is drawn to the operative side, allowing optimum expansion of the remaining lung. Mediastinal shift is assessed by tracheal displacement and the slight negative pressure necessary on aspiration. If excessive mediastinal shift is induced venous inflow may be hindered with a rise in jugular venous pressure and a fall in cardiac output. It is preferable to err on the side of caution and to be prepared to aspirate the pneumonectomy space again in the ward

once a chest X-ray is available. Nursing staff must be warned that in the absence of a drain greater vigilance is necessary to detect unexpected bleeding into the pneumonectomy space (*see* chapter on 'Resection of the lung', pp. 149–177.

For most intrathoracic procedures a single chest drain is inserted through a low stab incision. A stiff plastic catheter with a radiopaque line is preferable, and if a further basal hole is cut in the radiopaque line this catheter will function as an apical and a basal drain. If air leak is anticipated, as after lobectomy, two such drains are positioned, one anteriorly and one posteriorly, each connected to a separate underwater seal bottle.

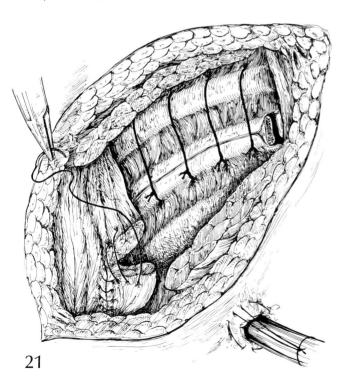

21

21

Closure

The ribs are approximated using five or six sutures, passing above the upper rib and below the lower one. These pericostal sutures should be of a strong braided material capable of sliding knots. Then progressive tightening of these sutures will draw the ribs together without the need for a brutal rib approximator. The sutures are tightened and the knots completed, taking care to lay the knots square to prevent later slackening.

Gentle pressure by the anaesthetist upon the shoulder then slides the scapula into its anatomical position and the muscles are sutured in layers using continuous absorbable sutures such as polyglycolic acid polymers. A continuous subcutaneous and subcuticular suture of similar material completes the closure giving a pleasant cosmetic result.

At the termination of the anaesthetic, a suction bronchoscopy is valuable where excessive sputum was present prior to surgery, especially in patients with limited pulmonary reserve. This must be skilled and expeditious.

Postoperative care

Drainage

Negative pressure applied to the drainage bottles will speed expansion of the remaining lung, tamponading any air or blood leak and promoting rapid obliteration of the pleural space. Suction of 15–20 mmHg may be delivered by a pump or wall suction capable of dealing with a large volume air leak and with suitable safety controls to prevent excessive vacuum. A large volume displacement pump such as the Vernon-Thompson or Clements pump is suitable, but the Roberts pump is obstructive if air leak is vigorous. Suction should never be applied to the chest drain in the pneumonectomy space.

Pain relief

Adequate pain relief is essential if the patient is to cooperate with the physiotherapist and yet any respiratory depression must be avoided. The use of the cryoprobe is gaining popularity but requires special equipment and expertise. An intravenous infusion of pethidine has proved safe, reliable and most effective in practice. Pethidine 2 mg/kg body weight is inserted into 100 ml of 5 per cent dextrose and 10–20 ml/hour are infused via a control mechanism such as an Ivac pump. The rate of infusion is varied by the nursing staff to provide satisfactory pain relief, but to leave the patient alert and cooperative. The rate may be increased temporarily just before and during physiotherapy.

Complications

Sputum retention

This is the commonest problem after pulmonary resection and if not recognized and treated quickly leads to retention pneumonia, hypoxaemia and the need for mechanical ventilation. The problem should be anticipated when extensive resections are performed on patients with limited pulmonary reserve, especially if additional predisposing factors such as chest wall resection or resection of the phrenic or recurrent laryngeal nerves have been necessary. Management consists of vigorous physiotherapy with adequate analgesia, but unless this succeeds rapidly suction bronchoscopy is advisable. Tracheostomy should be performed if the problem recurs or is expected to recur. Broad-spectrum antibiotics are useful but are of secondary importance.

Arrhythmias

Supraventricular tachycardias, most commonly atrial fibrillation, may occur at any time after thoracotomy, but most commonly occur 2–5 days after surgery. Such a complication is more prevalent after complicated operations, especially if the pericardium has been opened; it may also occur during a postoperative recovery complicated by sputum retention. Such a complication is often anticipated and the patient digitalized prophylactically.

Additional complications such as haemothorax or bronchopleural fistula are now rare and should be treated by reoperation (see chapter on 'Bronchopleural fistula after pneumonectomy and lobectomy, pp. 204–209). Dehiscence of the thoracotomy wound has not occurred in our practice using this method of closure.

Illustrations by Robert N. Lane

Resection of lung

Raymond Hurt FRCS
Thoracic Surgeon, Regional Thoracic Surgical Centre, North Middlesex Hospital, Edmonton, London and
St Bartholomew's Hospital, London, UK

TYPES OF RESECTION

Resection of lung may be by pneumonectomy, lobectomy (which may be combined with a segment of an adjacent lobe), segmental resection or wedge resection. The type of resection will depend on the pathology and extent of the disease. In some cases a resection of part of the chest wall may be required and it may be necessary to stabilize the resulting deficit by a prosthesis of Marlex mesh or tantalum gauze. In other cases a bronchoplastic procedure with 'sleeve' resection of the main bronchus will enable a lobectomy rather than a pneumonectomy to be carried out.

Indications for resection

Carcinoma

In Europe and the United States about 90 per cent of lung resections are carried out for carcinoma. Resection is the treatment of choice for this disease, including small cell carcinoma[1,2] (although some authorities would exclude tumours of small cell histology), provided that:

1. the patient is fit enough to undergo operation;
2. there is no evidence of spread of the growth outside the chest;
3. there is no clinical or investigatory evidence of inoperability.

Unfortunately only about one-third of patients in whom a diagnosis of carcinoma is made are found to be suitable for operation.

Resection for carcinoma may be by standard pneumonectomy (simple extrapericardial), extended pneumonectomy (radical intrapericardial), lobectomy or segmental resection. Pneumonectomy might seem to be the only logical operation for carcinoma of the lung but as many of these patients also have chronic bronchitis this operation is often unfortunately very disabling and many are never able to resume work, especially if they are over the age of 55 years. Because of this, lobectomy and, much less often, segmental resection are both carried out and both have provided excellent results in terms of cure rate as well as quality of life[3]. Lobectomy for peripheral carcinoma is as effective in curing the patient as pneumonectomy – and carries a lower operative mortality[4,5]. Segmental resection for small peripheral carcinoma in the elderly has also provided satisfactory results[6]. Lobectomy is sometimes combined with a segmental resection of an adjacent lobe, e.g. upper lobectomy with resection of the apical segment of the lower lobe, or lower lobectomy with resection of the lingular segment of the left upper lobe or the posterior segment of the upper lobe. It is often only possible to make the final decision at operation. In the three years 1975–1977 a total of 451 resections for carcinoma of the bronchus were undertaken by the author and his senior colleague – of these, 204 were pneumonectomies, 228 lobectomies and 19 segmental resections.

Benign tumours

Benign tumours such as carcinoid or hamartoma may be treated by local bronchial resection or enucleation unless they occlude a bronchus and cause distal infection or bronchiectasis, in which case a lobectomy or pneumonectomy will be necessary.

149

Bronchiectasis

The extent of the bronchiectasis must be assessed by complete bronchograms of both lungs so that the segmental involvement can be accurately defined. Surgical treatment should excise all the affected segments or lobes, and it is therefore essential that the disease is well localized and not scattered throughout both lungs. Removal of the affected area may be by pneumonectomy, lobectomy or segmental resection. If pneumonectomy is contemplated the contralateral lung must be normal. Bilateral lobectomy or segmental resection may also be undertaken. In patients with bilateral disease resection is contraindicated if more than seven to eight segments are involved.

Chronic infection

If the infection cannot be controlled by prolonged courses of an appropriate antibiotic, a lobectomy or even pneumonectomy will be necessary. In these cases hilar dissection is likely to be very difficult and this may make a more limited resection impossible.

Tuberculosis

Modern antituberculosis drugs have revolutionized the treatment of tuberculous but operation may still be required in patients who have developed drug resistance, who continue to be sputum-positive or who have non-tuberculous infection distal to a bronchostenosis. The assessment of these patients for surgery is often very difficult and the indications for operation controversial.

Secondary carcinoma

Secondary deposits in the lung from carcinoma and sarcoma occur frequently. They are usually multiple but may occur singly; if so, they should be excised, provided there is no evidence of any other metastases and the primary tumour has been treated two or more years previously.

Preoperative

Assessment

The preoperative assessment of patients undergoing lung resection is vitally important. Unfortunately there are no definite standards to establish whether a patient is sufficiently fit to tolerate operation and many factors must be taken into account. For example, whereas an obese bronchitic middle-aged patient may not survive a lung resection, a relatively thin man of 75 years or more may tolerate the procedure very well if not bronchitic. The clinical assessment must take into account the following:

1. *Chronic bronchitis* A long history of bronchitis always indicates a greatly increased risk for a patient undergoing lung resection, whether a lobectomy or pneumonectomy. Even if he survives the operation he may be left a respiratory cripple, especially after a pneumonectomy.
2. *Bronchospasm* This also indicates a greatly increased risk, though to some extent it may be controlled by antispasmodic drugs and steroids. However, patients with significant bronchospasm will usually not tolerate a lung resection. In a few patients the bronchospasm may be associated with the lesion for which operation is required (e.g. unilateral due to benign bronchial tumour or bilateral due to tracheal tumour) and will itself be relieved by operation. But this is very different from the bilateral bronchospasm so often associated with chronic bronchitis.
3. *Clinical examination* The chest movements and configuration of the chest must be assessed by clinical examination. Patients with a 'barrel-shaped' chest (large anteroposterior diameter) often suffer from chronic bronchitis and emphysema, and this will be confirmed by the radiological absence of lung markings and a depressed diaphragm. Excessive obesity also increases the operative risk.
4. *Lung function studies* It is customary to undertake extensive lung function studies in patients considered for lung resection[7]. However, although these tests provide valuable confirmatory evidence of impaired lung function, they are often very difficult to interpret and do not replace the simple tests of asking the patient how short of breath he is on exercise and of walking with him up two flights of stairs.

Preparation of the patient

This is of vital importance and 2–3 days of intensive preoperative treatment will often shorten the patient's stay in hospital by 2–3 weeks – and may even be life-saving. The aims of treatment are:

1. reduction of bronchial infection by the appropriate antibiotic and postural drainage if necessary;
2. reduction of bronchospasm by antispasmodic drugs such as ephedrine or salbutamol (Ventolin), together with steroids if necessary;
3. correction of anaemia; and
4. instruction in deep breathing exercises by the physiotherapist.

Surgical anatomy

1

Bronchopulmonary segments

The two lungs are basically very similar, despite the fact that on the right side there are three lobes and on the left two. The classification of the bronchopulmonary segments adopted by the Thoracic Society of Great Britain[8] is as follows.

Right lung
Upper lobe:	(*1*) apical, (*2*) posterior, (*3*) anterior.
Middle lobe:	(*4*) lateral, (*5*) medial.
Lower lobe:	(*6*) apical, (*7*) medial basal (cardiac), (*8*) anterior basal, (*9*) lateral basal, (*10*) posterior basal.

Left lung
Upper lobe:	(*1*) apical, (*2*) posterior, (*3*) anterior, (*4*) superior division of lingula, (*5*) inferior division of lingula.

Lower lobe: (*6*) apical, (*8*) anterior basal, (*9*) lateral basal, (*10*) posterior basal. (N.B. Segment 7 is omitted in the left lung).

Each lung has an *upper lobe,* which is divided into anterior, apical and posterior segments. On the right side these segmental bronchi branch as a trifurcation, but on the left side there is usually an apicoposterior stem bronchus and a separate anterior segmental bronchus.

The right *middle lobe* lies anteriorly and is a branch of the intermediate bronchus. In the left lung, however, the middle lobe is represented by the lingular segment, the first segmental bronchus of the left upper lobe which passes anteriorly and inferiorly.

The *lower lobe* on each side is composed of three basal segments, together with an apical lower segment lying posteriorly, which in the right lung arises immediately opposite the middle lobe. In the right lower lobe there is, in addition, a medially placed cardiac segment arising between the apical lower lobe bronchus and the basal divisions.

The portion of bronchus between the right upper lobe and the middle lobe is described as the intermediate bronchus.

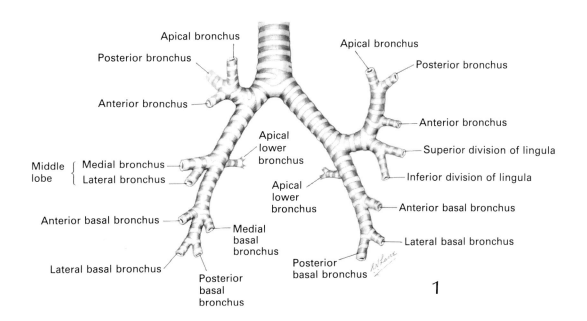

1

2 & 3

Pulmonary vasculature

Each segment functions as an individual unit and has its own bronchus, artery and vein. The segmental arteries run very close to the bronchi, usually on their superior or lateral aspect, whereas the *segmental veins* run between the segments from which they receive tributaries. The segments are held together by loose connective tissue and no bronchi or arteries cross the intersegmental plane. The *pulmonary arterial branches* are closely related to the corresponding bronchi. These usually follow a regular pattern[9], but variations are common and they must always be carefully dissected and identified during lobar or segmental resection.

The lung has a systemic as well as a pulmonary blood supply, and will survive ligation of a main pulmonary artery. The *bronchial arteries* arise from the descending thoracic aorta or upper intercostal arteries and run along the corresponding bronchi. They become very much dilated in any long-standing condition associated with chronic infection (e.g. bronchiectasis). The bronchial veins drain into the systemic and pulmonary circulations.

The following anatomical points must be borne in mind when resecting lung.

1. The origin of the right upper lobe is *very* close to the carina. Indeed, at bronchoscopy the right upper lobe orifice and the carina appear to be almost the same distance from the upper jaw.
2. The middle lobe and the apical segment of the right lower lobe arise from the intermediate bronchus immediately opposite each other. This is of importance in right lower lobectomy.
3. The middle lobe vein drains into the right superior vein and when performing a right upper lobectomy it is most important to preserve this vein.

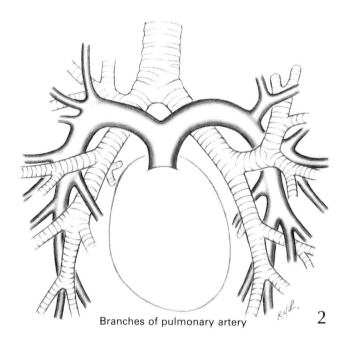

Branches of pulmonary artery   2

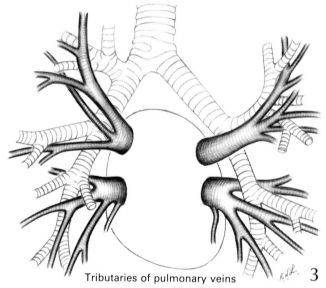

Tributaries of pulmonary veins   3

Surgical approach

A posterolateral thoracotomy through the bed of the fifth rib provides the best exposure for all lung resections and allows the hilum to be approached from both in front and behind, which is extremely useful if the growth is advanced and the dissection difficult. The 'face-down' position is no longer necessary or advisable now that a wide range of effective antibiotics is available for preoperative preparation – it precludes access to the pulmonary vessels from in front, makes the operation unnecessarily difficult and makes early ligation of the superior pulmonary vein in carcinoma resections impossible.

Sequence of dissection

In all cases of resection for carcinoma it is advisable first to divide the vein draining the affected lobe in order to prevent tumour embolization during manipulation of the lung. Thereafter it does not matter in which order the hilar structures are divided, though if there is an excessive amount of sputum or haemoptysis it is preferable at least to clamp, if not actually divide, the bronchus first. With all due respect to modern anaesthetic technique, it is not possible or wise to rely on control of bronchial secretions by the anaesthetist, however expert he may be in positioning the various types of endobronchial tubes or blockers. Except in such cases it is usually convenient to divide the bronchus last.

Division of the main pulmonary artery and veins

The dissection and control of the pulmonary vessels during lung resection is often very difficult, mainly because *both* arteries and veins are very fragile and tear easily. The O'Shaugnessy right angled clamp and the Crafoord uncovered curved coarctation clamp are suitably rounded at their ends and are very useful and safe instruments for the hilar dissection.

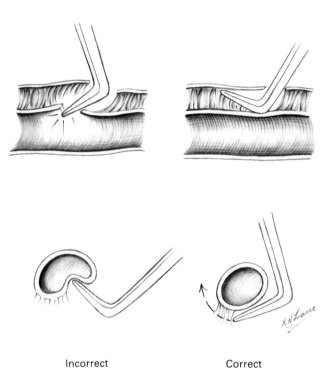

Incorrect   Correct

4

The pulmonary artery and veins, together with their branches and tributaries, are all enclosed in a sheath of fascia. This fascia must be deliberately picked up with fine-toothed forceps (Stille's forceps are ideal) and cut with scissors. It will then be very much easier, and certainly very much safer, to isolate and divide the vessel. The two proximal ligatures should be tied so that they overlap. There should be a cuff at least 1 cm long distal to the two ligatures – if this is not possible then it is wise to apply a Satinsky clamp and suture the divided vessel with a continuous 4/0 Mersilene suture. A transfixion suture may cause problems and is not required if an adequate cuff of vessel is available or if a Satinsky clamp is used. The ligature material must be reasonably thick – a thin ligature may cut through the vessel. No. 1 Mersilene is suitable. The distal ligatures may be multiple ligatures on the branches or tributaries of the vessel rather than on the main vessel itself. Alternatively, if there is insufficient length of vessel for a distal ligature, a clamp may be used distally and the vessel divided with a knife flush with the clamp. It is most important to make sure that the assistant relaxes on the lung retraction at the moment when the ligatures are being tied.

Dissection of lobar pulmonary arteries and veins

5

When ligating an arterial branch of the pulmonary artery it is important to avoid 'tenting up' of the main vessel and subsequent slipping of the ligature (slightly exaggerated in this illustration).

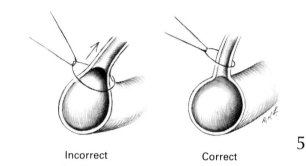

Incorrect   Correct

5

6

It is sometimes difficult to mobilize an arterial branch completely before its ligature, and the method illustrated usually overcomes this problem.

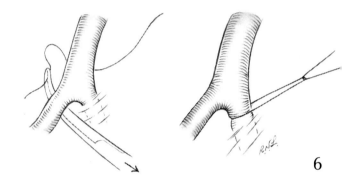

6

Closure of bronchus

There are several acceptable methods for closure of the bronchus, none of which completely avoids the complication of a bronchopleural fistula. The American automatic stapler (Auto Suture Model TA 30) is being increasingly used (*see* chapter on 'Use of stapler in lung surgery', pp. 185–188 and appears to be a quick and safe (though expensive) moethod of bronchial closure.

7

A long bronchial stump is an important contributory factor in the formation of a bronchopleural fistula. It must therefore be avoided and the bronchus divided close to the trachea or adjacent lobar bronchus.

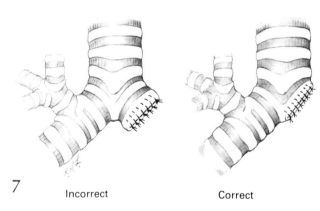

7

Incorrect   Correct

8

The author's preferred technique is to use the Brock non-crushing clamp with the handles towards the patient's head so that the membranous (posterior) wall of the bronchus is brought against the concavity of the C-shaped cartilage. Care must be taken not to place the clamp too proximal as the opposite main bronchus may be narrowed or the anaesthetist's tube compressed and subsequently caught in the sutures. The bronchus is divided with a long-handled angled knife and the stump closed with interrupted figure-of-eight No. 2 SWG stainless steel wire sutures on atraumatic needles about 1.5 mm apart so that the proximal loop is inserted under the blades of the clamp. For a left pneumonectomy the needles should be curved, but for all other resections straight needles are easier to use. The clamp is slipped out of the suture loops after first separating the blades, and the sutures are then tied. It is important to cut the bronchial sutures short to avoid the danger of the ends of the wire suture perforating adjacent structures, e.g. the oesophagus after a right pneumonectomy or the pulmonary artery after a left pneumonectomy. It is best to tie three knots and to cut flush with the third knot. Airtight closure may be confirmed by pouring saline on to the stump and requesting the anaesthetist to apply gentle pressure.

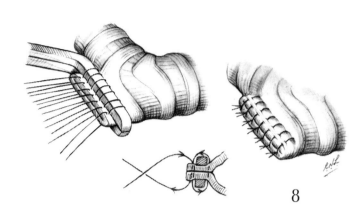

8

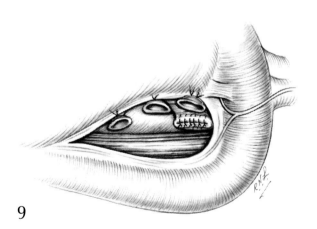

9

9

Open technique

A clamp is placed on the bronchus distally, and the bronchus is incised, divided and then closed with interrupted 3/0 Ethibond non-absorbable sutures on an atraumatic needle. These may be simple sutures or figure-of-eight sutures (as in this illustration). The membranous posterior wall of the bronchus is very thin and great care must be taken when tying the sutures. Anaesthesia is by a cuffed tube into the opposite lung so there is no escape of anaesthetic gases while the bronchus is open.

The operations

PNEUMONECTOMY

This may be a *standard pneumonectomy*, with division of the pulmonary vessels outside the pericardium and removal of carinal, paratracheal, pretracheal and para-oesophageal lymph nodes if they appear to be involved, or an 'extended' *radical pneumonectomy*, with division of the vessels inside the pericardium and removal of all the involved lymphatic glands described above. This extended operation must of necessity be more limited on the left than on the right because of the interposition of the aortic arch. Operability is decided by vision and palpation, though a final decision may not be possible until the pericardium has been opened and a hilar dissection attempted. Mediastinal lymph node involvement must be assessed and a decision made whether to open the pericardium in order to divide the pulmonary artery and veins. The liver should be palpated for possible secondary deposits and if necessary the diaphragm opened.

All of the following indicate that the tumour is inoperable.

1. Inability to separate the tumour from the aorta or superior vena cava.
2. Inability to separate the tumour from the lower end of the trachea.
3. Spread of growth along the pulmonary veins and to the left atrium so that the vein cannot be divided, even by 'pinching up' a portion of atrial wall.
4. Spread of growth along the pulmonary artery to such an extent that it cannot be divided even proximal to the obliterated ductus arteriosus on the left side or medial to the superior vena cava on the right side.
5. Inability to separate the tumour from vertebral bodies.
6. Involvement of oesophageal mucosa – if the growth involves only the muscle it may still be removable.

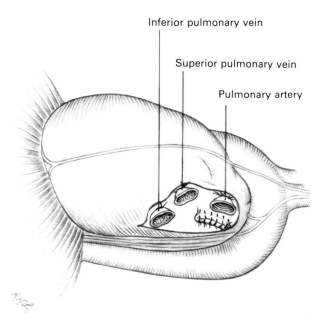

Inferior pulmonary vein

Superior pulmonary vein

Pulmonary artery

Left standard pneumonectomy (extra pericardial)

10

The left main bronchus is just below and behind the pulmonary artery, the superior pulmonary vein is immediately below the pulmonary artery and in front of the bronchus, and below them both is the inferior pulmonary vein.

10

Exposure

11

The periosteum is stripped from the upper border of the fifth rib, the rib bed is incised and the pleural cavity opened. The apex of the lung is mobilized and drawn downwards so that the aortic arch and hilum are clearly seen. If the lung is very adherent to the chest wall an extrapleural strip should be carried out over the adherent area, and care must be taken to avoid damage to the aorta and its branches posteriorly and superiorly or the internal mammary artery or phrenic nerve anteriorly.

The superior or inferior pulmonary vein is divided first, depending on the position of the tumour.

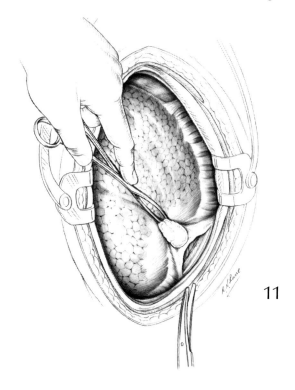

11

12

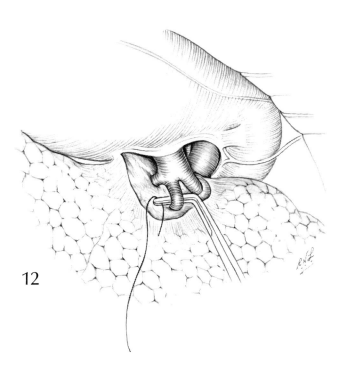

12

The *superior pulmonary vein* is approached from in front and the lung retracted backwards. The pleura and adventitia around the vein are incised and the vein is separated from the artery which is situated posteriorly. The vein is then divided between two proximal ligatures and another distal ligature or clamp, or as shown in this illustration, in which the tributaries are ligated separately.

13

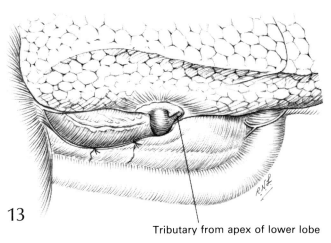

13

Tributary from apex of lower lobe

The *inferior pulmonary vein* is exposed by retracting the lower lobe upwards and forwards so that the vein is approached from behind. This is usually easier than approaching it from in front. The pulmonary ligament is divided (it often contains a small artery which requires ligation) and the dissection is carried up between its two layers until the inferior pulmonary vein is reached. Immediately below the vein there is often a lymphatic gland (of Brock) to mark its position. The adventitia around the vein is incised, and the vein is isolated and then divided between two No. 1 silk ligatures proximally and a clamp or another ligature distally, ensuring that an adequate cuff of vein remains. The vein may be approached from in front or behind, or a combination of both. Not infrequently the tributary from the apex of the lower lobe enters the pericardium separately from the main vein to join it *inside* the pericardium. This requires separate ligation and division. In this illustration it joins the inferior vein outside the pericardium.

14

The *pulmonary artery* is next isolated and divided between double proximal ligatures and another ligature or clamp placed distally. A Crafoord clamp or finger is passed from above downwards behind the artery and between the artery and the main bronchus. Some firm tissue (fold of pericardium over the vestigeal vein of Marshall) must be divided on the inferior aspect of the artery before the clamp can be passed round completely. The artery is divided between double proximal ligatures and another ligature or clamp placed distally.

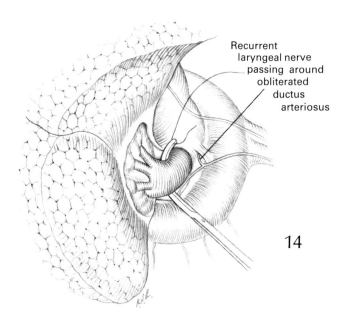

Recurrent laryngeal nerve passing around obliterated ductus arteriosus

14

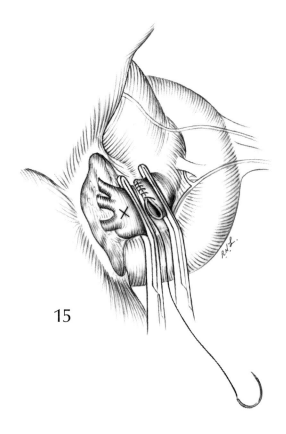

15

15

If an adequate cuff of pulmonary artery is not obtained the artery should be clamped and sutured with a continuous suture. In this illustration there is sufficient length of artery to permit the application of a distal clamp or ligature. But if tumour is situated over the area marked with a X then the proximal end of the artery will need to be sutured.

16

Finally, the bronchus must be defined. The surrounding adventitious tissue containing bronchial arteries and pulmonary branches of the vagus must be divided between clamps. Care must be taken to preserve the recurrent laryngeal nerve as it hooks around the obliterated ductus. The bronchus must be divided flush with the carina and is closed over a non-crushing clamp or by an 'open' technique, or with an automatic stapler, as already described. The bronchial stump retracts into the mediastinum under the aortic arch.

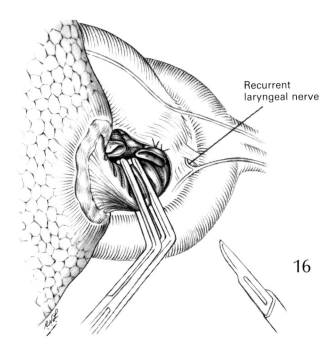

Recurrent laryngeal nerve

16

Left extended pneumonectomy (intrapericardial)

If the growth is extensive, with considerable mediastinal lymph node enlargement, an early decision must be made whether to open the pericardium. If so it is opened around the whole lung root, both anteriorly and posteriorly. It is preferable to retract the phrenic nerve anteriorly and not divide it so as to avoid paradoxical movement of the diaphragm and consequent difficulty in expectoration in the postoperative period. The situation of the growth, however, may make divison of the nerve necessary.

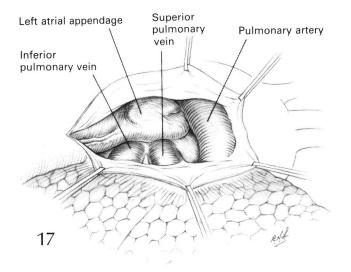

Left atrial appendage
Superior pulmonary vein
Pulmonary artery
Inferior pulmonary vein

17

17

The lung is retracted posteriorly, the pericardium opened anterior to the superior pulmonary vein and the incision extended superiorly towards the pulmonary artery and inferiorly towards the pulmonary ligament. The superior vein is divided between two proximal ligatures and a distal clamp. If necessary a Satinsky clamp can be placed on the left atrial wall, the vein clamped distally and divided, and the atrial wall then closed with a continuous 3/0 Mersilene suture. The inferior vein is divided separately in a similar way.

It may be preferable to divide the common pulmonary vein rather than the superior and inferior vein separately, in which case a Satinsky clamp should be placed on the common vein or atrial wall and the vessel closed with a continuous suture, as shown in *Illustration 26*.

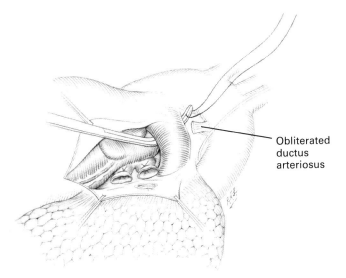

Obliterated ductus arteriosus

18

18

The pulmonary artery is generally divided distal to the obliterated ductus arteriosus (*see Illustration 14*) but it is sometimes necessary to divide the obliterated ductus in order to obtain an adequate cuff on the pulmonary artery. The artery is shown being doubly ligated but if there is insufficient cuff the ligatures are very likely to 'roll off' the divided pulmonary artery because of continued pulsation and in such a case the artery must be closed with a continuous 4/0 Mersilene suture.

19

The dissection is continued to expose the oesophagus posteriorly and care must be taken not to damage it on the medial side of the main bronchus or in the region of the inferior pulmonary vein. A small portion of oesophageal muscle may be removed, provided the mucosa is preserved. The vagus may need to be divided, preferably distal to the recurrent laryngeal nerve, though if there are numerous involved glands in the subaortic fossa the vagus may have to be divided above the aortic arch and the recurrent laryngeal nerve sacrificed.

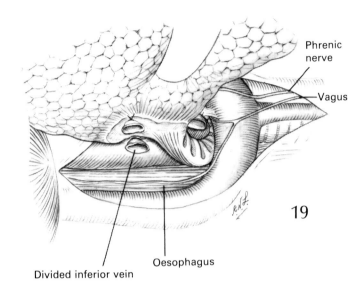

Phrenic nerve

Vagus

Oesophagus

Divided inferior vein

19

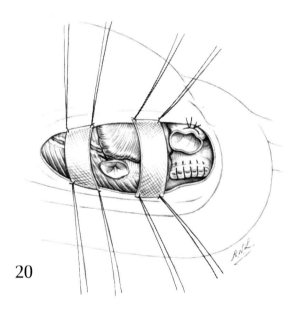

20

20

Management of pericardium

The pericardium should not be closed – indeed this would only rarely be possible. If any bleeding occurs it is much better for the blood to drain into the pleural cavity rather than to remain within a sutured pericardium and possibly cause cardiac compression from tamponade. If the pericardial defect is large the serious and usually fatal complication of herniation of the heart may occur – this should be prevented by suturing 1 cm wide Teflon strips to the edge of the pericardium across the defect.

*Right standard pneumonectomy
(extrapericardial)*

21

The pulmonary artery is immediately in front of the bronchus, with the superior pulmonary vein just below and a little in front, and the inferior pulmonary vein lower still.

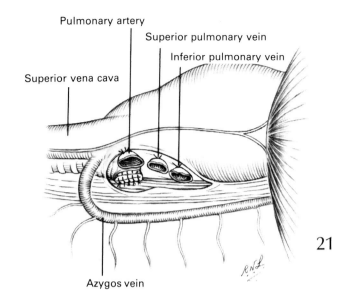

21

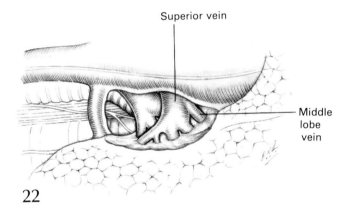

22

22

The *superior pulmonary vein* is exposed by retracting the lung backwards, when the vein will be seen entering the pericardium. The overlying pleura is divided before isolation, ligation and division of the vein and its tributaries. The most inferior tributary drains the middle lobe.

23

The *inferior pulmonary vein* is exposed by retracting the lung anteriorly and dividing the pulmonary ligament between clamps (there is often a small artery in the ligament which requires ligation). The dissection is carried up between its layers until the inferior vein is reached. Immediately below the vein there is often a lymphatic gland (of Brock) – this will aid its identification. The adventitia around the vein is incised, and the vein isolated and then divided between two No.1 silk ligatures proximally and a clamp or another ligature distally, ensuring that an adequate cuff remains. The vein may be approached from in front or behind, or a combination of both. Not infrequently the tributary from the apex of the lower lobe enters the pericardium separately from the main vein to join it *inside* the pericardium. It will require separate ligation and division. In this illustration it joins the inferior vein outside the pericardium.

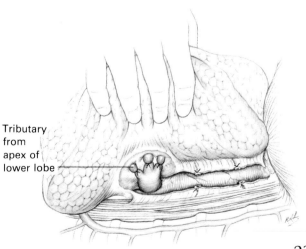

23

24

The *pulmonary artery* must next be divided – and the previous division of the superior pulmonary vein makes this easier. There is a condensation of tissue between the superior vena cava and pulmonary artery (shown by the dotted line) which should be deliberately cut with scissors. This frees a considerable *additional length* of pulmonary artery. It is then very easy to encircle the artery; this is carried out most safely by the right index finger from below upwards. The artery is divided between double ligatures placed proximally and a clamp or ligature distally. In this illustration the inferior and superior veins are shown undivided.

Finally the bronchus is divided flush with the carina (*see Illustrations 7–9*).

The lung is removed, together with the subcarinal lymph nodes.

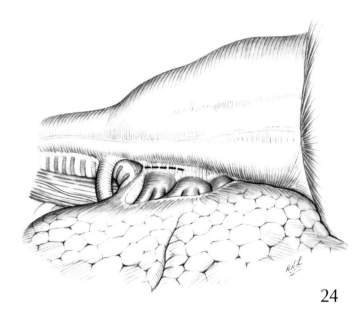

24

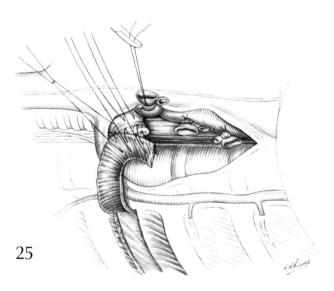

25

25

A bronchopleural fistula is almost unknown after left pneumonectomy but unfortunately occurs in a number of cases after right pneumonectomy, however careful the technique and even though care is taken to avoid a long bronchial stump. It is most likely to occur in those cases of advanced carcinoma in which there has been extensive excision of enlarged paratracheal glands and consequent impairment of blood supply to the sutured bronchus.

It is sometimes possible to cover the bronchial stump with adjacent pleura. A pedicled intercostal muscle bundle, with careful preservation of its blood supply, is recommended by some surgeons and is shown in this illustration. A second row of sutures is placed between the posterior border of the muscle bundle and the posterior edge of the sutured bronchus.

Right extended pneumonectomy (intrapericardial)

26

The lung is retracted posteriorly, the pericardium opened anterior to the superior pulmonary vein and the incision extended superiorly over the pulmonary artery towards the superior vena cava and inferiorly towards the pulmonary ligament. The veins are divided between two proximal ligatures and a distal clamp. The inferior vein is often best approached from below and behind (*see Illustration 13*). In some cases the growth will be so close to the atrium that it will be necessary, as in this illustration, to divide the common vein between a Satinsky clamp placed on the wall of the left atrium and two clamps (not shown) on the distal ends of the veins. The atrial wall is then closed with a continuous 3/0 Mersilene suture.

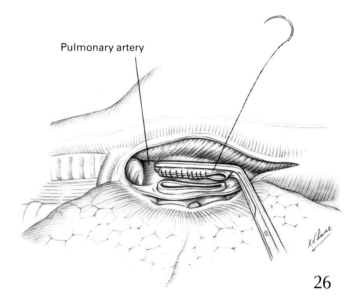

Pulmonary artery

26

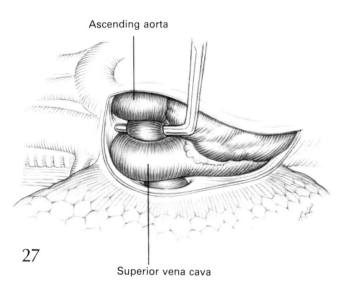

Ascending aorta

Superior vena cava

27

27

The right pulmonary artery is usually isolated and divided as shown in *Illustration 24*. It is possible, however, to ligate it *medial* to the superior vena cava and this may be necessary because of the extent of the growth. If the pulmonary artery is torn during its initial dissection, it may occasionally be life-saving. The superior vena cava is retracted laterally, horizontal incisions are made in the pericardium immediately above and below the pulmonary artery, and an O'Shaugnessy clamp can then be gently passed around the artery.

28

Once the artery and veins have been divided and the lung has been retracted anteriorly, the azygos vein is divided and the areolar tissue containing the paratracheal and pretracheal lymph nodes is removed completely, exposing the side of the trachea, the superior vena cava and the ascending aorta. The dissection is carried from the oesophagus behind to the internal mammary artery in front. The oesophagus is exposed posterior to the lung root and any lymph nodes are excised with the lung. The vagus nerve may need to be divided.

The main bronchus is then isolated and divided as already described.

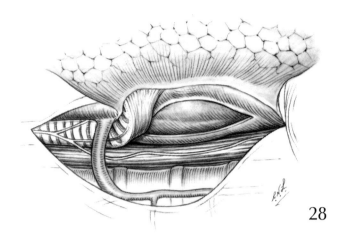

28

Drainage after pneumonectomy

There is a surprising difference of opinion amongst thoracic surgeons concerning the advisability of draining the pleural space after pneumonectomy, and at a recent meeting of the Society of Thoracic and Cardiovascular Surgeons of Great Britain and Ireland members were equally divided in their views. It is the author's opinion that a basal intercostal tube connected to an underwater seal should always be inserted after a pneumonectomy. This tube should be clamped but be released every hour for one minute only and the drainage noted. Suction must *never* be applied as this would lead to too much mediastinal displacement and cause hypotension by impairing venous return to the heart. The tube is removed after 24 hours. If this routine is used any postoperative haemorrhage will be obvious – this complication is not always easily diagnosed after pneumonectomy and patients who have not had a drain in place are known to have died without the cause being recognized. There is no risk of infection if the tube is removed after 24 hours and, moreover, the need for postoperative aspiration is avoided.

If the space is not drained the intrapleural pressure should be adjusted to a slightly negative level at the end of the operation by an intercostal catheter inserted through the third space anteriorly. This is then connected to an underwater seal and left in place until the patient has been placed on his back. It is then removed.

LOBECTOMY

Indications

Lobectomy is indicated in carcinoma of the bronchus if:

1. the growth is relatively peripheral and confined to one lobe (or middle and right lower lobe) – in the case of an upper lobe growth, especially on the right, it is possible to obtain almost as good a clearance of lymphatic glands as by pneumonectomy.

2. the patient is considered unfit for pneumonectomy because of age or impaired lung function.

The final decision whether to carry out a lobectomy or pneumonectomy must remain until the operation because the growth may be more extensive than anticipated.

Lobectomy is also carried out for bronchiectasis, lung abscess, benign tumours and other miscellaneous conditions.

Anatomy

The subsequent illustrations depict the anatomy of the vessels commonly found but there are many variations in the bronchovascular pattern, and these have been admirably described by Boyden[9]. All lung resections are 'voyages of discovery' with certain well-defined landmarks. Abnormal positions of the arterial and venous branches and tributaries are often encountered and it is always necessary to be prepared for this. It is most important to expose the hilar vessels adequately before any actual division is made in order to be sure which vessels lead to and from the part of the lung to be removed.

In all cases of lobectomy or segmental resection it is wise to request the anaesthetist to inflate the lung after the bronchus has been clamped and *before* it is divided to ensure that the proposed division is not too proximal – a mistake surprisingly easy to make.

Upper lobectomy is a more difficult operation than lower lobectomy because of the more complex arrangement of the upper lobe arterial branches as they leave the main arterial trunk and the close proximity of the superior pulmonary vein to the main pulmonary artery to the lower lobe (the 'upper lobectomy trap'). This artery lies immediately posterior to the vein, and damage to the artery will jeopardise the preservation of the lower lobe. The pulmonary vein, which lies in front of the hilum, should be divided first in cases of carcinoma, opening the pericardium if necessary.

Right upper lobectomy

29

The lobe is retracted posteriorly to expose the venous drainage. It is most important to preserve the middle lobe vein, which drains into the superior vein. The division of the veins to the upper lobe must therefore be distal to the middle lobe vein, which must first be identified. Division of these veins will expose the apical and anterior segmental arteries. These are divided. The posterior segmental artery to the upper lobe arises lower down below the upper lobe bronchus and often *quite close* to the middle lobe artery. It may not easily be visible until the bronchus has been divided. It is not visible in this illustration in which the veins to the upper lobe would usually have been divided *before* the arterial branches are ligated.

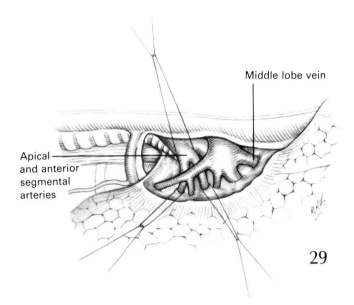

Middle lobe vein

Apical and anterior segmental arteries

29

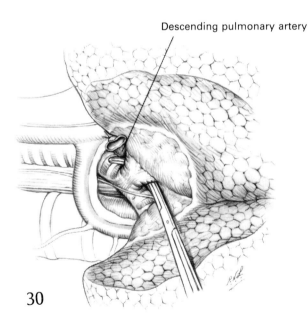

Descending pulmonary artery

30

30

The lobe is retracted forwards to expose the upper lobe bronchus. Only two of the segmental divisions are visible. The margins of the bronchus are defined, the adventitia containing bronchial arteries is divided between clamps and the upper lobe bronchus is clamped with a non-crushing clamp. Note that the descending pulmonary artery is immediately anterior to the upper lobe bronchus.

31

The bronchus is divided close to the main bronchus but not so close that the lumen is narrowed. This is most important to prevent postoperative lower lobe collapse. The bronchial stump is closed as described under pneumonectomy, or with simple interrupted 2/0 Ethibond (Ethicon) sutures on a 25 mm half-circle eyeless needle. The *posterior segmental* arterial branch to the upper lobe is not visible – it is deep to the blades of the distal bronchial clamp and will become visible when traction is applied to this clamp.

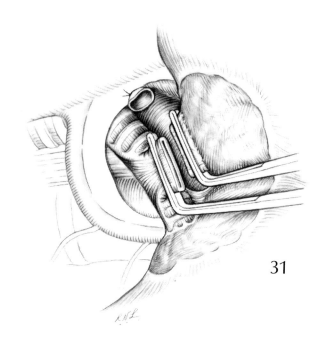

31

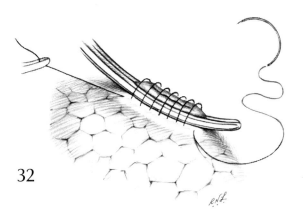

32

32

The hilar structures have now all been divided but the lobe may not yet be completely free – it may still be partially attached to the apex of the lower lobe and there may also be an incomplete fissure or no fissure between the upper and middle lobes. Any attachment to the apex of the lower lobe is managed by division of lung tissue between clamps. The apex of the lower lobe is closed with a continuous suture over the clamp. The lobe is then separated from the middle lobe by traction on the divided upper lobe bronchus and gentle blunt dissection with the index finger in the relatively avascular interlobar plane, as in segmental resection (*see Illustration 45*) commencing at the hilum and working towards the periphery. Inflation of the lung by the anaesthetist will help in the identification of the correct plane. Small air leaks and bleeding points are controlled by ligation. Finally the pulmonary ligament should be divided so as to allow the lower lobe to swing upwards to fill the upper part of the chest.

Left upper lobectomy

33

After division of the superior pulmonary vein (*see Illustration 12*) the lobe is retracted anteriorly to expose the arterial branches, of which there are three to five. These branches are divided separately. The lingular artery often arises from a basal branch to the lower lobe (as in this illustration) and not from the main artery itself. The division must therefore not be too proximal. The arterial branch to the apex of the lower lobe is visible *proximal* to the lingular branch.

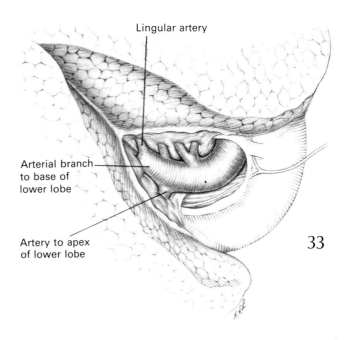

33

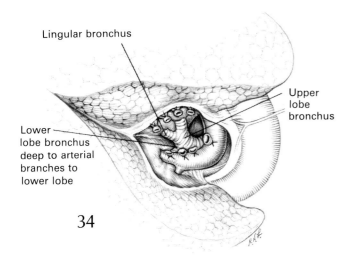

34

34

The artery to the lower lobe is retracted posteriorly to expose the upper lobe bronchus. The margins are defined, the adventitia containing bronchial arteries is divided between clamps and the upper lobe bronchus is clamped with a non-crushing clamp. The bronchus is divided and closed as described for right upper lobectomy. Any attachment to the apex of the lower lobe is managed by division of lung tissue between clamps. The apex of the lower lobe is then closed with a continuous suture over the clamp (*see Illustration 32*). Finally the pulmonary ligament should be divided to allow the lower lobe to swing upwards to fill the upper part of the chest.

Right lower lobectomy

The inferior vein should be divided first in resection for bronchial carcinoma. The lower lobe is retracted upwards and the pulmonary ligament divided between clamps. The vein is divided outside or inside the pericardium, as appropriate (see *Illustration 23*). The fissure between the two lobes should be exposed and developed if necessary to reveal the arterial branches to the lower lobe, which are situated in the depths of the fissure immediately overlying the bronchus. All the branches must be displayed before any division is carried out.

35

Care must be taken to preserve the right middle lobe artery, which arises opposite the artery to the apex of the lower lobe. There may be two branches. The arteries to the apex of the lower lobe and the basal segments must all be divided separately.

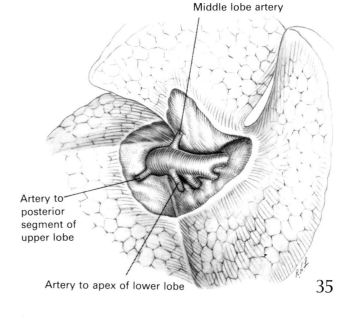

Middle lobe artery

Artery to posterior segment of upper lobe

Artery to apex of lower lobe

35

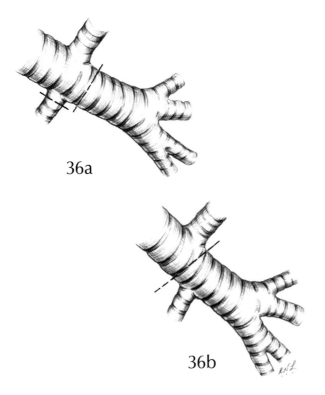

36a

36b

36a & b

The bronchus to the middle lobe must be preserved and not narrowed – it usually arises opposite the bronchus to the apical segment of the lower lobe. It is usually necessary to divide the apical lower segmental bronchus and the lower lobe bronchus separately (*a*). If the middle lobe bronchus is more proximal than usual this separate division may not be necessary (*b*).

If there is an incomplete fissure between the apex of the lower lobe and the upper lobe, the separation is as described for upper lobectomy (see *Illustration 32*).

Left lower lobectomy

37

The inferior vein and arterial branches to the lower lobe are divided as described for right lower lobectomy. Care must be taken to preserve the lingular artery, which may arise from a basal branch artery or from the main artery. It is never possible to ligate the artery to the lower lobe as a single trunk.

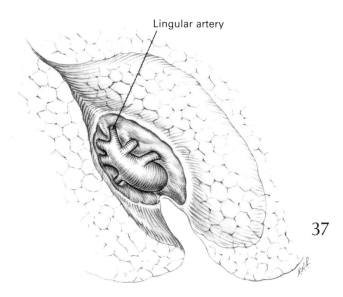

Lingular artery

37

38

The bronchus is defined by dividing the peribronchial tissue containing the bronchial arteries. The pulmonary artery is retracted anteriorly so that the upper lobe bronchus is identified. This identification of the upper lobe is important to prevent narrowing of the upper lobe bronchus by too proximal application of the bronchus clamp or even division of the main bronchus itself. The lower lobe bronchus is then clamped and divided close to the upper lobe, taking care not to narrow the origin of the upper lobe bronchus. The bronchial stump is closed as in upper lobectomy. A suture line flush with the upper lobe is important – a long stump is the usual cause of a bronchopleural fistula.

If there is an incomplete fissure between the apex of the lower lobe and the upper lobe, the lobe is separated as described for upper lobectomy.

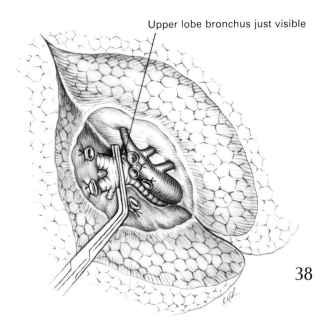

Upper lobe bronchus just visible

38

Middle lobectomy

The middle lobe is retracted posteriorly to expose the origin of the middle lobe vein, which is divided between ligatures close to its entry into the superior vein (see *Illustration 29*). The lobe is then retracted anteriorly, and the oblique and horizontal fissures between the upper, middle and lower lobes are developed to expose the arterial branches to the middle and lower lobes. The middle lobe is supplied by one or two arteries which pass anteriorly from the right main pulmonary artery opposite or just proximal to the branch to the apex of the lower lobe (see *Illustration 35*). The middle lobe artery is divided between ligatures and the middle lobe bronchus can then be seen and defined. It is divided and closed as in upper or lower lobectomy. The middle lobe can now be removed by traction on the middle lobe bronchus and gentle dissection with the index finger in the plane between the middle and upper lobes (see section on 'Segmental resection', pp. 172–175). Inflation of the upper lobe by the anaesthetist will help to define the correct plane. Small air leaks and bleeding points are controlled by ligatures.

Right lower and middle lobectomy

A right lower and middle lobectomy is frequently required for a carcinoma of the lower lobe which has extended to involve the middle lobe bronchus. It may also be required for bronchiectasis, which not infrequently involves both lobes. The technique for the venous and arterial ligation is as described for middle lobectomy and right lower lobectomy. The bronchial dissection is similar to a left lower lobectomy, i.e. the right upper lobe must be visualized before the bronchus clamp is applied so as to avoid a long bronchial stump or a narrowed right upper lobe bronchus.

SLEEVE RESECTION

Upper lobectomy with 'sleeve' resection of the main bronchus is a most valuable procedure in cases in which the growth involves the actual origin of the upper lobe bronchus at its junction with the main bronchus and where a standard upper lobectomy would not provide a complete removal of the growth. In these cases a 'sleeve' of main bronchus is removed with the upper lobe and the two ends of the main bronchus are re-anastomosed. This technique may be used for the left or right upper lobe, though it is technically more difficult on the left side because of the proximity of the aortic arch. The lymphatic drainage area can be removed as completely as by pneumonectomy. The technique is most valuable in older patients, or in younger patients with diminished respiratory reserve, in that it allows the tumour to be removed while preserving the right lower and middle lobes or left lower lobe. If necessary the resection may be extended to include a 'sleeve' of the main pulmonary artery. The final decision concerning the possibility of 'sleeve' resection must be taken at thoracotomy. The technique is best reserved for squamous carcinoma or for innocent tumours. It should not be used for anaplastic carcinoma.

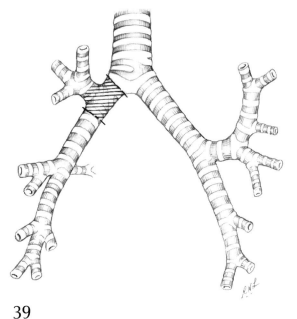

39

Right upper lobectomy with sleeve resection of main bronchus

39

Anaesthesia into the opposite lung must be by double-lumen tube. If the tumour is localized and it is decided that this technique can be carried out, the venous and arterial dissection is performed as already described. The shaded area represents the extent of resection of the main bronchus for a carcinoma at the origin of the right upper lobe bronchus. A standard right upper lobectomy could not be carried out as the site of division of the bronchus would be through tumour.

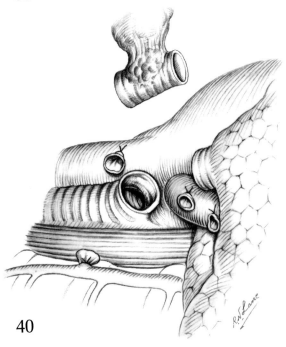

40

40

The arterial and venous dissection has already been completed. The azygos vein is divided. The pulmonary artery is separated by gentle finger dissection from the bronchus. A cylinder of main bronchus up to about 2.5 cm in length is isolated by division of the main bronchus proximally and distally. The proximal end of the bronchus may be left open but the distal portion should be temporarily occluded with ribbon gauze to prevent the entry of blood. The upper lobectomy may then be completed as already described. The lower and middle lobes must be mobilized by division of the pulmonary ligament.

41a & b

The two ends of the bronchus are anastomosed with interrupted 3/0 Ethibond on an atraumatic needle, with the knots on the outside of the bronchus. The sutures should be about 2 mm apart. Any discrepancy in size of the two portions of the bronchus can generally be overcome by placing the sutures closer together on the distal bronchus or by cutting the distal bronchus obliquely to increase its diameter. If this does not suffice, a wedge of main bronchus may be resected and a repair carried out as illustrated. Before final closure the lower lobe should be aspirated by a fine catheter. Airtight closure is easily obtained and the lower and middle lobes are readily inflated by the anaesthetist. A flap of pleura should be placed between the bronchus and pulmonary artery in order to prevent the rare but well-recognized late complication of secondary haemorrhage from the pulmonary artery.

Perhaps rather surprisingly there are no special immediate postoperative problems after this operation. The main late complication is a stricture at the site of the anastomosis, but the incidence of this is not high.

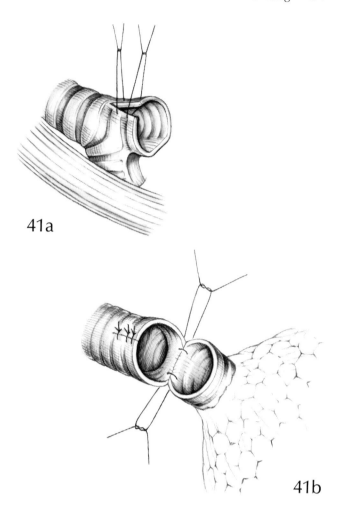

41a

41b

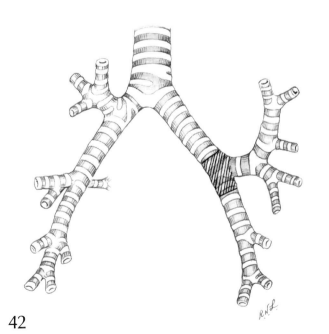

Left upper lobectomy with sleeve resection of main bronchus

42

The shaded area represents the extent of resection of the main bronchus for a carcinoma at the origin of the left upper lobe bronchus. The bronchial anastomosis is considerably more difficult on the left side because of the position of the aorta, but this may be retracted most efficiently by Cummings' shaped aortic retractor (G.U. Manufacturing Co. Ltd).

42

SEGMENTAL RESECTION OF LUNG

Any segment of the lung may be resected, though in the case of carcinoma it is the lingula or apical segment of the lower lobe that is most commonly removed[10], especially in the case of a localized peripheral tumour in an elderly patient with poor respiratory function. Other conditions requiring segmental resection are bronchiectasis, innocent tumours and congenital abnormalities.

General principles of segmental resection

Each bronchopulmonary segment has its own individual artery and bronchus. The vein runs *between* the segments in the intersegmental plane, receiving tributaries from both adjacent segments. When a segment is to be resected the appropriate segmental artery and bronchus are divided at the hilum. A clamp is then placed on the distal end of the bronchus. The segment can be separated from the adjacent lung by traction on this bronchus and gentle dissection with the index finger from the hilum outwards in the relatively avascular intersegmental plane. The correct plane is shown by the line of the intersegmental vein, which must remain in place undisturbed. Its tributaries from the segment to be removed are divided. Inflation of the remainder of the lung by increased endotracheal pressure will assist in defining the correct line of separation.

There is only minimal air leak from the damaged alveoli and these soon seal off with swab pressure. Very little, if any, lung suture is required. The raw surface of the lung should not be oversewn, as any attempt to do this will only increase the air leak. The bronchial stump is closed by an 'open' technique with two or three simple stainless steel or Ethiflex sutures.

Excision of apical and posterior segments of left upper lobe (apicoposterior segmental resection)

These two segments are a frequent site for tuberculosis and before the advent of modern antituberculous chemotherapy apicoposterior segmentectomy was a commonly performed operation. Although now rarely performed, it will be described in detail to show the principles of segmental resection.

43

The lung is approached from above and behind, as in left upper lobectomy. The pulmonary artery and its branches are exposed. The most proximal branch supplies the anterior segment. The next two branches have been identified as those supplying the segments to be removed and have therefore been divided. The fourth (undivided) branch can be seen passing inferiorly to the lingula.

44

The apical and posterior segmental bronchi usually arise from a single branch of the left upper lobe (*see Illustration 1*). This must be identified first by palpation and then by dissection deep to the divided arteries. It is advisable to confirm its identity by clamping the bronchus with a non-crushing clamp and requesting the anaesthetist to inflate the lung. The lack of aeration will usually be obvious, though transsegmental 'air drift' may make this less clear. Once the bronchus has been identified, it is clamped distally, divided, and closed by an 'open' technique with simple interrupted sutures. It is important to appreciate the close proximity of the anterior segmental bronchus, which is easily damaged if the apicoposterior bronchus is divided too close to its origin. In this illustration the anterior segmental bronchus is deep to the sutured bronchus and not visible.

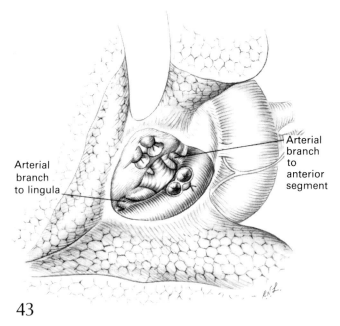

Arterial branch to lingula

Arterial branch to anterior segment

43

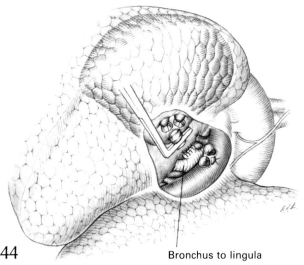

44

Bronchus to lingula

45

Once the arterial branches and bronchus have been divided, the correct plane for separation is identified by gentle traction on the bronchus clamp, possibly assisted by the anaesthetist applying gentle positive pressure. The separation is further assisted by gentle sideways movement of the pulp of the index finger. The correct plane is indicated by the intersegmental vein, which should remain undisturbed on the raw surface of the segment which is not being removed.

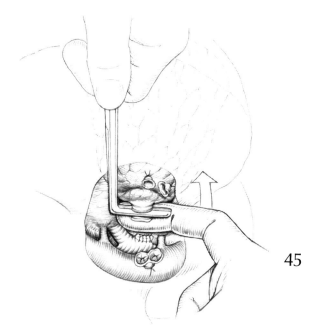

45

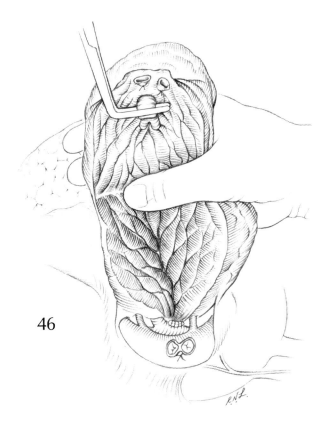

46

46

The separation is further helped by placing the hand under the segments to be removed and applying traction on the bronchus while at the same time applying gentle finger pressure to the plane of cleavage, making sure to leave the intersegmental vein intact. A few tributaries of the intersegmental vein require ligation and division.

47

The segments being removed are now held only by the visceral pleura, which should be cut with scissors. Bubbles show the site of a small air leak from the remainder of the upper lobe – this will cease with pressure from a swab.

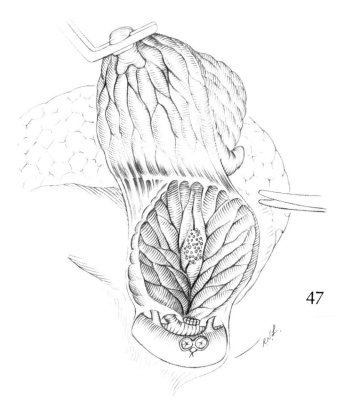

47

48

Sometimes an air leak from a bronchiole will require suture. The anaesthetist should inflate the lung fully to test for any other air leaks, but unless these are very large they will usually close during the first 48 hours after operation by the raw surface of the segment adhering to the parietal pleura or adjacent lung. It is unwise to suture the edges of the raw surface of the lung together as this will inevitably cause *increased* air leak.

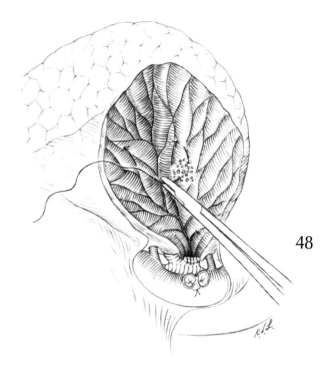

48

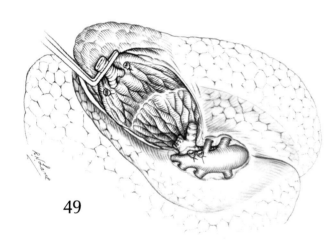

49

49

Lingulectomy

The lingular vein (situated anteriorly) is divided before the lingular artery and the origin of the lingular bronchus is then defined. It is the first inferior branch of the upper lobe bronchus (*see Illustration 1*). The lingular bronchus is divided and traction on the distal end, combined with finger dissection in the intersegmental plane, will complete the segmentectomy. In this illustration two arterial branches to the lingula are shown and have been divided.

50

Removal of apical segment of left lower lobe

The segmental vein is situated posteriorly (*see Illustration 13*). It usually drains into the inferior vein but may enter the pericardium separately. The artery is approached through the oblique fissure and divided (it has immediately divided into two branches in this illustration). The segmental bronchus will be seen immediately underneath. This too is divided and the segmentectomy completed as previously described.

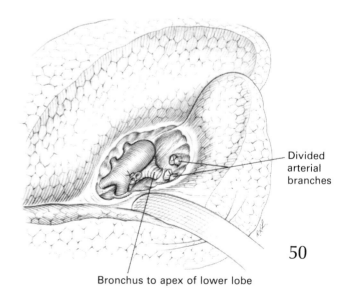

Divided arterial branches

50

Bronchus to apex of lower lobe

51

Removal of posterior segment of right upper lobe

The upper lobe bronchus is approached from behind after separating the upper and lower lobes. Its posterior division is identified by palpation and then by dissection. In this illustration, in which only the posterior and anterior segmental branches of the upper lobe bronchus are visible, a clamp has been passed under the posterior segmental bronchus. The posterior segmental artery arises as the most distal of the upper lobe branches of the main pulmonary artery, often quite close to the middle lobe artery. It has already been divided.

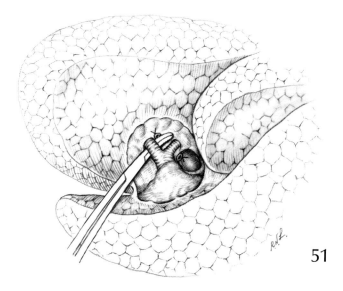

51

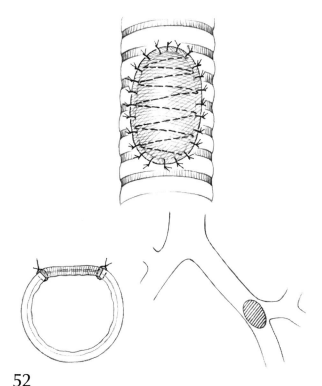

52

52

Gebauer skin graft

The use of a Gebauer skin graft[11], first described for the treatment of tuberculous strictures of the trachea and bronchi in 1950, is a valuable bronchoplastic technique for the local resection of benign bronchial tumours. The graft is full thickness skin and is taken from the edge of the thoracotomy wound. Fatty tissue is removed from the posterior surface and the graft is cut slightly larger than the defect in the bronchus to be closed. This is important as otherwise stenosis will occur later. The graft is strengthened by a lattice work of No.2 SWG stainless steel wire through its thickness and then sutured in place with interrupted 3/0 Mersilene sutures, with the epidermis inside. These grafts regain a blood supply and remain as viable tissue. The adjacent bronchial epithelium grows over the inner surface of the graft and the hair follicles gradually disappear.

Postoperative care

After lobectomy or segmental resection it is most important to obtain early expansion of the remainder of the lung. It is also vital to prevent tracheobronchial infection and its sequelae by enthusiastic and efficient physiotherapy. The following measures are important.

1. *Expectoration* must be actively encouraged, verbally as well as by manual support of the chest on the side of operation. If the sputum is thick and tenacious, 4-hourly inhalations of menthol, Friar's Balsam, or in severe cases tyloxapol (Alevaire), are advisable. A mucolytic agent such as bromhexine hydrochloride (Bisolvon) is also very useful.
2. *Analgesics* will relieve thoracotomy pain and increase the effectiveness of expectoration. But excessive analgesia must be avoided as this will reduce the cough reflex and lead to sputum retention and lobar collapse.
3. *Postural drainage* ('tipping') should be carried out for one-half to one hour three times daily immediately after inhalations, or more often if expectoration of sputum is inadequate.
4. *Antibiotic cover* is generally given for 10 days, as so often patients undergoing lung resection have associated chronic bronchitis. The sputum must be sent for bacteriological examination and the antibiotic changed if necessary. Chloramphenicol is often life-saving in elderly patients.
5. *Ambulation* is encouraged and the patient should be allowed out of bed on the second or third day, even though chest drainage tubes are still in place.
6. *Chest tube management* will depend on postoperative progress. The apical and basal drainage tubes drain air and blood-stained fluid respectively. They are both connected to suction via underwater drainage bottles. They should remain in place for a varying number of days, depending on the amount of drainage and the radiographic appearances.

Complications

1. *Sputum retention.* Collapse-consolidation of a lobe or lung, together with diffuse bronchopneumonia, will occur if expectoration of sputum is inadequate. This will lead to respiratory insufficiency and general weakness, which in turn will cause increased difficulty in expectoration. Bronchoscopy must be carried out, and if this has to be repeated frequently a tracheostomy will be necessary. A recent innovation is a mini-tracheostomy in which a small suction tube is inserted through the cricothyroid membrane[12].
2. *Atrial fibrillation.* Many patients over the age of 50 years will develop atrial fibrillation during the first 10 days after lung resection, especially if the pericardium has been opened. If the heart rate is fast, a shock-like condition may occur. The irregularity should be confirmed by electrocardiography and requires urgent digitalization.
3. *Bronchospasm.* This is best treated by ephedrine, salbutamol (Ventolin) or hydrocortisone.
4. *Surgical emphysema.* Surgical emphysema will occur if the drainage tubes become kinked or blocked or if the air leak from the raw surface of the lung is greater than the suction pump can handle. The tube must either be made patent or replaced by a new tube, or the sucker must be removed to allow the free escape of air through the bottle.
5. *Haemorrhage.* If this is severe, the chest must be reopened to secure haemostasis.

Late complications

Empyema after lobectomy or segmentectomy

The diagnosis will be suspected by the onset of fever and radiological evidence of increased fluid, aspiration of which will reveal its purulent nature. The empyema should be drained by rib resection. An empyema may be associated with a bronchopleural fistula. This should be suspected if the patient is expectorating blood-stained purulent sputum and may be confirmed by the injection of methylene blue into the empyema and its subsequent appearance in the sputum. The fistula will usually close spontaneously once the empyema is drained and the lung expands.

Post-pneumonectomy empyema

This complication may or may not be associated with a bronchopleural fistula. If there is no fistula an attempt should be made to sterilize the empyema cavity by daily aspiration and instillation of the appropriate antibiotic. The initial aspiration should be through a thoracoscope in order to remove all infected fluid and fibrin. After 14 days the interval between aspirations can be increased, provided the fluid remains sterile. Frequently, however, a permanent rib resection drainage is required as it may be impossible to sterilize the cavity. In some cases a thoracotomy and evacuation of the pneumonectomy space will result in permanent sterility of the space. After several months it may be wise to obliterate the pneumonectomy space by an extensive lateral thoracoplasty.

If associated with a bronchopleural fistula, the empyema should be drained by rib resection followed about 6 months later, when the infection has subsided and if the patient is fit enough, by a lateral thoracoplasty (with preservation of the first rib) together with a modified Roberts' flap operation in which the decostalized chest wall is sutured on to the open bronchial stump. Complete healing usually occurs within a few weeks.

Post-pneumonectomy bronchopleural fistula

This complication is extremely serious and very often requires permanent tube or stoma drainage of the pneumonectomy space, and may even lead to death. The pneumonectomy space may or may not be infected. The fistula almost always occurs on the right side, usually in those cases in which the blood supply to the bronchial stump has been reduced by the removal of enlarged paratracheal lymph nodes. Most often a fistula occurs 7–21 days after operation but it may occur after several months.

The sudden expectoration of blood-stained sputum, exacerbated by the patient lying towards the contralateral side and dramatically relieved by the patient lying on the pneumonectomy side, is diagnostic of this complication. The development of a fistula is a surgical emergency and it is vital for the patient to be instructed to lie on the pneumonectomy side until the pleural space is evacuated, either by intercostal tube or thoracoscopic suction. If the diagnosis is in doubt, methylene blue should be injected into the pneumonectomy space – its appearance in the sputum will be diagnostic.

The management of the fistula depends on whether the pleural fluid is sterile. In addition, bronchoscopy should be performed if the fistula has occurred late in order to exclude recurrence of the carcinoma. *If the fluid is sterile* the bronchus should be resutured. As the patient will be in the lateral position, it is most important to prevent aspiration of fluid into the remaining lung. It is dangerous to rely on a cuffed endobronchial tube to prevent this happening, however expert and persuasive the anaesthetist. The only safe procedure is to aspirate the pneumonectomy space dry through a thoracoscope immediately before thoracotomy in the operating theatre, with the patient in the sitting position. This will prevent any possibility of aspiration of fluid and a consequent inhalation pneumonitis in the remaining lung.

The pneumonectomy space is opened, fibrin and blood clot are removed and the fistula is identified. The bronchial stump must be mobilized and closed as described in the chapter on 'Bronchopleural fistula', pp. 204–209.

If the fluid is infected an attempt to resuture the bronchus will almost inevitably fail. In addition the thoracotomy wound itself will become infected. The empyema should initially be drained by rib resection. About 6 months later, when the infection has subsided, an extensive lateral thoracoplasty (with preservation of the first rib) should be performed, together with a modified Roberts' flap operation in which the decostalized portion of chest wall is sutured on to the open bronchial stump. In many cases complete healing of the fistula will eventually occur.

If a recurrence of carcinoma at the bronchial stump is the cause of the fistula, treatment can only be palliative and directed towards the prevention of aspiration of infected pleural fluid into the contralateral lung. A rib resection drainage should be carried out. Radiotherapy is not advisable.

References

1. Levison, V. What is the best treatment for early operable small cell carcinoma of the bronchus? Thorax 1980; 35: 721–724

2. Shore, D. F. E. and Paneth, M. Survival after resection of small cell carcinoma of the bronchus. Thorax 1980; 35: 819–822

3. Bates, M. Surgical treatment of bronchial carcinoma. Annals of the Royal College of Surgeons 1981: 63: 164–167

4. Belcher, J. R. Lobectomy for bronchial carcinoma. Lancet 1959; 2: 639–642

5. Flavell, G. Conservatism in surgical treatment of bronchial carcinoma – a review of 826 personal operations. British Medical Journal 1962; 1: 284–287

6. Bates, M. Segmental resection for bronchial carcinoma. Thorax 1975; 30: 235

7. Saunders, K. B. The assessment of respiratory function. British Journal of Hospital Medicine 1975; 14: 228–238

8. Thoracic Society of Great Britain. The nomenclature of broncho-pulmonary anatomy. Thorax 1950; 5: 222–228

9. Boyden, E. A. Segmental anatomy of the lungs: a study of the patterns of the segmental bronchi and related pulmonary vessels. New York: McGraw-Hill, 1955

10. Le Roux, B. T. Management of bronchial carcinoma by segmental resection. Thorax 1972; 27: 70–74

11. Gebauer, P. W. Reconstructive surgery of the trachea and bronchi: late results with dermal grafts. Journal of Thoracic Surgery 1951; 22: 568–584

12. Matthews, H. R. and Hopkinson, R. B. Treatment of sputum retention by minitracheotomy. British Journal of Surgery 1984; 71: 147–150

Illustrations by Margot B. Mackay

Resection of the trachea for stricture

F. G. Pearson MD, FRCS(C), FACS
Professor of Surgery, University of Toronto;
Surgeon-in-Chief, Toronto General Hospital, Toronto, Ontario, Canada

Indications

Diseases of the trachea requiring segmental resection and reconstruction by primary anastomosis are relatively uncommon. The lesions most frequently encountered are postintubation strictures, primary tumours of the trachea and the sequelae of blunt or penetrating trauma.

POSTINTUBATION STRICTURES

The commonest indication for tracheal resection today is stricture due to injury from a cuffed tracheostomy tube or endotracheal tube. Strictures may develop at the level of the tracheostomy stoma in the cervical trachea, or at the level of the inflatible cuff in the mediastinum[1,2]. The pathogenesis of these lesions is well summarized in a monograph by Grillo[2].

Postintubation strictures are usually short, no more than 2–4 cm in length, and extensive mobilization techniques to achieve a tension-free primary anastomosis are infrequently required.

Certain features of the preoperative assessment are critical to obtaining optimal results. The precise length and level of the stricture should be determined by rigid bronchoscopy and either tomography or contrast tracheography. Such definition will avoid resection of unnecessary segments of healthy, adjacent trachea. Whenever possible, the tracheal mucosa should be free of inflammation and ulceration at the levels of transection and subsequent anastomosis. During the early acute stages in the evolution of postintubation strictures, inflammatory changes may extend for some distance on either side of the actual site of ulceration and wall destruction. In this situation it is desirable, if possible, to delay resection and reconstruction until the adjacent inflammatory changes have resolved. On occasion, this may be achieved by extubating the patient and allowing the tracheostomy stoma to close, and maintaining the airway by intermittent endoscopic dilatation.

The operation

1

In most patients, the airway between the hyoid bone above and the junction between middle and lower thirds of the mediastinal trachea below is easily accessible through a generous collar incision. Resection of strictures at this level (unshaded area) rarely requires a median sternotomy, except in patients with a very short neck or in older patients with a dorsal kyphus and a rigid inelastic trachea. With the neck extended, a bolster between the shoulders and a traction suture placed in the anterior tracheal wall below the stricture, it is almost always possible to elevate a long segment of mediastinal trachea into the operative field afforded by a collar incision.

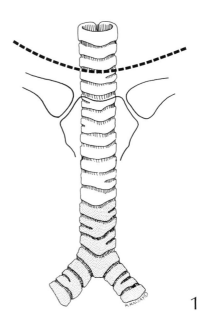

1

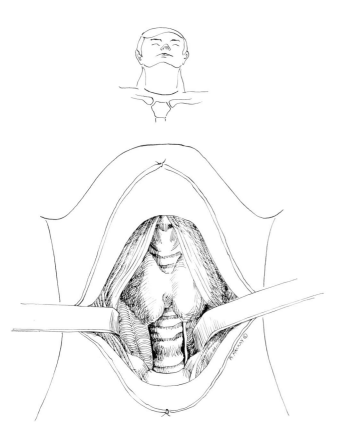

2

2

Skin flaps are elevated in the plane deep to the platysma and retracted to expose the airway from the level of thyroid cartilage to the suprasternal notch. The strap muscles are separated in the midline and retracted to expose the anterior tracheal wall. With the neck in full extension, the upper mediastinal trachea is then elevated into the operative field and the stricture is identified at the level of the seventh tracheal cartilage. At the level of the stricture, the tracheal wall is often deformed and enveloped by fibrous tissue which may be densely adherent to adjacent structures. The strictured segment is mobilized circumferentially by sharp dissection, which is maintained as close to the tracheal wall as possible, particularly at the tracheo-oesophageal angles in which the recurrent laryngeal nerves run. In most cases, no effort is made to identify the recurrent nerves.

3

The stenotic segment is freed circumferentially, but this mobilization should not extend for more than 1 cm above and below the segment to be resected (indicated by interrupted lines) in order to preserve maximum blood supply. The anterior and lateral walls of the trachea may be freed from the cricoid cartilage above to the bifurcation below without jeopardizing the circulation.

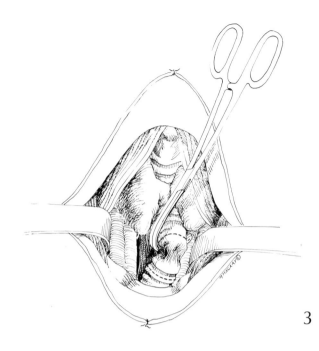

3

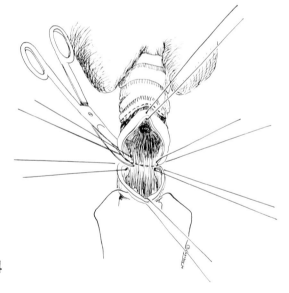

4

4

The airway is divided transversely through healthy trachea immediately below the damaged segment. Following incision of the cartilaginous wall anteriorly and laterally, stay sutures are placed in the midline anteriorly and on each side at the junction between cartilaginous and membranous trachea. Traction on these sutures will accurately display the tracheal lumen and membranous tracheal wall, which may otherwise be deformed and contracted. These stay sutures also prevent retraction of the distal tracheal stump into the mediastinum once the membranous trachea is divided.

5, 6 & 7

Following division of the airway distal to the stricture, anaesthesia is maintained with sterile connections carried across the operative field. The distal stump is intubated with a cuffed, armoured endotracheal tube.

The anastomosis is begun by placing a row of interrupted sutures in the posterior membranous trachea. These sutures are spaced at 2–3 mm intervals, taking a generous bite of trachea on each side of the anastomosis, and the entire posterior row is placed before any suture is tied. Suturing the membranous trachea with fine gauge (No. 35) stainless steel wire sutures with the knots on the inside permits precise approximation of the posterior tracheal wall under direct vision. Using appropriate traction on the stay sutures, all tension is removed from the tracheal ends while the posterior sutures are being tied.

The anastomosis is completed with similarly spaced interrupted sutures of 2/0 or 3/0 chromic catgut in the anterolateral cartilaginous wall. Once the sutures in the membranous trachea have been tied, anaesthesia may be maintained by advancing the original orotracheal tube across the anastomosis from above. Tension on the completed anastomosis should be minimal, and approximation should be easily maintained by relatively fine suture material. Unfortunately, there is as yet no practical method to quantitate tension at the anastomosis, and this evaluation must be learned through experience.

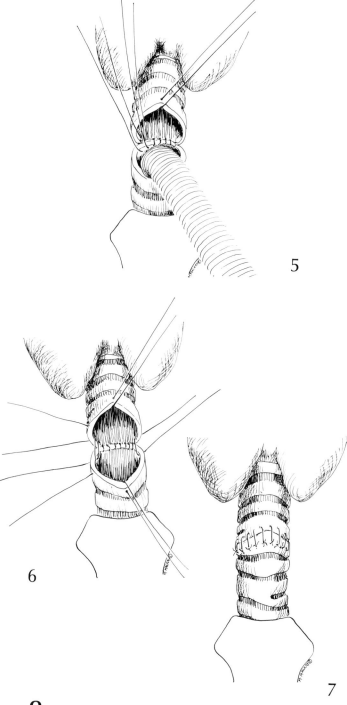

5

6

7

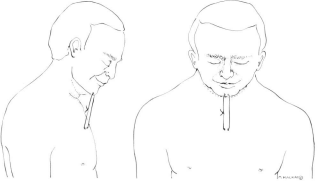

8

8

The wound is closed and the operative area drained with a closed system. Cervical flexion undoubtedly reduces tension at the anastomosis and should be maintained for 7–10 days after operation. This can be done very effectively with a stout silk suture tethering the skin of the chin to the skin of the chest. This apparently barbaric technique is remarkably well tolerated by the patient and is completely dependable in maintaining flexion at all times.

RESECTION OF TRACHEA FOR TUMOUR

Most primary tumours of the trachea are malignant. Squamous cell carcinoma and adenoid cystic carcinoma are the cell types most frequently encountered[2,3]. In most instances squamous cell carcinoma of the trachea is inoperable at the time of presentation because of invasion of local stuctures and mediastinal lymph node metastases. Adenoid cystic carcinoma of the trachea infrequently invades vital structures adjacent to the airway, and mediastinal lymph node metastases are less common than with squamous cell carcinoma. This tumour is more often amenable to resection and reconstruction[4].

Tracheal tumours are rarely recognized before the patient develops significant symptoms of upper airway obstruction. At this stage, most tumours have grown to such dimensions that extensive segments of trachea have to be removed. Mobilization procedures are then almost always required to reduce tension on the subsequent anastomosis. In most individuals it is possible to resect up to 3 cm of trachea and obtain a primary anastomosis with minimal tension without the addition of special mobilization techniques. The laryngeal release operation described by Dedo and Fishman[5] permits resection of an additional 2–3 cm of trachea by dropping the larynx and reducing tension at the anastomosis. Mobilization of the right pulmonary hilum permits resection of a further 2 cm. With the addition of these techniques it is therefore possible to resect circumferential segments up to 7 cm in length and approximate the divided tracheal ends without undue tension or critical interruption of the tracheal blood supply.

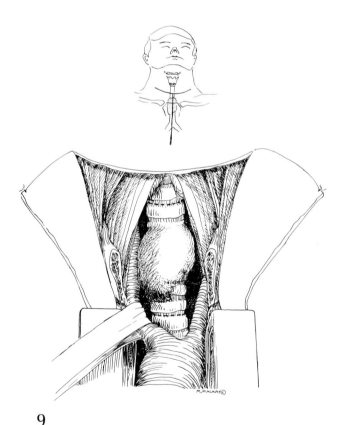

The operation

PRIMARY ADENOID CYSTIC CARCINOMA OF THE LOWER CERVICAL AND UPPER MEDIASTINAL TRACHEA

9

Exposure is obtained through a collar incision with the addition of a median sternotomy. The strap muscles are separated and retracted, exposing the trachea from the level of the thyroid cartilage to the aortic arch. The innominate artery is retracted inferolaterally. The gross boundaries of the tumour on the external aspect of the trachea are defined above and below. The interrupted lines represent the proposed level of the segmental resection and lie about 1 cm beyond the gross limits of the tumour. Since adenoid cystic carcinoma may extend well beyond the visible and palpable limits of the tumour, the resection lines must be assessed by frozen section.

9

10

The mediastinal trachea is divided transversely on the distal side of the tumour, and three stay sutures are placed in the distal stump to provide control of the lumen and prevent retraction inferiorly. The distal stump is intubated with a sterile armoured orotracheal tube for maintenance of ventilation and anaesthesia.

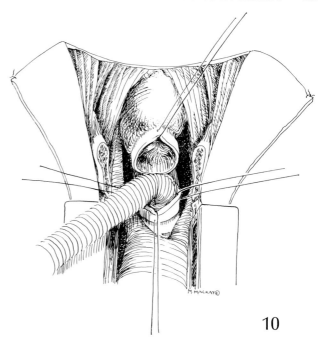

10

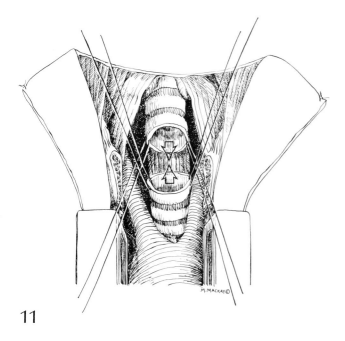

11

11

The trachea is then divided proximally above the tumour, completing segmental resection of a 7 cm length of trachea. This represents approximately half of the length of the average adult trachea. If either resection line is found to be involved by tumour on frozen section assessment, an additional segment of trachea is resected whenever possible.

At this stage in the procedure the bolster is removed from between the shoulders, and the neck is flexed in order to shorten the trachea and reduce tension. If, after applying appropriate traction on the stay sutures which have been placed in the upper and lower tracheal stumps, it is evident that the ends cannot be approximated without excessive tension, additional mobilization of the trachea is required.

Laryngeal release

12

The upper cervical skin flap is elevated to the level of the hyoid bone above. In the illustration, the sternohyoid muscles have been retracted laterally to expose the underlying soft tissues behind the hyoid and thyroid cartilages. The thyrohyoid muscles on each side are freed and divided transversely along the interrupted lines, exposing the thyrohyoid membrane and central thyrohyoid ligament.

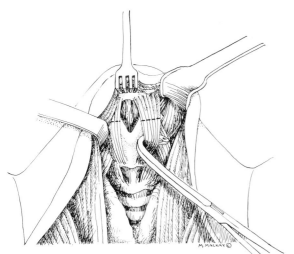

12

13a & b

The membane and ligament are then divided anteriorly and laterally between the superior cornua of the thyroid cartilage. The tips of the superior cornua are amputated, taking care to avoid injury to the superior laryngeal nerves and their accompanying vessels, which are usually readily identified on each side.

After division of the thyrohyoid membrane and ligament, the submucosa of the anterior pharyngeal wall is exposed. This is easily recognized by its rich submucosal plexus of vessels. It is now possible to 'drop' the larynx for at least 2–3 cm below its original position. The divided tracheal ends can then be anastomosed without excessive tension. The anastomosis is done as for the benign tracheal stricture (see *Illustrations 5, 6 and 7*).

Recent experience (Grillo, personal communication; Payne, personal communication) suggests that the *suprahyoid* laryngeal release originally described by Montgomery[6], results in a laryngeal 'drop' of similar magnitude and avoids the common complication of transient difficulty in swallowing which is associated with the thyrohyoid release described here.

The wound is closed leaving a large-bore catheter in the anterior mediastinum behind the sternotomy for closed drainage. A stout suture between the skin of the chin and the anterior chest wall is used to maintain neck flexion for 7–10 days after operation.

If the upper resection line lies at or above the level of the inferior border of the cricoid cartilage, there is a significant hazard from laryngeal or subglottic obstruction due to haemotoma or oedema. In such cases, a small-bore tracheostomy tube may be inserted distal to the anastomosis to ensure a safe airway during the early postoperative period. In most cases, however, a tracheostomy is neither necessary nor advisable.

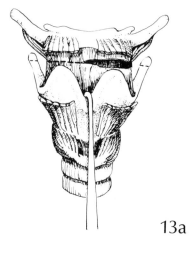

13a

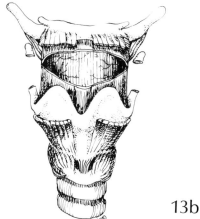

13b

References

1. Pearson, F. G., Goldberg, M., DaSilva, A. J. A prospective study of tracheal injury complicating tracheostomy with a cuffed tube. Annals of Otology 1968; 77: 867–882

2. Grillo, H. C. Surgery of the trachea. Current Problems in Surgery 1970; July: 3–59

3. Houston, H. E., Payne, W. S., Harrison, E. G. Jr., Olsen, A. M. Primary cancers of the trachea. Archives of Surgery 1969; 99: 132–140

4. Pearson, F. G., Thompson, D. W., Weissberg, D., Simpson, W. J. K., Kergin, F. G. Adenoid cystic carcinoma of the trachea: experience with 16 patients managed by tracheal resection. Annals of Thoracic Surgery 1974; 18: 16–29

5. Dedo, H. H., Fishman, N. H. 'Laryngeal release and sleeve resection for tracheal stenosis. Annals of Otology, Rhinology and Laryngology 1969; 78: 285–296

6. Montgomery, W. W. Surgery of the upper respiratory system, Vol. II. Philadelphia: Lea and Febiger, 1973

Use of stapler in lung surgery

Stuart C. Lennox FRCS
Consultant Surgeon, The Brompton Hospital, London;
Senior Lecturer, Cardiothoracic Institute, University of London, UK

Instruments

The automatic staplers used in this section are manufactured by the United States Surgical Corporation.

1a & b

The TA30 (a) and TA55 (b) are intended for thoracoabdominal work (hence the description TA) and use a cartridge of staples either 30 mm or 55 mm long. Two sizes of staples are available for bronchial closure, the 3.5 mm and the 4.8 mm, and the 30V staples are used for vascular work.

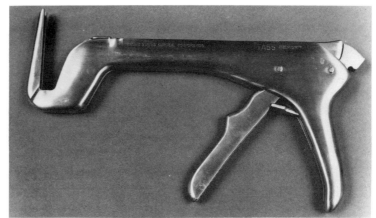

1a

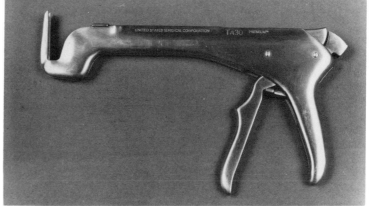

1b

2

The third stapler used is the GIA (gastrointestinal anastomosis). This places two, double, staggered rows of stainless steel staples and, if desired, simultaneously divides the tissue between the two double staple rows. The size of the staples and whether or not the dividing cut is made is determined by the Disposable Loading Unit selected. At present, three types of loading units are available: the GIA, the PGIA and the SGIA.

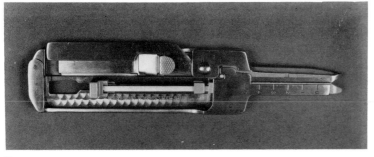

2

Basic applications

3

Closure of the bronchus

The bronchus is prepared as described in the chapter on 'Resection of lung' (pp. 149–177). The TA30 stapler is applied to the bronchus in the same way as a proximal clamp would be used, that is flush with carina for a pneumonectomy or as proximal as possible for a lobectomy. For a pneumonectomy 4.8 mm staples are generally used. For a lobectomy either 4.8 or 3.5 mm staples are used according to the thickness of the tissues. After discharging the staples the bronchus is divided flush with the stapler. Bronchial stump closure should then be tested. It is unusual to have to insert any further sutures. The bronchus is seen (*insert*) to be closed with two rows of interdigitating staples.

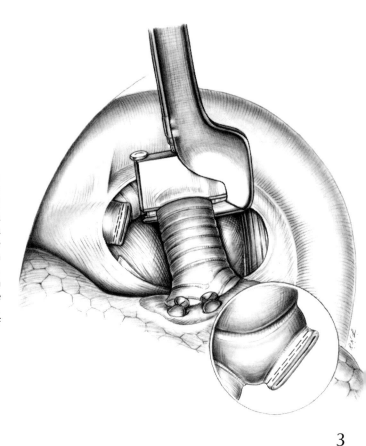

3

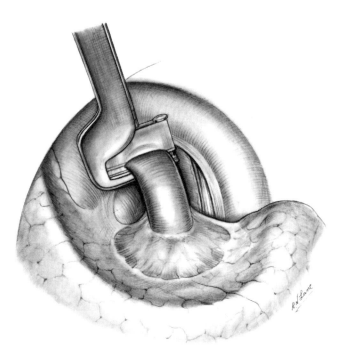

4

4

Closure of the pulmonary artery

The pulmonary artery can be closed safely with the TA30 stapler using 30 V staples. The main indication for their use is when there is insufficient length of the artery to allow it to be tied safely. The stapler is used in the same way as for closure of the bronchus.

5

Closure of the left atrium

The stapler is particularly useful for those patients with involvement of the pulmonary veins. The TA30 with 30 V staples is applied to the left atrium, distal to the tumour. After discharging the staples the left atrium is cut flush with the stapler.

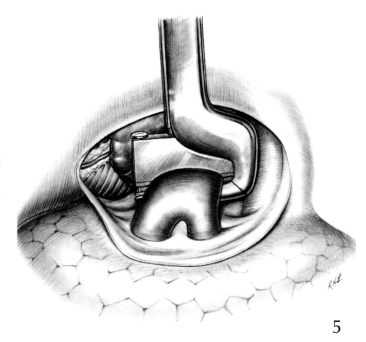

5

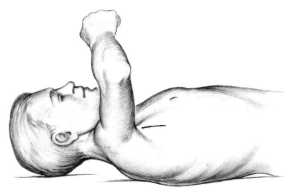

6a

6a & b

Open lung biopsy

This can be carried out through a small cosmetic incision either in the axilla or through the auscultatory triangle. The incision need only be large enough to allow palpation of the lung, thereby enabling the appropriate tissue to be biopsied.

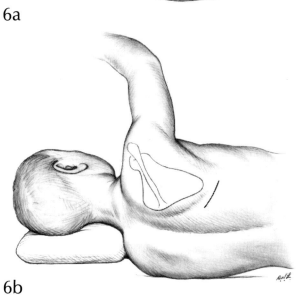

6b

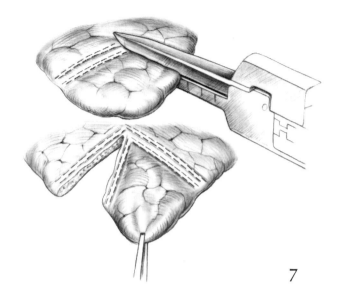

7

7

Through the small incision a stapler can be introduced and the biopsy performed. If the material to be biopsied is peripheral then the TA30 or TA55 can be used with 3.5 mm staples as shown.

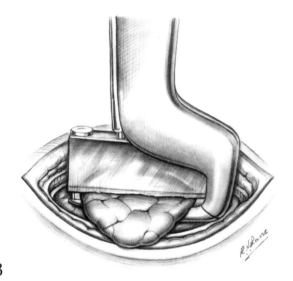

8

8

If, however, the tissue to be biopsied is deeper in the lung, then it is more suitable to use the GIA which enables a deep wedge of tissue to be removed. Incomplete fissures in the lung can be similarly divided with this instrument during resection of a lobe.

Surgical treatment of pulmonary cysts and bullous disease

E. R. Townsend FRCS
Consultant Thoracic Surgeon, North West Thames Regional Health Authority and Oxford Regional Health Authority, and Harefield Hospital, Middlesex, UK

Introduction

Air-filled pulmonary cysts are commonly referred to as bullae. They can be divided into two major groups, depending on aetiology: (1) those associated with emphysematous disease, and (2) those resulting from infective processes.

In infants and children, simple cysts, or pneumatoceles, may occur as the result of infection, particularly staphylococcal pneumonia. Such cysts usually disappear once the underlying condition has been brought under control. In adults, cysts may be associated with tuberculosis or bronchiectasis, and usually do not disappear even if the disease process is controlled.

Small simple cysts (pleural blebs) are possibly the commonest cause of spontaneous pneumothorax, the management of which is described in detail in the chapter on 'The management of spontaneous pneumothorax', pp. 118–123). Rupture of a cyst, particularly if associated with infection, may result in a pyopneumothorax with subsequent empyema formation (see chapter on 'Decortication of the lung and excision of empyema', pp. 218–225).

Bullae may be single or multiple (unilateral or bilateral), and may be difficult to distinguish from generalized lobar emphysema. It is important to differentiate a large single cyst from generalized emphysema, which is clearly not amenable to operative therapy. Large bullae are usually obvious on chest radiographs, but in some cases may be extremely difficult to distinguish from a pneumothorax. As the treatment of a bulla is different from that of a pneumothorax, every attempt should be made to diagnose the condition accurately; computerized axial tomography may be helpful in this respect.

Preoperative

Anaesthesia

The technique of induction and maintenance of anaesthesia is of extreme importance. Paralysis of the respiratory muscles and manual ventilation of the lungs can be dangerous, as there is a high risk of causing increased tension within the cyst which may prove fatal by compressing other intrathoracic structures. (Intubation under local anaesthesia followed by inhalation anaesthesia is the method of choice in some centres – *Editor*). Although general anaesthesia is preferred, cyst decompression in seriously ill patients may be carried out under local anaesthesia. Nitrous oxide should not be used until either the affected lung has been isolated with a double-lumen tube or an appropriate bronchus blocker, or the chest has been opened.

The insertion of an arterial cannula to enable frequent monitoring of blood gases during the operation and in the immediate postoperative period is valuable in all patients and essential in those with respiratory failure. An ear oximeter may prove a useful adjunct as an indicator of the patient's state of oxygenation.

The operations

Two operative techniques are available: excision (bullectomy) and decompression. The choice of operation remains controversial and is frequently decided by the personal preference of the surgeon. However, the author believes that decompression is the procedure of choice for patients who are respiratory cripples and who have more than one bulla in one lung, in other words, those who are perhaps more likely to develop further bullae as time goes go by. Younger patients with a single bulla are probably best treated by excision, although some surgeons would advocate decompression even in these cases.

BULLECTOMY

The purpose of the operation is to remove any mechanical interference with respiration and expansion of functioning lung tissue caused by large cysts. If there are multiple cysts or bullae, it is not essential to remove them all. If a whole lobe is extensively destroyed, it may be preferable to perform a lobectomy. A general rule, however, in patients with bullous emphysema, is to retain as much functioning lung tissue as possible; this point cannot be over emphasized.

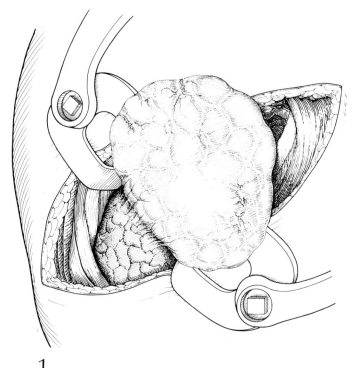

1

The incision

A standard posterolateral thoracotomy is preferred.

1

Each bulla to be removed is first opened near the point where it merges with normal lung tissue, and the redundant wall of the cyst is then excised. Transillumination of the tissue may help to clarify where the wall merges with underlying normal lung.

When the cyst arises from a narrow pedicle, simple ligature and excision is all that is required.

2

Multiple air leaks are oversewn with a monofilament suture such as 5/0 polypropylene, and an attempt is made to reconstitute the underlying lung, which is often extremely fragile. (Tissue adhesives may prove to be of value in the future.) Resection of emphysematous lung tissue is easily performed with an appropriate stapling machine. The author prefers the GIA stapler, as illustrated.

At least two drains should be inserted, one apical and one basal. Some surgeons advocate performing a pleurectomy or pleural abrasion in order to encourage subsequent adhesion formation between the raw pulmonary surface and the chest wall, and thus minimize the length of time of air leakage.

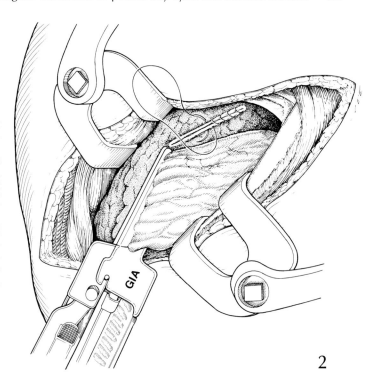

2

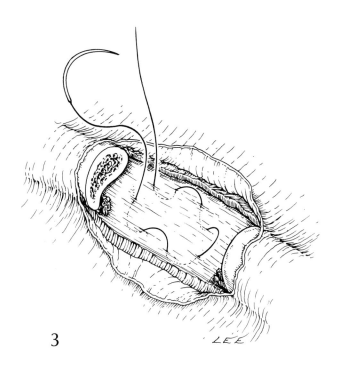

3

MONALDI-TYPE DECOMPRESSION OF A GIANT BULLA BY INTRACAVITARY SUCTION

This operation may be performed under local anaesthesia.

The incision

The incision should be placed over the bulla. In apical bullae, it should be as high as possible and in basal bullae as low as possible. A transverse or vertical incision may be used.

3

A portion of rib is excised and the neurovascular bundle ligated with an absorbable suture. With the parietal pleura intact, a 4/0 or 5/0 monofilament suture is inserted in order to hold the parietal and visceral pleural layers together. This suture passes through the parietal pleura and then through the wall of the bulla.

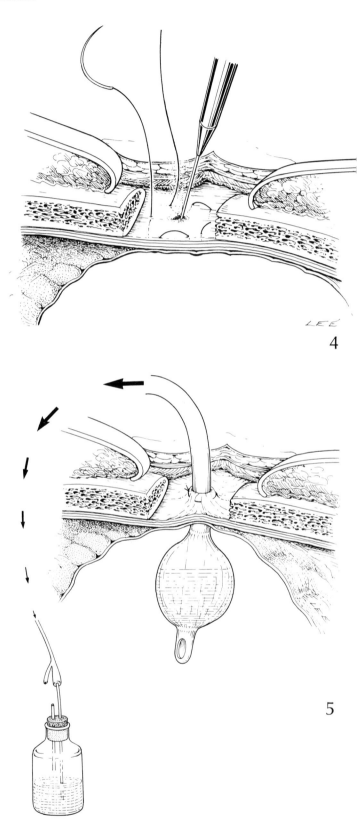

4 & 5

The bulla is then opened and explored digitally or with a suitable sterile telescopic instrument, and a large Foley or similar self-retaining balloon catheter is inserted and connected to an underwater drainage system. The balloon of the Foley catheter is inflated with water and air, and the catheter is pulled back so that the inflated balloon stops any air leaking from the bullous sac and thus prevents a pneumothorax developing. The catheter is firmly held in place with nylon sutures, which are first sutured to the skin and then tied around the catheter.

A pleural drain is usually not necessary, unless the pleural cavity has clearly been breached. The wound is then closed.

Before the patient leaves the operating theatre, a chest radiograph is taken. If this reveals a pneumothorax, a chest drain or drains are inserted as necessary and suction is applied to all of the drains. If there is no pneumothorax, the bulla is usually allowed to decompress slowly without the application of suction. During the next few weeks the bulla usually gradually deflates. (Infection of the bulla at this stage is fairly common and, indeed, may aid its eventual obliteration.) After about 3–6 weeks, even when an air leak persists, the catheter is clamped for 24 h, and, provided the bulla does not re-expand during this time, the Foley ballon is decompressed and the catheter removed.

Postoperative care and complications

Two major postoperative problems are leakage of air, particularly after bullectomy, and abnormalities of blood gases. Whenever the pleural cavity has been drained, it is essential that the drains remain patent until all air leakage has stopped.

Air leakage

Air leakage from the raw surfaces of the lung may be very considerable, particularly after bullectomy. The drainage tubes must therefore be attached to a high-volume (in excess of 20 l/min), low-pressure (20–30 cmH$_2$O, or 14–22 mmHg, or approximately 2–3 kPa) suction apparatus. Modified wall suction may be satisfactory in this respect, or an electric suction pump of the Vernon Thompson or Tubbs (UK) or Emmerson (USA) design may be used. Low-volume suction pumps such as the Roberts pump are inadequate, and may be positively dangerous in that they prevent adequate escape of air from the chest cavity and may result in a tension pneumothorax. If this high-volume, low-pressure suction system proves inadequate, then the pressure should be steadily increased over 48 h in an effort to facilitate expansion of the lung to fill the hemithorax and adhere to the chest wall. If the lung is not kept fully expanded, it may never become adherent to the chest wall and may never become efficient functionally. If the suction apparatus is not capable of matching the air leak from the lung, then no suction apparatus should be employed but the air allowed to escape from the chest through an underwater seal. In ventilator-dependent patients, the use of high-frequency (jet) ventilation may dramatically reduce the air loss.

Ideally, the tubes should only be removed when the leakage of air has ceased entirely, and the lung is fully expanded and adherent to the chest wall. If almost fully expanded, with only a small pocket of air surrounded by lung which is firmly adherent to the chest wall, then the tube drains may be removed even in the presence of a small air leak. This should cease if the surrounding lung is firmly adherent to the chest wall.

If a major air leak persists for more than 7–10 days, then reoperation may be necessary. The site of the residual leakage should be identified and dealt with by oversewing of lung tissue or closure of small bonchi. If not already performed at the first operation, pleurectomy (or insufflation of iodized talc) should be carried out to encourage adhesion formation between lung and chest wall.

Surgical emphysema

This condition, which is most frightening to the patient, may occur extremely rapidly. It frequently results if the drainage tubes are too small or the suction apparatus inadequate to deal with the air leak from the lung. In such cases, if the drainge tubes are large enough, suction should be discontinued and the air leak allowed to bubble out through the underwater seal drainage. It may also result from kinking of the tubes. Once the cause of the surgical emphysema has been corrected, the condition usually spontaneously subsides over the course of a few days. In extreme cases, where the skin is particulary tense over the neck and face, insertion of large-bore needles into the skin may help in the removal of air. A small transverse incision over the front of the chest may also prove helpful. In extreme, repeated or persistent cases, a tracheostomy may be needed in order to prevent the patient coughing and thus generating high intrathoracic pressures.

Abnormalities of blood gases

Many patients coming to operation have maintained a persistently high PCO$_2$. Adjustment of the respiratory centre towards the normal after operation may take some time. Excessive air leakage from the lungs may cause a dramatic reduction in the PCO$_2$, to levels well below normal. Blood oxygenation must therefore be carefully monitored by frequent blood gas analysis, and any hypoxia treated as soon as it occurs.

Infected tracheobronchial secretions

Infected tracheobronchial secretions should be rare if every effort has been made to treat respiratory tract infections preoperatively. Prophylactic antibiotics should be used, but frequent postoperative physiotherapy is probably more important in preventing infection. If a chest infection does occur, it must be treated promptly by administering the appropriate antibiotic(s). Secretions are frequently thick and tenacious, and, if the patient has difficulty in clearing them even with the help of the physiotherapist, bronchoscopy should not be delayed. A mini-tracheostomy may be helpful in allowing suction of the secretions. However, a formal tracheostomy may eventually prove necessary.

Empyema

If the residual lung is too small to fill the pleural cavity, empyema is liable to occur and has to be treated on its merit (see chapter on 'Decortication of the lung and excision of empyema', pp. 218–225).

In high-risk patients, that is those with giant gullae and emphysematous lungs who are already respiratory cripples, the risk of operation is high, with a mortality of up to 20–30 per cent. In successful cases, however, the patient's quality of life is often dramatically improved after operation.

Further reading

Fitzgerald, M. X., Keelam, P. J., Cugell, D. W., Gaensler, E. A. Long term results of surgery for bullous emphysema. Journal of Thoracic and Cardiovascular Surgery 1974; 68: 566–587

Laros, C. D., Gelissen, H. J., Bergstein, P. G. M. et al. Bullectomy for giant bullae in emphysema. Journal of Thoracic and Cardiovascular Surgery 1986; 91: 63–70

Macarthur, A. M., Founttain, S. W. Intracavity suction and drainage in the treatment of emphysematous bullae. Thorax 1977; 33: 668–672

Potgieter, P. D., Benatar, S. R., Hewitson, R. P., Ferguson, A. D. Surgical treatment of bullous lung disease. Thorax 1981; 36: 885–890

Illustrations by N. Krstić

Pulmonary hydatid cysts

E. Ginzberg MD
Professor of Thoracic Surgery, Military Medical Academy, Belgrade, Yugoslavia

Introduction

Aetiology

Hydatid disease or echinococcosis was known in ancient times and is still endemic in numerous countries. Moreover, as a result of increasingly frequent travel and migration, it may sporadically occur anywhere. It is caused by the larva of the 4 mm long canine tapeworm, *Taenia ecchinococcus*. *T. echinococcus* requires two hosts, most frequently dog and sheep, for both its existence and the survival of its species.

Infestation

The parasite's life cycle

The fertilized ova are passed out in the faeces of a dog with taeniasis, contaminating the pasture. The sheep ingests the contaminated food, the ova penetrate through the intestinal wall into the blood stream, and most frequently infest liver and lungs, with only 10–15 per cent being found in other tissues. An embryo lodged in the tissue develops into the primary hydatid cyst, within which scolices or the heads of tapeworms are formed. Cysts are usually solitary, but in 20–30 per cent of cases they may be multiple in one or several organs*. If a dog swallows infested organs of a sheep just slaughtered and containing live scolices, it will develop taeniasis; the parasite's life cycle is complete.

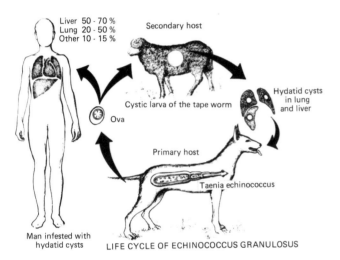

Liver 50 - 70 %
Lung 20 - 50 %
Other 10 - 15 %

Secondary host

Cystic larva of the tape worm

Ova

Hydatid cysts in lung and liver

Primary host

Taenia echinococcus

Man infested with hydatid cysts

LIFE CYCLE OF ECHINOCOCCUS GRANULOSUS

1

1

Infestations in humans

Humans are also infected by ingesting ova, and thus contract hydatid disease. Nevertheless, humans do not normally become part of the life cycle of the parasite because, in a civilized world, human organs are not accessible as dog food. A patient with a hydatid cyst cannot therefore infect other people, though the disease can spread further within his own body. In fact, following a spontaneous or iatrogenic rupture, scolices contaminate new tissue where they metamorphose and develop directly into secondary cysts. Rupture of the cyst may occur into body cavities, and rarely, the bronchial tree, bile duct and blood vessels, the site of rupture determining the location of the secondary echinococcosis and further course of disease.

---

* Numerical data from this chapter are derived from the author's own experience of 400 cases operated on during the past 20 years.

Pathology

The structure and appearance of both primary and secondary cysts are identical: white or bluish, shining, soft, elastic, but nevertheless friable so that they may be easily torn at the first impact of a sharp, hard object. The cyst wall is about 2–3 mm thick and consist of two layers: the external, protective, laminated membrane formed of semipermeable chitinous components; and the internal, germinative layer, whose cells produce scolices, clear hydatid fluid and the protective layer itself.

The cysts grow much faster in the lung than in any other organ. They may grow very large, but even in such cases they usually cause only a reversible compression of lung parenchyma. After removal of the cyst, loss of lung volume may be insignificant. In about 70–80 per cent of cases lung cysts are solitary. A pericyst (adventitia or capsule) forms around the cyst and consists of host fibrous tissue and compressed lung parenchyma. It is usually visible on the very surface of the lung in the form of a firm white membrane or bulge. The pericyst sticks to the cyst, but there is no fusion between them, so that the surgeon can separate them bloodlessly. The pericyst plays a dual role: first, it feeds the parasite and protects it against mechanical trauma; and second, it guards the host against dissemination of the hydatid disease. In some multivesicular cysts, many new generations of daughter cysts grow, originating directly from the scolices. Such cysts are a rare occurrence in the lung (5 per cent) though common in the liver. Calcified cysts are even rarer in the lung.

Rupture of the cyst

It is not the growth and the size but the rupture of a pulmonary hydatid cyst that is the main danger to the patient. About half the patients are referred to hospital with ruptured cysts. Rupture into the bronchus occurs most often. There is a long list of possible consequences, ranging from death caused by suffocation or anaphylaxis (rarely!) to spontaneous healing through expectoration of the contents of the hydatid cyst with subsequent obliteration of the residual cavity. Haemoptysis, pneumonitis, abscess, bronchiectasis, and, very rarely, secondary echinococcosis due to bronchogenic dissemination may occur. About 10 per cent of ruptures occur into the pleural cavity, which can produce pneumothorax, empyema, and pleural secondary echinococcosis.

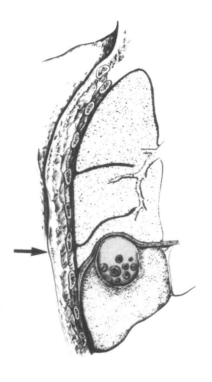

2

Subphrenic involvement

Hydatid cysts of the liver and other subphrenic organs are also of concern to the thoracic surgeon[1]. About 20 per cent of patients with lung hydatids also have cysts in the liver. As a rule, they are multiple primary cysts. Cysts in the upper part of the right lobe of the liver tend to grow upwards and, since they change the form, position, mobility and integrity of the diaphragm, they may lead to various pulmonary and other intrathoracic complications. The best surgical approach to these cysts is through thoracotomy, i.e. from above[2,3].

Surgical treatment

Indications

Spontaneous cure of pulmonary cysts, although possible, is unpredictable. Medical treatment is of unproven value, though the antifungal agent mebendazole may prove of some help in controlling the disease. Surgical treatment is, therefore, indicated as soon as a pulmonary cyst is diagnosed or even suspected. If there is a large number of small cysts in both lungs, however, operation may be inadvisable because the pulmonary tissue would be excessively mutilated. Such cases should be left to follow their natural course, and, if rupture occurs into the bronchial tree, intermittent bronchoscopic aspirations may be of value. An operation is urgent in impending or actual rupture of a cyst, especially if a pneumothorax, haemoptysis, or sepsis are also present. Similarly, urgent surgery is necessary in hepatic cysts penetrating through the diaphragm. Aspiration or marsupialization of a lung cyst may still be indicated occasionally in extremely poor-risk cases. Fears that such a procedure might lead to a persistent bronchocutaneous fistula are less justified than hitherto thought.

Anaesthesia

Endotracheal anaesthesia is used in all cases when thoracotomy is to be performed. For large or bilateral cysts, a double lumen tube should be inserted so that if the cyst ruptures, aspiration of hydatid content into the other lung can be avoided.

Thoracotomy

Wide lateral thoracotomy at the level of the fifth to the ninth rib, depending on the number and location of the cysts, provides ideal exposure for the surgical treatment of pulmonary and other thoracic hydatids. It facilitates both atraumatic freeing of the lung and detailed exploration for undiagnosed cysts in the lung and in other structures both above and below the diaphragm. Through this exposure hydatid cysts can be removed easily and the residual cavity dealt with.

The wound edges should be protected by sterile towels.

PULMONARY CYSTS

In 80–90 per cent of cases, pulmonary cysts are removed by cystectomy (hydatidectomy); in the remainder, resecttion of lung tissue may be required.

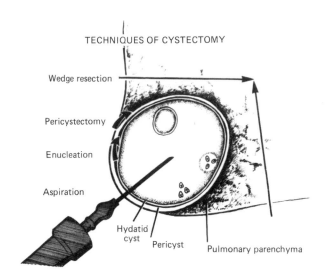

TECHNIQUES OF CYSTECTOMY

Wedge resection

Pericystectomy

Enucleation

Aspiration

Hydatid cyst   Pericyst   Pulmonary parenchyma

3

Cystectomy

The term cystectomy or hydatidectomy includes four conservative surgical methods which allow the radical removal of pulmonary cysts and the maximal saving of normal lung tissue. They differ according to the method of removal and the level of detachment of the cyst from the lung, but often are combined in the same operation. The term also covers wedge resection and other small excisions of damaged pulmonary tissue in which the loss of normal parenchyma is insignificant.

3

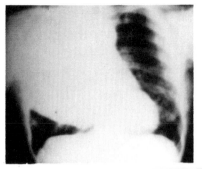

4a

4a–e

One particular case of a giant cyst (mass 1.8 kg) is shown. The postoperative bronchograms (c,d), which show all segmental bronchi preserved and complete decompression of all essentially normal lung tissue (e), clearly illustrate why surgery for pulmonary hydatid should be conservative whenever possible.

Resection

Resection, usually by lobectomy, is indicated for pulmonary hydatids in less than 20 per cent of all cases; in unruptured cysts, it is necessary in only 5–8 per cent[1,4]. If the indication for resection is not immediately evident, it is preferable first to enucleate or aspirate the cyst, to expand the lung, and then decide whether a resection is unavoidable; if the cyst is large, its preliminary removal or decompression will considerably facilitate the lobectomy[5].

Multiple pulmonary cysts

Multiple cysts in one or both lungs occur in about 20 per cent of cases, and in a majority are primary. Even when bilateral, they should be removed if possible through two separate lateral thoracotomies[3]. The more diseased lung should be operated on first. Bilateral operation in one stage is highly desirable for, if only unilateral thoracotomy is performed, the contralateral cyst which has been left *in situ* may burst after operation leading to serious complications or even death.

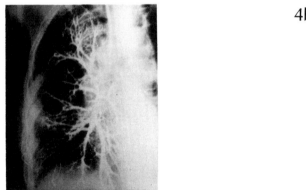

4b

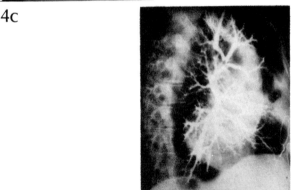

4c

4d

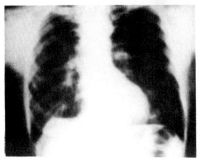

4e

NON-PULMONARY INTRATHORACIC CYSTS

Primary cysts of the chest wall, diaphragm, mediastinum, pericardium and myocardium are rare. They can usually be removed by extirpation or aspiration. Secondary cysts of the parietal pleura, usually originating from a primary cyst in the lung or liver, may be removed without any major mutilation; pleuropneumonectomy should be performed only if there is no other means of removing the parasite.

Cysts of the myocardium

Sometimes myocardial cysts, unrecognized before the operation, are found at thoracotomy. In most cases they can be removed without the need for cardiopulmonary bypass[6]. If, after puncture, it is revealed that the cyst does not communicate with a heart chamber, the pericyst is incised, its contents aspirated; the remaining part of the pericyst is sutured to reinforce the thinned myocardium, thus hopefully preventing the development of a ventricular aneurysm.

'RECURRENT' CYSTS

These cysts may, in fact, be *primary*, resulting either from a failure to detect them at previous thoracotomy or from reinfestation, or *secondary*, as a result of contamination during previous surgery. With meticulous attention to preventing spillage of cyst contents at operation, the incidence of secondary cyst from contamination should be relatively low.

Depending on the number and location of the cysts, wide thoracotomy is not always necessary. Local minor incisions may suffice.

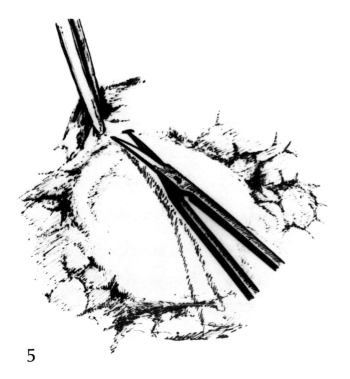

5

THORACOABDOMINAL CYSTS

In approximately 30 per cent of thoracotomies performed for thoracic hydatids, the cysts may be found located below the diaphragm, or extending through the diaphragm. The pathology of these thoracoabdominal cysts and the associated clinical pictures are diverse. However, they can be grouped according to their location, as follows.

1. Cysts in the upper and posterior part of the right lobe of the liver.
2. Cysts penetrating through the diaphragm into the pleura, lung or pericardium.
3. Multiple primary cysts of lung and liver as well as other subphrenic organs and structures.

Lateral thoracotomy at the correctly chosen level, extended by phrenotomy or performed as thoracolaparotomy, secures an excellent approach for every operation on the lung, liver and other adjacent abdominal organs. All cysts can be removed easily in one stage from the chest and abdomen, especially if they are ipsilateral[1-3,7]. Multiple cysts in both lungs and liver can be removed at one operating session, through two separate lateral thoracotomies. A spleen, greatly enlarged by hydatid, may be removed safely and simply through a thoracotomy[8]. (Using a laparotomy, it is difficult to prevent bursting of the spleen and subsequent contamination of the abdominal cavity.) If intra- or extrahepatic drainage is required, the drainage tube can be placed through the pleural sinus and an intercostal space, instead of through the abdominal wall.

The operation

Enucleation, aspiration and pericystectomy are among the specific surgical procedures for pulmonary hydatids. Each operation has two phases: (1) removal of the cyst; and (2) dealing with the residual cavity. Total enucleation must be used for all intact cysts.

ENUCLEATION

5

To enucleate a hydatid cyst intact, the pericyst should be opened widely. The visceral pleura is incised by scissors along the borderline between the exposed pericyst and normal lung (i.e. extrapericyst). If the cyst is more deeply situated, the parenchyma is incised where the cyst is nearest to the surface. By advancing both sharp and blunt dissection with scissors in a plane close to the pericyst, the denuded part of the pericyst may crack spontaneously at one or several places, since the pericyst is thinner and more frail within the lung than on the surface. (It may, however, be possible to remove the entire cyst and pericyst intact.)

6

While the opening in the pericyst is small, abrupt protrusion and subsequent rupture of the cyst may occur. This is effectively prevented by pressing and pushing back the protruding cyst with a finger, whilst dissection of the pericyst continues. Once the endocystic pressure is eased, which can clearly be felt by the pressing finger, the edge of the opening in the pericyst is grasped with two fine forceps placed next to each other. By pulling them aside simultaneously, the pericyst tears and, after repeating the same manoeuvre in several directions, the opening in the pericyst will be enlarged to its maximum. For solid structures, scissors are used.

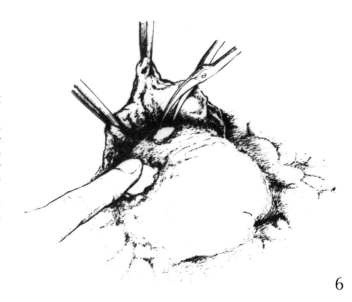

6

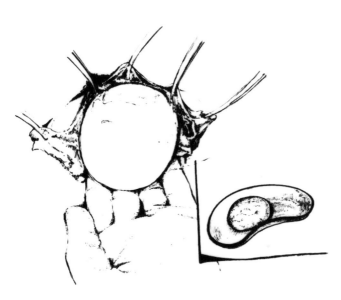

7

7

When the cyst is from one-third to one-half exposed in this way, the hand is gently pushed beneath the cyst and the remaining part of it is separated from the pericyst by careful finger dissection, until the cyst lies in the palm of the surgeon's hand. It is then placed in a basin. On occasions, both hands are required to lift out a large cyst. The cyst is delivered by tilting the operating table, which is sometimes all that is required, and applying gentle outside pressure on the lung. Inflation of the lung by the anaesthetist to 'assist' in enucleation of the cyst is not recommended. In fact, an intensified air jet through a wide bronchial opening may tear the cyst, and the expanded lung also narrows the passage way, rendering delivery of the cyst more difficult.

Many[3–5, 9, 10] incise the pericyst by knife. We have abandoned this method, since the use of scissors, as described above, makes enucleation of an intact cyst much easier and safer. In the last 10 years no surgical rupture of a hydatid has been experienced by the author. If this does occur, the pleural cavity should be filled for 5 minutes with acriflavine 1:1000 or sodium chloride 10 per cent, which provides reliable decontamination.

ASPIRATION

Needle aspiration is a useful adjunctive procedure in the surgical treatment of pulmonary echinococcosis. It should be used if there are more than three or four cysts in one lung, particularly if some are already ruptured. This method is recommended for the less experienced surgeon.

8

The part of the lung containing a cyst is exposed. The pleural cavity is protected with gauze packs against contamination by spillage of hydatid contents. The pericyst is punctured by a large-bore needle, and all the hydatid fluid is aspirated with a syringe. A rubber or plastic tube is used to connect needle to syringe, and may be clamped off during aspiration; this is simpler than using a three-way tap. A trocar mounted on an aspirator can also be used for the same purpose. The surgical sucker is also held close, ready to aspirate every drop accidentally spilt. Indeed, leakage of hydatid fluid around the needle is common.

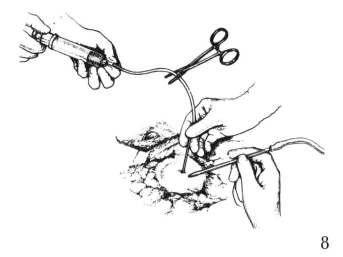

8

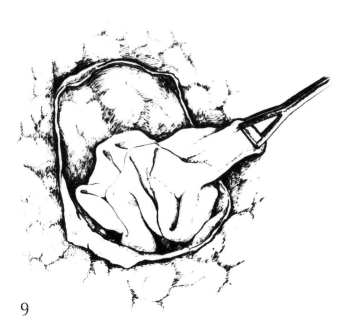

9

9

The pericyst is then incised broadly, the collapsed laminated membrane is extracted, and the remaining hydatid fluid and debris are thoroughly aspirated. A scolicide (acriflavine 1:1000 or NaCl 10 per cent) is poured into the pericystic cavity and left there for 5 minutes. The whole pericyst should be well explored and palpated to discover other possible cysts nearby; if any are found they too are punctured and removed as described above. Daughter cysts are best removed with a kitchen spoon.

Ruptured cysts

In 70 per cent or more of such cases conservative surgery, as outlined above, is possible. If parts of adjacent lung tissue have been destroyed, they must be excised. As the presence of pyogenic organisms is always possible, the residual cavity must be thoroughly cleaned, preferably by 3 per cent hydrogen peroxide solution.

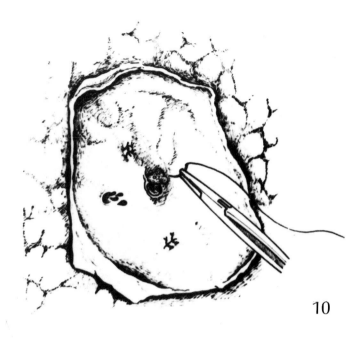

10

RESIDUAL CAVITY

10 & 11

Leaving the pericyst in the lung is entirely harmless if air leaks are effectively arrested, and lasting persistence of a pulmonary cavity is prevented. First, all visible bronchial openings are individually sutured with non-absorbable material. Small bronchial openings are best found by filling the residual cavity with water while insufflating the lung. The cavity itself is obliterated in many layers by running or interrupted sutures of chromic catgut. Prior to closure of the cavity, redundant flaps of the pericyst which have lost broad contact with the lung should be trimmed. Alternatively, if the flaps are well preserved, they can be inverted into the cavity before closure, to serve as a living pack.

Obliteration of the pericystic cavity is not necessary if, after lung expansion, spontaneous reduction of the space is achieved. However large the residual cavity may be, if it is shallow the adjacent lobes can be approximated and fixed to the remaining pericyst or raw surface of the lung with a few sutures. Whatever form of anatomical restoration of the lung is chosen, it is vitally important to avoid strangulation of the hilar structures of the remaining lobes.

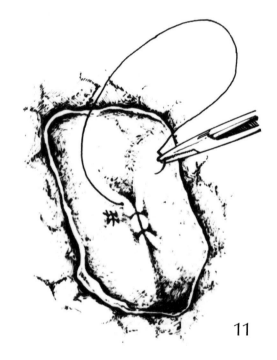

11

PERICYSTECTOMY

Some surgeons feel it is essential to remove the pericyst in all cases, particularly if the cyst were large. Others feel that pericystectomy (extirpation), or wedge resection, is only indicated for minor and peripheral cysts, especially when the diagnosis of echinococcosis is not esablished and the presence of a tumour is possible.

Excision of the parasitic cyst, together with its capsule, is performed by sharp and blunt dissection through the lung tissue, close to the pericyst. The larger bronchial or vascular structures are ligated. The operation can also be performed by first removing the parasite by enucleation or aspiration, and then excising the empty pericyst only. The residual space can, if necessary, be reduced by approximation of the edges with a few sutures.

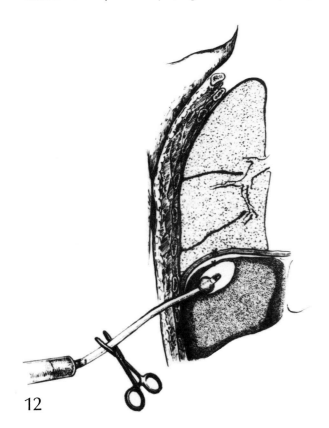

12

Postoperative care

12

The postoperative problems are the same as for any thoracotomy. Following thoracoabdominal procedures, intrahepatic drainage requires special care. The drain is maintained clamped, but is aspirated once or twice daily. The drainage fluid is examined, and, if necessary, antibiotics or other drugs should be administered. The drain may also be used for radiographic examination with contrast media. It can usually be removed within a few days or a week, except in the case of sepsis or copious bile flow.

References

1. Susman, M. P. Hydatid disease as it affects the thoracic surgeon. Journal of Thoracic Surgery 1953; 26: 111

2. Cleland, W. P. Pulmonary hydatid disease. In: Perry, K. M. A., Sellors, Sir Thomas Holmes, eds. Chest Diseases, Vol II. London: Butterworths, 1963: 386

3. Crausaz, P. H. Surgical treatment of hydatid cysts of the lung and hydatid disease of the liver with intrathoracic evolution. Journal of Thoracic and Cardiovascular Surgery 1967; 53: 116

4. Xanthakis, D., Efthimiadis, G. et al. Hydatid diseases of the chest. Thorax 1972; 27: 517

5. Lichter, I. Surgery of pulmonary hydatid cysts – the Barrett technique. Thorax 1972; 27: 529

6. Papo, I., Ginzberg, E., Albreht, J., Martinović, N., Sokolić, J. Surgical treatment of cardiac echinococcosis: report of nine cases. Texas Heart Institute Journal 1982; 9: 3

7. Heslop, J. H. (1978) Hydatid cysts of the liver. In: Dudley, H., ed. Operative Surgery: Alimentary Tract and Abdominal Wall 2, 4th ed. London: Butterworths, 1983

8. Smith, R. Abbey. Pulmonary hydatid disease. In: D'Abreu's Practice of Cardiothoracic Surgery, 4th ed. London: Edward Arnold, 1976: 153 (Eds.)

9. Barrett, N. R. Pulmonary hydatid cysts. In: Jackson, J. W., ed. Operative Surgery: Cardiothoracic Surgery 3rd ed. London: Butterworths, 1978: 300

10. Valdoni, P. Excision of pulmonary echinococcus cysts. In: Cooper, F., ed. The Craft of Surgery, 1st ed. Vol. I. Boston: Little, Brown, 1964: 326

Bronchopleural fistula after pneumonectomy and lobectomy

M. F. Sturridge MS, FRCS
Consultant Thoracic Surgeon, The Middlesex Hospital, London;
Consultant Surgeon, London Chest Hospital;
Honorary Consultant Thoracic Surgeon, The National Hospital for Nervous Diseases, London, UK

Introduction

Bronchopleural fistula is the commonest cause of morbidity and mortality following pneumonectomy. The seriousness of the condition is due to the large volume of fluid that normally accumulates in the pleural space after pneumonectomy, entering the airway rapidly to produce sudden drowning or more gradually to interfere with the function of the remaining lung. In the long term, infection of the pleural space and of the respiratory tract leads to chronic debilitating illness.

The fistula is caused by an abscess in the suture line. Predisposing factors are infection which is generally present in the lung of patients requiring pneumonectomy and interference with the blood supply of the bronchial stump by mediastinal dissection. Unusually, bronchopleural fistula may result from technical problems associated with closure of the bronchus.

A bronchopleural fistula may form at any time following pneumonectomy, but most cases present between the seventh and twenty-first days after operation. The mode of presentation and the management of this complication is dependent upon the size of the fistula and is described accordingly.

VERY SMALL BRONCHOPLEURAL FISTULA

The very small fistula produces no clinical manifestation. The patient, who recovered normally from the operation, is found on routine follow-up X-ray to have an increased amount of air present in the pneumonectomy space as assessed on straight postero-anterior chest X-ray. There is no alteration of temperature, pulse or respiratory rate, no cough, haemoptysis or increase in sputum. The patient is completely unaware of the event.

The condition is brought about by a pinhole leak in the suture line which allows air to pass into the pneumonectomy space but does not permit the fluid to pass back into the airway. Alteration of pressure in the space towards atmospheric arrests transudation of fluid into the space and may lead to reabsorption of the fluid across the pleura.

The passage of air into the space is synonymous with the presence of a bronchopleural, oesophagopleural or pleurocutaneous fistula. The first is most common and the last most easily excluded. The oesophagopleural fistula is usually associated with mucus and saliva in the pleural effusion and the presence of Gram-negative organisms. If this is suspected, radiographic examination with a barium swallow will confirm or refute the diagnosis in most cases.

Patients with a very small bronchopleural fistula need to be kept under careful observation, although their clinical state causes no alarm. Untreated, the fistula may heal spontaneously and, following reabsorption of air from the pleura, transudation will progressively replace it, with an end result identical to that following uncomplicated pneumonectomy.

In some patients, particularly those in whom the fistula develops late, the fistula may close spontaneously but the pleura loses its ability to transude fluid. The space remains empty with a high negative pressure, and this, plus contraction of fibrous tissue, may lead to progressive, and perhaps, gross mediastinal displacement, with over-distention of the remaining lung. Provided the pleura is sterile, once the fistula has closed and the intrapleural pressure is negative, the space can be filled artificially by instilling normal saline at body temperature through a drip apparatus while at the same time allowing any gas within the space to escape through a separate small cannula. This procedure seems to arrest mediastinal displacement.

If infection enters the space while the fistula is present, even though the fistula subsequently closes, a post-pneumonectomy empyema may develop. (The management of this is dealt with in the chapter on 'Post-pneumonectomy empyema', pp. 210–211.

SMALL BRONCHOPLEURAL FISTULA

These fistulae measuring 2–3 mm in diameter and often valvular in type are the most difficult to diagnose and produce the most severe symptoms and rapid deterioration in the patient's condition. The patient becomes distressed, often cyanosed with peripheral vasoconstriction. The pulse rate is elevated and atrial fibrillation often occurs. The patient develops a cough which may be unproductive, or may produce moderate quantities of clear, frothy sputum. A small streak of red blood may precede or accompany the onset of symptoms. The respiratory rate rises and moist sounds can be heard over the lung. The diagnosis is easily confused with a primary cardiac arrhythmia, myocardial infarction, infection of the remaining lung, pulmonary embolism or respiratory insufficiency.

The possibility of a bronchopleural fistula should be foremost in the clinician's mind and must be disproved before accepting any alternative diagnosis. Clinical evidence of development of a fistula can be obtained by listening for vocal resonance over the gas in the pneumonectomy space. Under normal circumstances the pressure in the space is negative and vocal resonance is poor. As soon as the pressure becomes atmospheric or above, vocal resonance is markedly accentuated and the sudden change is almost diagnostic.

1a & b

Diagnosis is confirmed by comparison of consecutive chest X-rays; an alteration in the airspace can be appreciated. A normal triangular outline, formed at the apex by the chest wall, the mediastinum and the fluid level, becomes 'dome-shaped' with widening of the fluid level, which will progressively fall as long as the fistula persists.

The positive objective radiological evidence described is all that is required to make the diagnosis. Neither pleurocutaneous nor oesophagopleural fistulae will produce so profound a systemic disturbance. Other investigations including measurement of intrapleural pressure, injection of indicator fluids into the pleura, bronchoscopy and bronchography, for diagnostic purposes are unreliable and serve only to reduce the clinician's confidence and thus the likelihood of the patient receiving the correct treatment.

The patient's condition is explained by the gradual passage of the hypotonic contents of the pleural space into the respiratory tract. Large volumes of this fluid may be absorbed, giving rise to hypervolaemia, and an inflammatory reaction is produced in the airway, causing respiratory embarrassment and anoxia. Cardiac irregularities are probably secondary to these causes. Fluid does not enter rapidly enough to cause postural coughing or recognizable amounts of pleural fluid in the sputum.

The treatment of these patients is a surgical emergency. The patient should be laid on his side with the pneumonectomy space dependent and the chest aspirated. The patient is then transferred to the operating theatre as soon as possible for closure of the fistula.

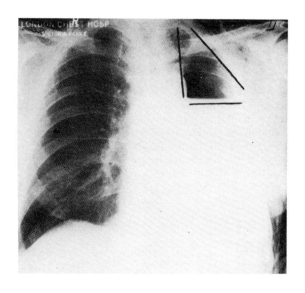

1a

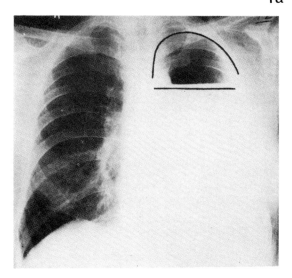

1b

LARGE BRONCHOPLEURAL FISTULA

The development of a large bronchopleural fistula, that is one greater than 3 mm in diameter, is usually heralded by the production of a small amount of fresh blood-staining in the sputum. Further events will depend on how much fluid is present in the pneumonectomy space. If the amount is large, the patient may drown from a sudden rush of pleural fluid into the airway. The only hope of saving this patient is to turn him immediately onto the side of the pneumonectomy. Endotracheal intubation and aspiration may be needed to restore the airway provided the heart is still beating, but if cardiac arrest has occurred the chances of successful resuscitation are remote. External cardiac massage, which is normally effective only because the lungs support the heart in the midline, cannot be relied upon after pneumonectomy, as the ventricles easily move aside on compression of the sternum. Immediate thoracotomy will provide the only hope.

If the pneumonectomy space is less full, the patient may cough up a volume of characteristic pleural fluid, so large that it may appear to have been vomited. This alarming occurrence will be repeated any time that the patient leans away from the pneumonectomy side. As long as the patient remains upright or inclined towards the operated side he is perfectly well, without cough and undistressed. The diagnosis is confirmed by chest X-ray which shows a gross increase of air in the pneumonectomy space and reduction in the height of the fluid level, but the mediastinum remains central.

The explanation for this event is that fluid only enters the airway when the patient leans over and then enters at such a rate that it immediately stimulates a cough reflex. As long as the patient is not overwhelmed by the amount of fluid entering, the airway is rapidly cleared. Absorption is minimal and it appears that respiration is only intermittently affected.

The ideal treatment is aspiration of the chest to remove as much fluid as possible followed by early elective operation to close the fistula. These fistulae are now rare except following unsuccessful attempts to repair a bronchopleural fistula. Such patients and those who are grossly debilitated *before* they develop a fistula or require resuscitation at the time of development can be successfully treated by initial drainage, followed by education in postural drainage via the fistula and then closure of the pleurocutaneous drainage wound. The end result, however, is never as good as that following successful operative closure of a fistula.

Closure of bronchopleural fistula

Position of patient

The patient is brought to theatre, well propped-up on a trolley, inclined towards the side of pneumonectomy and breathing oxygen from a mask.

Anaesthesia

The principle of anaesthesia is to achieve isolation of the fistula from the airway without further spillage occurring in the process. This is best achieved by the passage of a double-lumen endobronchial tube under local anaesthesia. Once the tube is correctly and securely situated, general anaesthesia can be induced, and the patient is carefully positioned on the operating table in the lateral position, with the pneumonectomy space uppermost, remembering that however successfully the pleural space has been emptied beforehand, there is likely to be at least 500 ml of fluid remaining. If difficulty is encountered, and doubt remains about the correct siting of the tube, it is safer to operate on the patient in the prone position.

The exposure

The pneumonectomy wound is reopened, removing all suture material layer by layer. The ribs are spread very gradually to avoid breaking them and the pleura is then sucked dry. The parietal pleura below the level of the wound is stripped from the chest wall as far as the diaphragm and is excised. This serves the dual function of removing any infected granulation tissue and promoting a healthy blood supply to the pleural space from the underlying muscle. The apical and mediastinal pleura are then cleared of any infected material and granulation tissue by gently rubbing the surface with a nylon mesh, and the pleura is then washed out with a dilute solution of Flavine in water, which acts as a mild antiseptic and assists clearance of remaining debris.

Mobilization of the bronchial stump

In patients treated soon after their original operation there is no difficulty in locating the bronchial stump. Fistulae occurring later, when the mediastinum is covered by a layer of fibrous tissue, are more difficult. Usually there is a tract leading down from the surface of the pleura into the fistula, but in some cases this may be obliterated by granulation tissue. The method of dissection varies on each side.

2

Right-sided bronchopleural fistula

Dissection is begun posterior to the fistula by making a longitudinal incision in line with the oesophagus. This is carried through the fibrosed pleura with care until the muscle of the oesophagus can be identified. Usually, it is slightly distorted and adherent to the bronchial stump. Great care must be exercised not to perforate the mucosa. The incision is gradually extended until a finger can be insinuated between the oesophagus and the trachea above the level of the bronchial stump. The azygos vein is divided between ligatures to facilitate this procedure. The tissues of the mediastinum are usually relatively normal despite previous dissection, and the oesophagus can be separated from the bronchial stump by gradually working downwards in this plane until the carina is reached. Starting back above the level of the stump, the pleura is separated from the trachea until a finger can be passed between the trachea and the superior vena cava, and this plane is developed until it reaches the previous one below the level of the fistula. Care is necessary when separating the stump from the right pulmonary artery at the lower end of the bronchial suture line.

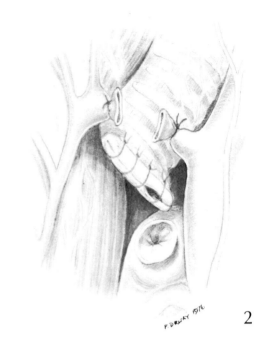

2

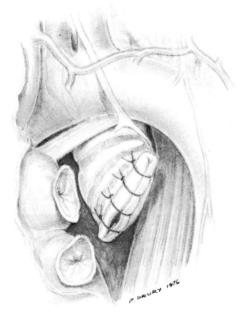

3

3

Left-sided bronchopleural fistula

Because of the important structures closely surrounding the bronchial stump on the left side, including the recurrent laryngeal nerve, the left pulmonary artery and superior pulmonary vein, all of which tend to adhere to the bronchial stump after pneumonectomy, it is safest to approach the bronchus along the fistula tract and to open it completely by removing all sutures, excising the overlying fibrous tissue as vision is obtained. Once the stump is fully opened, an incision can be made in the fibrous tissue surrounding it and the stump is mobilized by separating the neighbouring tissues from it. As on the right side, it will be found that once the mediastinal tissues are entered they can be separated quite easily from the bronchus by careful dissection.

Closure of the fistula

No matter how tempting it may appear, the fistula should not be closed by an extra stitch or two as this inevitably results in recurrence of the fistula within a remarkably short period of time.

The end of the bronchial stump, including all the tissues that have borne sutures, should be amputated completely to give a clean, fresh bronchus for suture. Usually the tissues are hyperaemic owing to the influences of infection and healing. The bronchus is closed in the manner usual to the surgeon, care being taken only to preserve the blood supply and avoid undue tension on the stitches.

Closure of the chest

Now that the fistula has been closed, the pneumonectomy space must be considered as a potential empyema cavity and will require sterilization by antibiotics in the ensuing days. A plastic nasogastric tube is introduced into the pleura obliquely through a separate incision in the chest wall at a dependent site. (It is convenient to amputate the indwelling end of the tube to enlarge its orifice.) This is firmly fixed to the skin by a surrounding stitch, and the end of the tube is spigoted.

The chest wall is reclosed as accurately as possible. Careful separation and suture of the muscle layers is important in obtaining a good end result. The skin is closed with interrupted sutures, after careful haemostasis.

Postoperative care

Care of these patients is essentially that following pneumonectomy, except for the management of the pleura. Every 24 hrs after operation the spigot-containing end of the 'nasogastric' tube is amputated. A sample of pleural fluid is aspirated with a syringe for culture. If a specific antibiotic is indicated for a known infection in the pleura, this is injected via the tube and a fresh, sterile spigot applied. If no infecting organism has been identified, 2 mega-units of benzyl-penicillin are injected. This process is repeated every 24 hrs until three consecutive sterile cultures have been reported. This normally takes 7 days at least. The nasogastric tube is then withdrawn and sterility in the pleural space is checked by aspiration of specimens twice in the following 7 days, and again 7 days later. If sterility is maintained it is safe for the

patient to leave hospital. Whatever antibiotic is used in the pleura is also given systemically for 7 days or until the pleura and sputum are sterile.

Persistent infection or re-infection of the space must arouse suspicion of recurrence of the fistula and confirmation of this is sought in the same way as after the initial pneumonectomy. If there is no evidence of recurrence of the fistula the empyema should be treated in the same manner as described in the chapter on 'Postpneumonectomy empyema', pp. 210–211.

Bronchopleural fistula following lobectomy

Bronchopleural fistula is a rare complication of lobectomy perhaps because of the small number of resections for pulmonary tuberculosis and bronchiectasis now performed in the UK.

The significance of this complication depends upon the state of the residual lobe. Provided that this is healthy and expanded the patient is usually unaware that a bronchopleural fistula has developed. Occasionally a little blood-stained sputum is produced followed by a small amount of pleural fluid or pus. The diagnosis is made by the appearance in the chest X-ray of a pneumothorax which is usually in the site previously occupied by the resected lobe.

If the pneumothorax is localized and small (less than 5 cm in diameter) it can often be managed conservatively and will become obliterated spontaneously over a period of a few weeks. If a fluid level persists or the pneumothorax is larger, it is best treated by closed drainage followed after a few days by open drainage. The space will then obliterate slowly by expansion of the underlying lung and contraction of the overlying chest wall until only the fistulous track remains. The tube is then withdrawn and the fistula will close spontaneously.

The complication is extremely serious if the residual lobe is infected and atelectatic at the time of fistula formation. There is, in these circumstances, a considerable volume of transudate in the pleura which forms in response to the high negative pleural pressure. The presentation is then identical to that of a bronchopleural fistula after pneumonectomy (see above) and the management is the same except that it is nearly always necessary to resect the residual lobe if the patient's life is to be saved.

Postpneumonectomy empyema

M. F. Sturridge MS, FRCS
Consultant Thoracic Surgeon, The Middlesex Hospital, London;
Consultant Surgeon, London Chest Hospital;
Honorary Consultant Thoracic Surgeon, The National Hospital for Nervous Diseases, London, UK

Introduction

Infection of the pleural space following pneumonectomy is an uncommon complication except in association with a bronchopleural fistula (see chapter on 'Bronchopleural fistula after pneumonectomy and lobectomy', pp. 204–209); it probably results from opportunist bacteria left in the pleura at operation. Empyema usually presents within the first year after operation.

Infection should be suspected in the early postoperative phase if rapid accumulation of fluid in the pneumonectomy space causes mediastinal displacement towards the remaining lung. Such fluid, formed in the presence of positive intrapleural pressure, is an exudate and the stimulus to its formation may be infection. Aspiration of the fluid to correct mediastinal displacement allows microscopy and culture. The presence of numerous pus cells and the culture of pyogenic bacteria confirm the diagnosis. Untreated, the empyema will usually track through the recent wound to the surface and discharge.

Patients presenting later after operation usually have general malaise, pyrexia and loss of appetite. The course may start slowly and insidiously but eventually there is a rapid deterioration in health with severe toxaemia and sometimes septicaemia. The pus in the pleura tracks towards the chest wall and presents as a painful tender area with surrounding inflammation. Fluctuation develops and palpation may elicit an expansile cough impulse. This condition is known as empyema necessitans. Aspiration of the chest wall abscess yields an undue volume of pus and rapid refilling of the abscess cavity occurs. The diagnosis is confirmed when the pleural fluid is separately aspirated and pus of the same quality and cultural characteristics is obtained.

Treatment

The initial treatment is to reduce the patient's toxicity. Early drainage of the pleura is mandatory. Fluid replacement by intravenous infusion and intravenous administration of a broad-spectrum antibiotic may be indicated before the culture results are ready.

Intercostal drainage of the pleura through either the presenting abscess on the chest wall or at a fresh site if this seems more appropriate is perfectly adequate in the first stage of treatment. Drainage should be performed in an operating theatre. A generous incision is made over the elected site and blunt dissection carried down to the pleura. The pleura is entered with the index finger and pus is evacuated with a wide-bore sucker. All sloughs and any residual blood clot are removed. Thoracoscopy may be a useful adjunct to this procedure. Great care must be taken to avoid damage to the diaphragm since this may spread the infection to the subphrenic space, a complication which must always be considered iatrogenic in aetiology.

In order to evacuate all the pus it is necessary to introduce air into the pleura but once the fluid has been displaced the drainage tube can be connected to an underwater seal. Pleural washouts may be performed using flavine 1:5000 in water or Noxyflex (noxytiolin) 1 per cent solution. The fluid is introduced by catheter through the drainage tube with the patient lying on his unaffected side. Air in the pleura can escape around the catheter. After 3–4 hours' retention the fluid is allowed to drain out, if necessary letting air into the pleura to displace it.

Samples of pleural fluid should be collected daily for bacterial culture and sensitivity to antibiotics; subsequent management is dependent upon these results and the patient's progress.

If the fluid cultured is consistently sterile and the patient's condition is good, the drainage tube can be removed when the daily drainage becomes less than 100 ml/24 hours. Fluid should then gradually collect in the space as after pneumonectomy and samples should be aspirated for bacterial culture at intervals of 3, 4 and 7 days. If all of these are sterile the patient can be discharged.

If bacteria are identified, the patient should be treated with the specific antibiotics orally and by instillation *every 24 hours* into the pleura. As soon as the fluid from the pleura becomes thin and serous a narrow plastic catheter can be introduced into the pleura through the drainage tube which is then withdrawn. Each day a sample is obtained for culture via the catheter and the antibiotics are instilled, until three consecutive daily cultures have been reported sterile. The tube is then removed and continuing sterility checked by aspiration and culture of fluid samples at intervals during the following 2 weeks.

Continuing infection must raise the possibility of a persistent source of infection such as a foreign body, bronchopleural or oesophagopleural fistula. In debilitated patients it may be preferable to perform dependent rib resection and drainage and to leave this for a period until their general condition is improved before re-admitting them to hospital for sterilization of the pleura as described above. It should never be necessary to accept permanent drainage for uncomplicated pleural infection.

Illustrations by Gillian Lee

Rib resection for empyema

Vernon C. Thompson FRCS
Consulting Thoracic Surgeon to The London Hospital and London Chest Hospital, London, UK

Preoperative

Indications and contraindications

Rib resection for empyema should only be employed when more conservative methods have failed. It should never be employed as the primary treatment. Rib resection is essentially an open method of drainage, and the size of the empyema cavity must be reduced to the smallest possible dimensions by aspiration and possibly intercostal drainage beforehand.

The primary treatment of empyema is by aspiration and the instillation of suitable antibiotics. A sterile empyema of a persistent nature is best treated by resection. A pure tuberculous empyema should never be treated by open drainage.

It is only when conservative measures have failed or are doomed to fail that rib resection should be employed. The causes of failure of conservative measures are: (1) infection with an organism resistant to all antibiotics; (2) loculation of the empyema by massive deposits of fibrin or blood clot; (3) persistent reinfection by a bronchopleural fistula or by an oesophageal fistula; (4) postoperative infections of the pleural cavity by bronchial fistula after lung resection or by oesophageal fistula after oesophago-gastric resections; (5) underlying lung disease such as bronchiectasis or tumour.

Anaesthesia

If there is no bronchial fistula the patient may be given a general anaesthetic, but if a fistula is present local anaesthesia should be employed. The technique is a little more elaborate than that for intercostal drainage. The line of incision should be infiltrated together with the subcutaneous and deep fascial planes. The intercostal spaces above and below the rib to be resected can be infiltrated after they have been exposed.

Site of drainage

It is essential that drainage should be at the lowest point; but this requires some qualification. The lowest point should be in relation to the patient's normal position in bed, which is semirecumbent. The site for gravitational drainage should therefore almost invariably be posterior. Another consideration which must be borne in mind is that the diaphragm always rises in the obliteration of an empyema space. Allowance must be made for this, and the tube should be introduced one rib space above the diaphragm, otherwise the rising of the diaphragm may seal off the end of the tube.

The site of drainage must be determined after a study of posteroanterior and lateral X-rays and a careful rib count. The lowest point of the empyema can be most clearly demarcated by preliminary injection of propyliodone (Dionosil) into the empyema space.

Finally the site is confirmed by aspiration above and below the rib selected for resection, after exposure by a vertical incision.

The operation

Position of patient

1

If there is no bronchopleural fistula and the patient is able to lie on the contralateral side without distress, the operation can be carried out in the lateral position under a general anaesthetic.

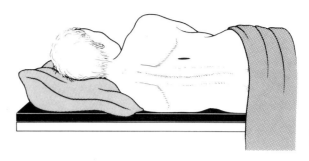

3

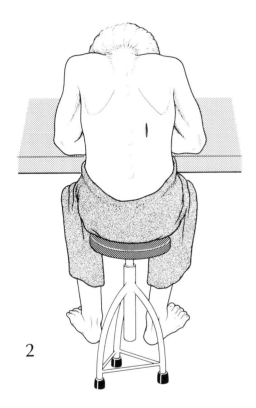

2

2

If there is a bronchopleural fistula and the patient is unable to lie on the contralateral side, the operation should be carried out under local anaesthesia, with the patient sitting on a stool and leaning forward with the arms resting on the operating table.

3

The incision

The incision should be vertical and about 7.5 cm (3 inches) in length. This allows extension upwards or downwards if it is not quite correct as shown by aspiration above and below the rib previously selected for resection. The incision is carried through skin, subcutaneous tissues, deep fascia and muscle to the ribs and intercostal muscles.

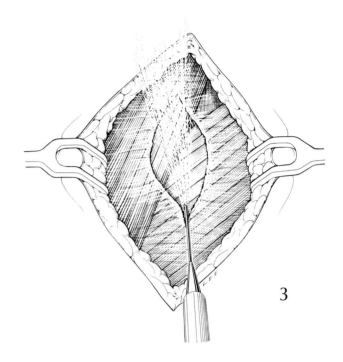

3

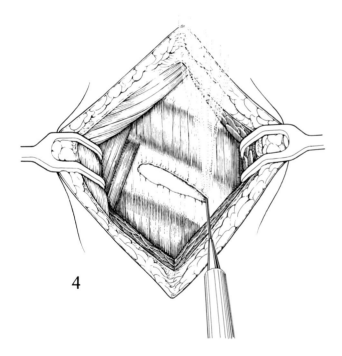

4

4

Incision of periosteum

When the rib has been exposed and selected for resection, the edges of the wound are retracted along the line of the rib and the periosteum is incised for 5–7.5 cm (2–3 inches) with the diathermy knife.

Before resecting the rib, aspiration should be performed above and below the rib once again to confirm that the site is well chosen.

A specimen of pus should be sent to the laboratory to identify the organisms present and to determine their sensitivities to antibiotics.

5

Elevation of periosteum

The periosteum is separated from the rib with a rougine. On the upper surface of the rib the rugine should be carried forwards in the direction of the intercostal muscle fibres and on the lower surface it should be carried backwards. In this way the part of the rib to be resected should be completely freed from its periosteum.

Care should be taken to keep close to the rib and not to tear the periosteum, which should be left intact. If this procedure is not carried out carefully there is a risk of tearing the intercostal vessels and causing troublesome haemorrhage which will require ligation of the vessels after the segment of rib is removed.

If the vessels are ligated care must be taken to preserve the intercostal nerve as it has an important motor and sensory supply to the anterior abdominal wall.

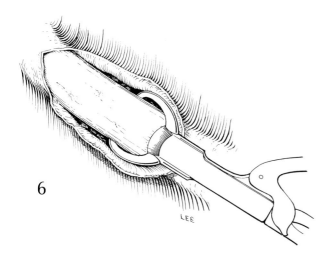

6

Resection of rib segment

With a costotome, of which there are many varieties, and almost any can be employed provided it cuts the rib cleanly, a portion of the rib 5–7.5 cm (2–3 inches) in length should be resected.

7

Opening of pleura and cleaning of empyema space

The periosteum and pleura deep to the rib should be incised keeping well above the leash of intercostal vessels and nerve. The contents of the empyema are removed with a sucker. The empyema cavity is inspected with a Nelson light and great care should be taken to remove all fibrinous deposits from the surface of the pleura with the sucker, leaving the space quite clean. A portion of parietal pleura is excised and sent for histological examination.

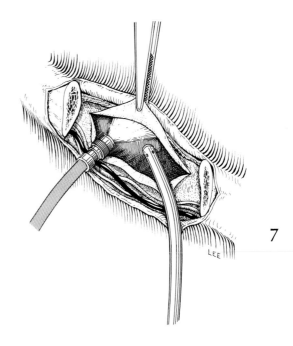

8

Insertion of tube

A wide-bore rubber or plastic tube is then inserted into
the pleural cavity; its external diameter should be about
2 cm, and it should project into the cavity about the same
distance. The pleura and deep periosteal layer should
then be sutured round the tube as closely as possible.

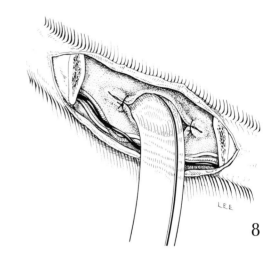

8

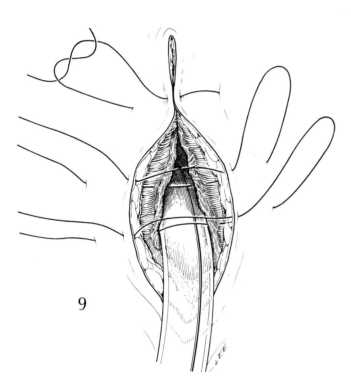

9

9

Wound closure

The muscles, deep fascia, subcutaneous tissue and skin
are then loosely sutured round the tube, using catgut for
the muscles and unabsorbable sutures for the skin.

No attempt should be made to suture the tissues tightly,
as some drainage to the wound itself must be allowed.
Tight suture will cause oedema of the wound and possibly
cellulitis; this may tend to withdraw the tube from the
empyema space.

10

Fixation of tube

The tube should be anchored by the insertion of a safety
pin through the upper wall of the tube (not through the
middle of the lumen, as this may cause obstruction by
clots) and the safety pin should be fixed to the skin by
adhesive strapping taken round the arm of the safety pin
that pierces the tube. The length of each piece of
strapping should be 20 cm (8 inches), the width 1 cm (0.5
inches), and the angles between the arms of the strapping
90°.

The tube should be connected to an underwater seal
bottle.

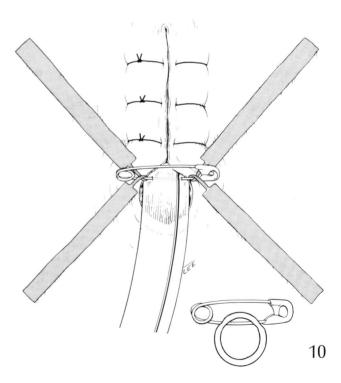

10

Postoperative care

Breathing exercises of the inspiratory type should be instituted from the day after operation. Suction at about 30 cmH$_2$O should be applied to the exit tube from the bottle. The patient should be allowed out of bed and encouraged to take exercise as soon as possible; on such occasions the tube can be disconnected from the suction apparatus, but this should be reconnected whenever the patient is in bed.

X-ray examination should be repeated weekly at first to show the diminution in size of the pleural space. When this is no longer visible on direct radiography the space can be outlined by filling it with a radio-opaque material such as Dionosil.

The technique is to remove the tube, to lie the patient so that the wound in the chest wall is uppermost and to fill the space with Dionosil with a syringe and catheter until it overflows. The sinus is then packed with gauze, all Dionosil on the skin is cleaned off, a metal marker is placed on the sinus at skin level, which is then sealed off with adhesive strapping, and radiographs are taken in the erect lateral and posteroanterior positions.

The fundamental points in the management of the tube are that the end of the tube should be at the bottom of a cavity, but when a long track exists the end of the tube should be about 2.5 cm (1 inch) from the end of the track. If the end of the tube is kept at the bottom of a long track it is highly probable that a bottle-neck will seal off the top of the track.

Once an empyema has reduced itself to a long track, it may be necessary to lengthen the tube. A good rule is to remove the tube once a week, to measure the length of the track with a gum elastic bougie and to adjust the tube so that it is 2.5 cm (1 inch) shorter than the track.

The tube should not be finally removed until the pleural space has become completely obliterated and only the tube track in the chest wall remains.

Causes of chronic empyema

The commonest causes of chronic empyema are mismanagement of acute empyema, e.g.:

1. drainage too soon or too late;
2. drainage in the wrong place;
3. drainage tube too small;
4. tube removed too soon;
5. foreign bodies (for example tubes) lost in the pleural cavity;
6. development of a bottle-neck in the empyema cavity, leaving a persistent undrained space.

Other causes of chronic empyema are:

1. serious underlying disease in the lung such as tuberculosis, carcinoid or carcinoma;
2. specific infections of the pleura, such as tuberculosis or actinomycosis;
3. persistent bronchopleural or oesophageal fistula;
4. osteomyelitis of rib or spine.

Illustrations by Gillian Lee

Decortication of the lung and excision of empyema

Mary P. Shepherd MS, FRCS
Consultant Thoracic Surgeon, Harefield Hospital, Harefield, Middlesex, UK

Introduction

Decortication means 'the removal of the cortex or external covering from any organ or structure'. In thoracic surgery decortication indicates the removal of thickened pleura – both visceral and parietal layers if necessary – from the surface of the underlying restricted lung.

Decortication is an elective procedure. Preparation should be unhurried, careful and meticulous.

Aim of the operation

The operation should result in full mobilization and expansion of normal lung, obliteration of the 'pleural space' and restoration of normal respiratory movements and function.

Ideally, any space enclosed by thickened pleural layers should not be breached.

If underlying lung tissue is diseased or destroyed, decortication can be combined with lobectomy or pneumonectomy.

Preoperative

Indications

Decortication is indicated when thickened pleura so reduces movements of the lung, chest wall and diaphragm that respiratory function is restricted to the extent of interfering with that patient's normal activity. Thickened pleura may result from the following.

1. A previous tuberculous infection which has left fluid enclosed by thickened pleura, with or without calcification. The fluid may become acutely infected or there may be recrudescence of tuberculous infection. Concomitant lung resection and/or thoracoplasty may be necessary.
2. Failure of conservative measures to resolve completely acute empyema thoracis (defined as pus between the pleural layers). It should be noted that decortication can be done in the presence of a previous rib resection.
3. Organized and unresolved haemothorax.
4. Idiopathic mediastinal and pleural fibrosis, asbestosis and similar conditions.
5. Previous lung resection.
6. Plombage and other collapse techniques used in the treatment of pulmonary tuberculosis. Removal of plombage material is usually accompanied by thoracoplasty.

Contraindications

The operation is a severe one. It should not be done in the following circumstances.

1. In the presence of active infection, either intrathoracic or systemic.
2. If the operation will not improve the patient's quality of life.
3. In the frail.
4. In the elderly.
5. In those whose general condition is poor. The decision can be reconsidered at a later date if necessary.

Preoperative investigations

Preoperative investigations are directed at establishing the nature of the underlying pathology and the condition of the underlying lung.

The following investigations can be repeated as often as necessary before operation.

1. Bacteriological and cytological examination of pleural fluid and sputum.
2. Full blood count and electrolyte estimation.
3. Chest radiographs – posteroanterior and the appropriate lateral. Tomography and/or bronchoscopy may also be indicated.
4. Bronchoscopy. Unless there is any suspicion of endobronchial pathology, this may be done immediately prior to the operation.

Preoperative preparation

Preparation of the patient is aimed at improving his or her general condition and respiratory function to the optimum possible.

Pleural fluid is removed, preferably by aspiration. An infected space must be sterilized by repeated aspiration and instillation of the appropriate antibiotic.

Anaemia is corrected by blood transfusion. The operation is very traumatic and blood loss can be considerable.

Systemic effects of infection are eliminated by systemic administration of antibiotics.

Intensive chest physiotherapy, with emphasis on rib and diaphragmatic movements, is necessary for as long as possible before operation.

Anaesthesia and position of the patient

After suitable premedication, a general anaesthetic is given. Though it is possible to use a standard endotracheal tube, a double lumen tube is usually used as one-lung anaesthesia may be required.

The patient is placed on the operating table in the lateral position with the affected side uppermost.

An intravenous infusion is established to allow immediate blood replacement during mobilization of the lung. A central venous line may also be considered useful. Hypotensive drugs may be used to diminish blood loss.

The operation

1

The incision

A standard lateral thoracotomy is made through the bed of the sixth rib. There is usually considerable rib crowding and it is often necessary to resect one rib. At the level of the sixth rib, access to the apex of the hemithorax as well as the posterior costophrenic recess is gained, these being the areas where subsequent dissection may be the most difficult.

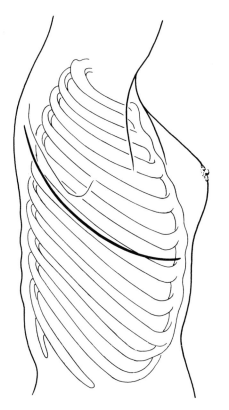

1

2 & 3

Incision of the periosteum of the rib bed reveals the fibres of the innermost layer of the intercostal muscles. The extrapleural plane is entered by division of these fibres and the thickened parietal pleura is stripped, often with great difficulty, from the chest wall above and below the incision. If possible, the fingers are used but it may prove necessary to use the curved closed blades of a Roberts forceps. Some rib spreading with the Sellors rib approximator with the rib hooks reversed will become possible. The extrapleural stripping is continued until a rib spreader can be inserted.

The thickened parietal pleural surface frequently shows indentations made by the ribs. If intercostal muscle fibres are also seen on the surface, the stripping is not proceeding in the right plane. This must be corrected to avoid damage to extrapleural structures including the following.

1. The internal mammary blood vessels anteriorly.
2. The intercostal blood vessels in the paravertebral gutter.
3. The vena azygos and superior vena cava on the right.
4. The aorta, innominate vein, recurrent laryngeal nerve and thoracic duct on the left.
5. The phrenic and vagus nerves.
6. The oesophagus. Identification is facilitated by the presence of a bougie or nasogastric tube in the oesophageal lumen.
7. The diaphragm.

Stripping of thickened parietal pleura from the chest wall results in considerable bleeding. As much haemostasis as possible must be maintained using coagulation diathermy. Blood must be replaced as it is lost.

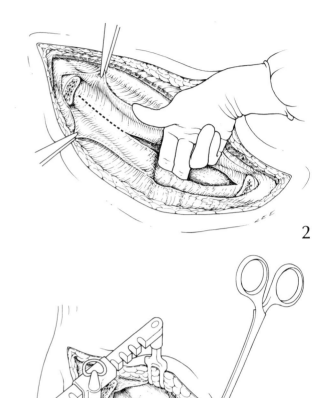

2

3

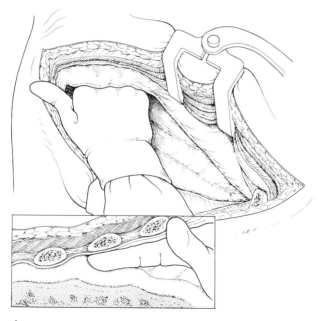

4

4

The overall strategy of the dissection is to find the regions where pleura is relatively normal and to dissect towards the most adherent areas. To this end, the extrapleural stripping is carried out anteriorly in the lower part of the hemithorax where the edge of the thickened pleura usually forms a ridge where the abnormal layers meet. Beyond this ridge normal lung is seen under thinner pleura covered by loose areolar tissue. Having identified this, attention is directed to completing the mobilization of the lung, separating the ribs a little further whenever possible. Pleural thickening over the upper lobe, if present, is greatest in the paravertebral gutter, at the apex and anteriorly. Extrapleural stripping of the pleura off the ribs should continue superiorly and posteriorly onto the mediastinum.

5a–d

When the vena azygos or posterior part of the aortic arch has been identified, the stripping is carried anteriorly to identify, at the same level, the phrenic nerve on the superior vena cava or pericardium. Stripping is finally extended towards the apex. If the apex of the lung mobilizes readily, the mediastinal pleura can be stripped from the apex down towards the hilum, leaving the identified phrenic and vagus nerves *in situ*.

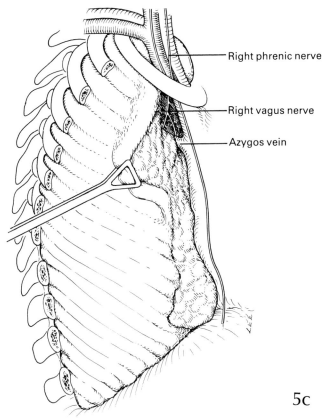

Right phrenic nerve

Right vagus nerve

Azygos vein

5c

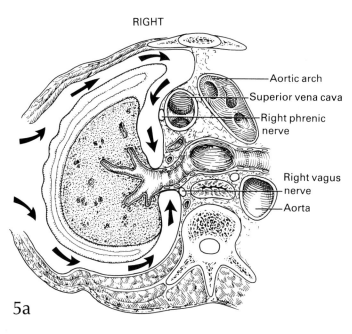

RIGHT

Aortic arch

Superior vena cava

Right phrenic nerve

Right vagus nerve

Aorta

5a

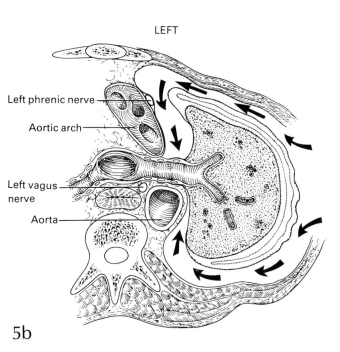

LEFT

Left phrenic nerve

Aortic arch

Left vagus nerve

Aorta

5b

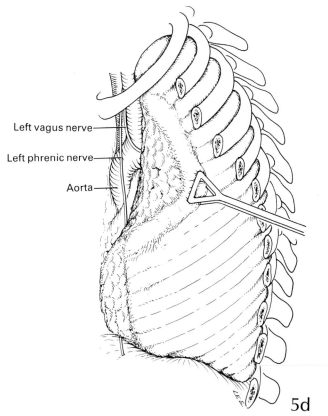

Left vagus nerve

Left phrenic nerve

Aorta

5d

6

If the apex is very adherent, a tunnel must be made under the mediastinal pleura at the level of the vena azygos or aortic arch to join up the anterior limit of mobilization with the posterior limit. This may have to be done blindly with the finger – or *very* gently with a closed curved clamp. The tunnel is then enlarged upwards taking particular care to preserve the phrenic and vagus nerves.

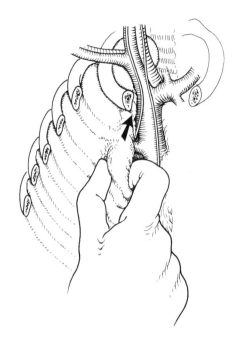

6

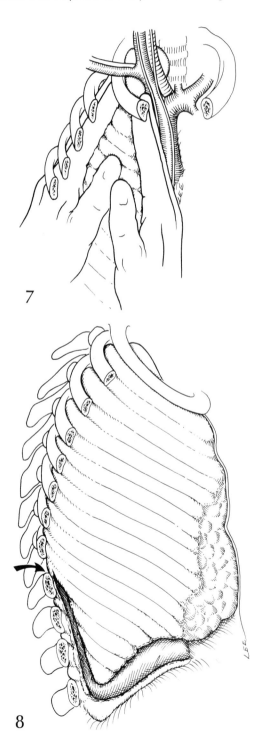

7

8

7

To mobilize the adherent apex, gentle traction is applied to it using both hands, one having been passed up the mediastinal aspect and one over the costal surface of the lung. With the traction and 'pinching' movements of the fingers of the two hands against each other the apex will be freed. Sharp dissection should be avoided if possible and should never be used blindly or above the level of the first rib.

8

The greatest pleural thickening is found in the paravertebral gutter and posterior costophrenic recess. Adhesion to the diaphragm can also be considerable. Mobilization of the lower lobe is commenced by dissecting anteriorly. Here pleural thickening is often minimal and the diaphragm can be recognized. If the diaphragm cannot be recognized, the mediastinal aspect of the lobe is freed from the pericardium taking care to preserve the phrenic nerve. When the pericardiophrenic junction is reached the dissection, using a scalpel or scissors, is carried outwards over the diaphragm. In the presence of dense adhesions, holes in the diaphragm can readily be made. These must be recognized and repaired immediately. The extrapleural stripping from the ribs is then carried posteriorly and may be facilitated by the surgeon working from the front of the patient. During this part of the operation, it is very easy to detach the diaphragm. To avoid this the extrapleural stripping process should stop at the level of the ninth rib posteriorly. Using sharp dissection, a layer of the fibrous pleura is left on the chest wall and in the posterior costophrenic recess, so preserving the posterior diaphragmatic attachments. As any space enclosed by thickened pleura is most easily breached at this stage of mobilization, contained fluid must be sterile.

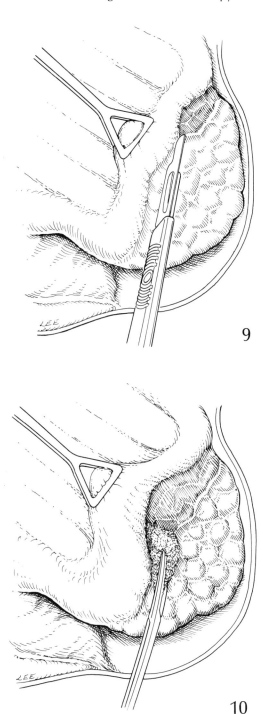

9 & 10

When the lung with its thick pleural covering has been mobilized, the pleura is dissected off the lung. This process is commenced at a previously identified point where normal lung is visible through relatively normal pleura. If adhesion to the lung is dense, less damage to the lung will result if the visceral pleural layer is also removed. To achieve this, a precise plane must be found. The thickened edge of pleura adjacent to recognizable lung is held up in tissue forceps, slightly stretching the lung. The relatively normal visceral pleural layer is carefully incised, exposing lung tissue. With a dissecting swab, the lung is gently wiped off the deep surface of the visceral pleura. When the correct plane is found, normal lung will usually separate readily and can be swept off by gentle, firm movements of the fingers. Great care must be taken not to deviate from the correct plane, as considerable damage to the lung can otherwise be caused.

11

If this manoeuvre does not prove successful, the lung is slightly stretched as before and with *very* light strokes of a scalpel which is held almost parallel to the lung surface, the lung is separated. This method avoids serious damage to lung tissue but has to be a slow meticulous process.

The mass of thickened pleura, which may enclose a fluid-filled space, is removed leaving, if necessary, portions in the posterior costophrenic angle and on the diaphragm. The lung is inspected. Mobilization and full inflation are completed by removing any residual restricting islands of pleura and opening the fissures, where the pleura is frequently normal. The process is assisted by the anaesthetist who applies positive pressure to inflate the lung fully. An assessment of the air leak from the lung surface is made and all bronchial or bronchiolar leaks are oversewn. Every effort must be made to close all but alveolar air leaks. Haemostasis is achieved by coagulation diathermy and washing out the hemithorax with warm saline. Hydrogen peroxide may also be used as this has the additional value of countering possible contamination by fluid from a breached empyema cavity.

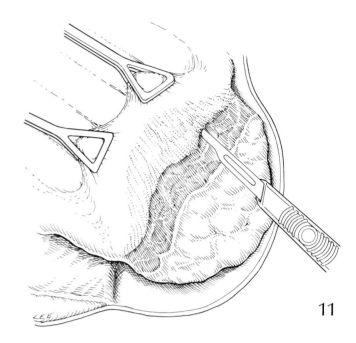

11

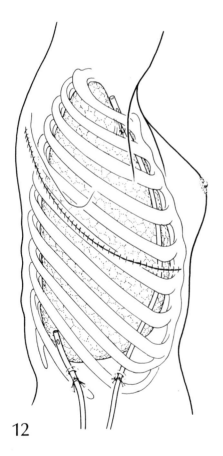

12

12

Apical and basal intercostal drains are placed carefully through separate stab incisions. The apical drain passes anterolaterally to the apex. The tip of this tube should lie about 1 cm above the border of the first rib about 3 cm lateral to the costochondral junction. It must not impinge on the autonomic nerve chain as a permanent Horner's syndrome can result. This tube is kept in position by a catgut stitch which picks up some of the internal intercostal muscle of the first or second space before being tied around the tube. The tip of the basal tube lies posteriorly in the costophrenic recess.

The thoracotomy is closed in layers and adequate suction applied to the underwater drainage tubes as soon as the incision is closed.

Postoperative management

Management is aimed at achieving early and complete expansion of the decorticated lung with obliteration of all 'dead space' in the hemithorax.

1. If the air leak is only alveolar, suction on the drainage tubes at a flow rate greater than the rate of total air leakage from the lung surface probably will not exceed the patient's respiratory tidal flow and will produce early and complete expansion of the lung. This may require a negative pump pressure of several mmHg via a Tubbs Barrett or Vernon Thompson pump. A Roberts pump should *not* be used as the flow rate is unlikely to be high enough.
2. If with adequate suction the air leak is greater than the patient's spontaneous respiratory tidal flow, the underwater seal drains should not be subjected to suction but a partially collapsed lung accepted. Adequate suction to the tubes is reapplied at 24 hourly intervals and the effect reassessed. It will usually prove possible to achieve full lung expansion within 3 or 4 days of operation. If this does not occur, either reoperation and closure of the large air leak, or intermittent positive pressure ventilation must be considered. Artificial ventilation must also be considered if, in the early postoperative period there is a large air leak and the patient's respiratory reserve is insufficient to tolerate partial collapse of one lung.
3. Vigorous chest physiotherapy is essential to assist full lung expansion and achieve full movements of the released ribs and diaphragm. It must be instituted as early in the postoperative period as possible.
4. A full course of prophylactic antibiotics is given.
5. Early mobilization of the patient is desirable.
6. The intercostal drainage tubes are removed when fluid loss and air leak have stopped. This may be at any time up to 10–12 days postoperatively. Usually the basal drain can be removed first. Apical intercostal drainage must be maintained until all air leakage in the presence of aerated lung has ceased for 24 hours.

Complications

Atelectasis and/or bronchopneumonia Bronchopulmonary secretions may give rise to atelectasis and/or bronchopneumonia. If these do not respond to vigorous physiotherapy with postural drainage, orotracheal catheter aspiration or bronchoscopy may be required. In extreme cases tracheostomy may be necessary.

Haemorrhage If blood loss through the intercostal drainage tubes exceeds 200 ml/hour on more than one occasion within the first 12 hours postoperatively and/or there is clinical and radiological evidence of blood collecting in the hemithorax, rethoracotomy may be required. If large amounts of blood have been transfused a haematological check of the clotting factors is wise before a decision regarding reoperation is taken.

Persistent large air leak (*See above* under 'Postoperative management').

Persistent air space This will require obliteration by aspiration or tube drainage. Rib resection drainage may be required. In rare instances thoracoplasty may be indicated.

Further reading

Arom, K. V., Grover, F. L., Richardson, J. D., Trinkle, J. K. Post-traumatic empyema. Annals of Thoracic Surgery 1977; 23: 254–258

Beck, C. PS to thoracoplasty in America and visceral pleurectomy with report of a case. Journal of the American Medical Association 1897; 28: 58

Benfield, G. F. A. Recent trends in empyema thoracis. British Journal of Diseases of the Chest 1981; 75: 358–366

Cohn, L. H., Blaisdell, E. W. Surgical treatment of non-tuberculous empyema. Annals of Surgery 1970; 100: 376–381

Dietrick, R. B., Sade, R. M., Pak, J. S. Results of decortication in chronic empyema with special reference to paragonimiasis. Journal of Thoracic and Cardiovascular Surgery 1981; 82: 58–62

Fishman, N. H., Ellertson, D. G. Early pleural decortication for thoracic empyema in immunosuppressed patients. Journal of Thoracic and Cardiovascular Surgery 1977; 74: 537–541

Le Roux, B. T. Empyema thoracis. British Journal of Surgery 1965; 52: 89–99

Malier, H. C. The pleura. In: Sabiston, D. C., Spencer, F. C., eds. Gibbon's surgery of the chest. 3rd ed. Philadelphia: W. B. Saunders 1976: 370–405

Mavroudis, C., Symmonds, J. B., Minagi, H., Thomas, A. N. Improved survival in management of empyema thoracis. Journal of Thoracic and Cardiovascular Surgery 1981; 82: 49–57

Morin, J. E., Munro, D. D., MacLean, L. D. Early thoracotomy for empyema. Journal of Thoracic and Cardiovascular Surgery 1972; 64: 530–536

Nohl-Oser, H. C., Nissen, R., Schreiber, H. W. Surgery of the lung, Stuttgart and New York: George Thieme, 1981

Pecora, D. V. The surgical treatment of chronic pleural empyema. Journal of Thoracic Surgery 1958; 36: 92–101

Thomas, C. P., Cleland, W. P. Decortication in clotted and infected haemothoraces. Lancet 1945; 1: 327–334

Samson, P. C. Empyema thoracis: essentials of present day management. Annals of Thoracic Surgery 1971; 11: 210–221

Sarot, I. A. Extrapleural pneumonectomy and pleurectomy in pulmonary tuberculosis. Thorax 1949; 4: 173–223

Sellors, T. H., Cruickshank, G. Chronic empyema. British Journal of Surgery 1951; 38: 411–432

Shepherd, M. P. The management of acute and chronic empyema thoracis. British Journal of Clinical Practice 1979; 33: 307–322

Young, D., Simon, J., Pomerantz, M. Current indications and status of decortication of 'trapped lung'. Annals of Thoracic Surgery 1972; 14: 631–634

Illustrations by Gillian Lee

Thoracostomy for permanent chest drainage

John W. Jackson MCh, FRCS
Formerly Consultant Thoracic Surgeon, Harefield Hospital, Harefield, Middlesex, UK

Indications

Over the years, this operation has found intermittent favour with some surgeons as an alternative means of managing a troublesome empyema[1,2,3]. At best, it must be considered as a compromise and a way of coming to terms with a patient who does not have the patience to persist with tube drainage or whose prognosis is such that sufficient time will not be available for healing.

The indications for its use cannot be clearly defined because, given time, it should normally be possible to obtain complete healing with the measures described earlier (see chapter on 'Postpneumonectomy empyema', pp. 210–211). Possible exceptions may be underlying infection with an antibiotic-resistant organism such as *Actinomyces israeli* or *Aspergillus fumigatus* or where a bronchopleural fistula is associated with residual tumour. As Sturridge says in his chapter on 'Postpneumonectomy empyema'. 'It should never be necessary to accept permanent drainage for uncomplicated pleural infection'.

Possible indications include antibiotic-resistant infection, osteomyelitis of the spine, and bronchopleural fistula with residual tumour. It may also be indicated in patients refusing to persist with tube drainage; in those who are unable to attend for surgical supervision or prefer to manage the dressings themselves; and in patients whose prognosis is poor.

Aims

The principle of the operation is to establish a skin-lined opening of adequate size that will provide permanent open drainage at the base of the pleura. It should be sited in the axilla so that it is accessible to the patient for inspection (if necessary by using a mirror), cleaning and dressing and therefore not so far posteriorly as the usual site for tube drainage.

The initial opening must be sufficiently large to allow for contraction and fibrosis – 'twice as large as you think is necessary' is a good rule – and the rib resection must include equal lengths of two adjacent ribs.

Anaesthesia

The operation may be carried out under local or general anaesthesia, and special precautions with regard to position may be necessary if there is a bronchopleural fistula (see chapter on 'Bronchopleural fistula after pneumonectomy and lobectomy', pp. 204–209). General anaesthesia is to be preferred as this is a more extensive procedure than rib resection and likely to have been made more difficult because of chronic infection and previous surgery.

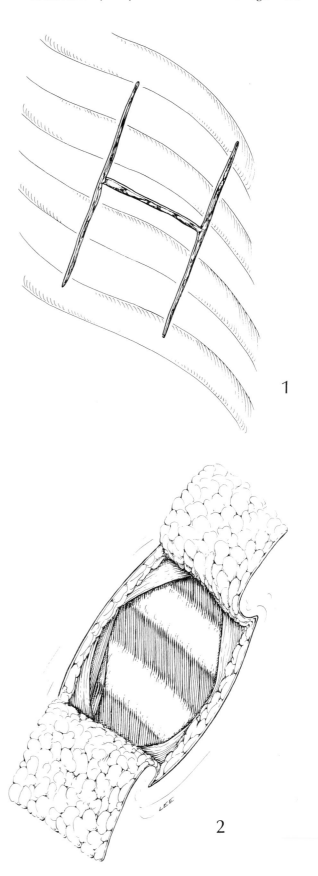

1

2

The operation

1 & 2

The incision

An H-shaped incision is made, with the transverse portion overlying the interval between the ribs that are to be resected. It should be at least 7.5 cm long and extend down to the intercostal muscle. The limbs of the H may need to be a little longer (7.5–10 cm) so as to overlap two ribs above and below, thus producing long rectangular rather than square flaps that can be attached to the pleura after the ribs have been resected.

Rib resection

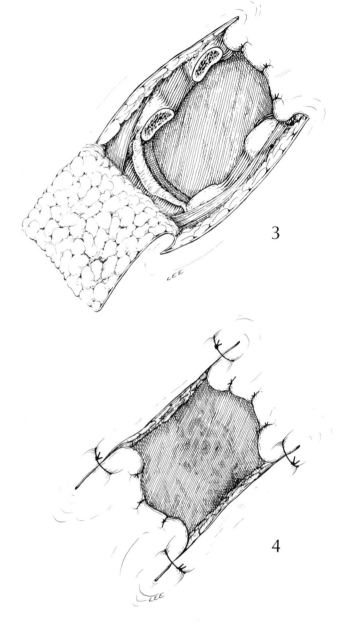

3

Equal lengths (7.5 cm) of adjacent ribs are removed with the rib raspatory and costotome as in the chapter on 'Rib resection for empyema' pp. 212–217). The intervening intercostal bundle is double ligated as it bridges the gap between the excised ribs and removed so as to establish a single opening approximately 7.5 × 7.5 cm in size.

4

The skin flaps are then sewn down to the pleura with non-absorbable sutures so that they become wrapped round the intact ribs above and below the opening. A single stitch may be required in the skin at each corner of the incision but there is no need to fix the skin to the sides of the opening on the chest wall.

Postoperative management

Once the stoma and flaps have become established the sutures are removed. The wound should be loosely packed with gauze and covered with an absorbant dressing. This will probably need to be changed twice a day. A mild antiseptic such as noxythiolin (Noxyflex), hypochlorite or dilute hydrogen peroxide will help to keep it clear of infection and remove debris.

If the original opening is as large as described there should be no question of stenosis of the stoma, and eventually the base of the empyema should become completely epithelialized so that dressings are no longer necessary.

References

1. Eloesser, L. An operation for tuberculous empyema. Surgery, Gynecology and Obstetrics 1935; 60: 1096–1097

2. Vieritz, H. D. Das Thorakostoma. (Eine Wertrolle Behandlungs methode bei der Sanierung von Pleuraempyema) Žentralblatt für Chirurgie 1973; 98: 1496–1500

3. Clagett, O. T., Geraci, J. E. A procedure for the management of post-pneumonectomy empyema. Journal of Thoracic and Cardiovascular Surgery 1963; 45: 141–145

Further reading

Kerr, W. F. Late onset, post-pneumonectomy empyema. Thorax 1977; 32: 149–154

Illustrations by Cathy Slatter

Thoracoplasty

R. P. Hewitson   FRCS, FRCS(Ed)
Associate Professor of Thoracic Surgery, Groote Schuur Hospital and
University of Cape Town Medical School, Cape Town, South Africa

THORACOPLASTY WITH APICOLYSIS FOR TUBERCULOSIS

Indications

The operation is designed to produce permanent concentric relaxation of the tuberculous upper lobe. In many centres, resection is the preferable procedure, but where chemotherapy has failed and the patient is considered unsuitable for resection, thoracoplasty can help control chronic fibrocaseous or cavitating upper lobe disease. It may be of particular value where the organisms are resistant to the available drugs.

Contraindications

Children are generally regarded as unsuitable for thoracoplasty, as, with growth, a considerable physical deformity may develop. Elderly patients may not tolerate the operation well. Operation should be delayed in the presence of active, progressive disease when toxicity is marked. Patients whose general condition is poor or whose respiratory reserve is low should not be submitted to operation. Associated conditions (asthma, chronic bronchitis, emphysema or ischaemic heart disease), if severe, add to the hazards of the operation. The effects of bronchiectasis may be made worse by collapse.

Preoperative preparation

Every patient should have an adequate period (4–6 months) of antituberculous therapy before consideration for operation. Diaphragmatic breathing exercises, coughing exercises and arm and shoulder movements should all be taught beforehand. Patients with excessive amount of sputum should be treated with the appropriate antibiotics.

Anaesthesia

Either general or local anaesthesia can be employed.
General anaesthesia is effected by thiopentone, a muscle relaxant, nitrous oxide and oxygen, using a cuffed endotracheal tube.
Local anaesthesia requires adequate premedication for which one of the benzodiazepines is satisfactory. An intravenous opiate can be given intraoperatively as necessary. The skin and muscles in the line of the incision are infiltrated extensively with 0.2 per cent lignocaine (xylocaine) with 0.5 ml 1:1000 adrenaline, using a total volume of about 400 ml. A paravertebral block of the upper 7 thoracic nerves is carried out using 0.4 per cent lignocaine and a lower brachial plexus block is sometimes performed in addition.

The operation

FIRST STAGE

1

The incision

The patient lies flat on the opposite side with a support in front of the chest so that the arm can be pulled well forward. A small bolster under the mid-thorax helps to extend the exposed chest. A periscapular incision is used, running midway between scapula and spine, from the level of the first spine, to the mid-axillary line below the scapula.

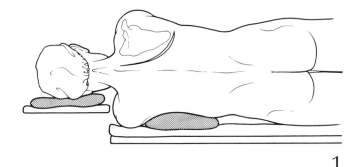

1

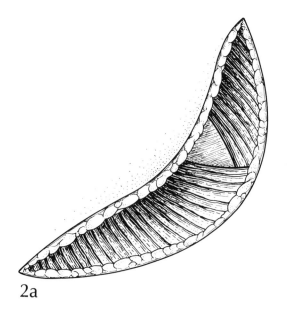

2a

2a & b

Division of muscles

The superficial (trapezius and latissimus dorsi) and deeper (rhomboids and serratus anterior) layers of muscle are divided in the line of the incision.

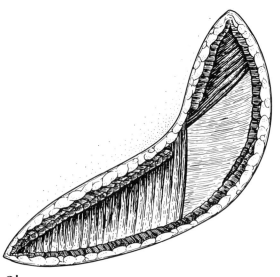

2b

3

Exposure of ribs

The scapula is elevated upwards and away from the chest wall as the areolar tissue is stripped and incised to expose the posterior aspect of the upper digitation of the serratus anterior muscle. The narrow gap between the scalenus medius and the uppermost digitation of the serratus is opened and developed by blunt dissection in the areolar plane on the anterior surface of the serratus (that is, in the axilla). In this way the digitations of the serratus arising from the upper ribs are isolated and can now be cut with scalpel or diathermy close to their origin from the ribs and intercostal spaces to the level of the fourth rib.

The serratus posterior superior is excised and the upper ribs are now completely exposed. The insertions of the scalenus medius and posterior are then detached from the first and second ribs.

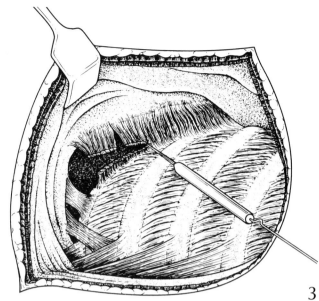

3

4a & b

Removal of second and third ribs

The periosteum of the third rib is incised with diathermy from its costotransverse joint to the anterior axillary line and is then stripped from the rib. The erector spinae muscle is retracted to expose the costotransverse ligament; this is divided with a sharp Semb's disarticulator and the neck of the rib is cut obliquely with bone shears. The rib is divided transversely at its anterior end and the second rib is dealt with similarly.

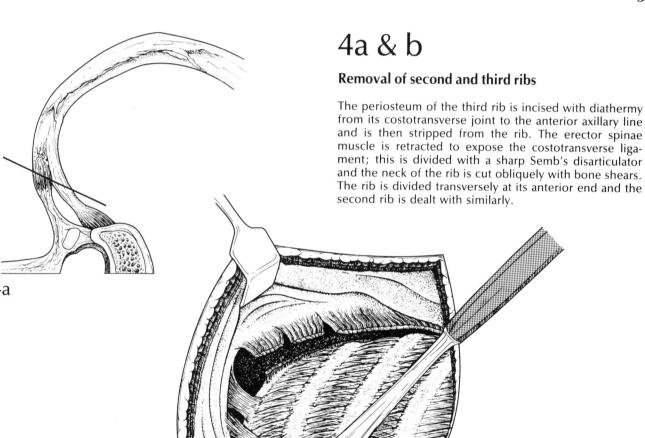

4a

4b

Removal of the first rib

5a & b

A broad raspatory is used to split the periosteum along the lateral margin of the rib; the undersurface of the rib is then denuded and so, finally, is the upper surface. Care is needed in avoiding injury to the axillary vessels and brachial plexus lying close to the inner and upper margins. The costotransverse ligament at the back and the costal cartilage in front are exposed. The ligament and the neck of the rib are cut as before.

The rib is then pulled downwards to expose the costoclavicular ligament which is divided with scissors or knife. The costochrondral junction is cut transversely. The first intercostal muscle and bundle are divided between ligatures at the posterior end.

Some surgeons prefer not to denude the periosteum of the upper surface of the first rib but instead detach the scalenus anterior at its insertion so that it retracts freely into the neck between vessels and nerves, thus avoiding a sling of periosteum pulling on these structures. The upper surface periosteum is then removed with the rib.

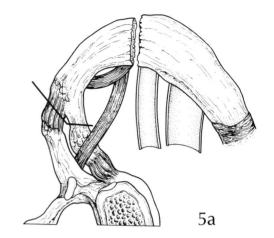

5a

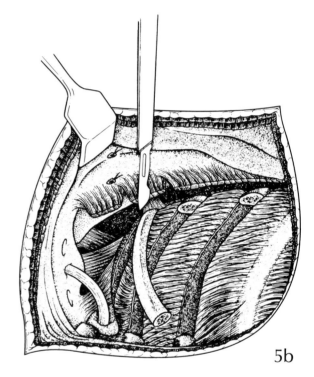

5b

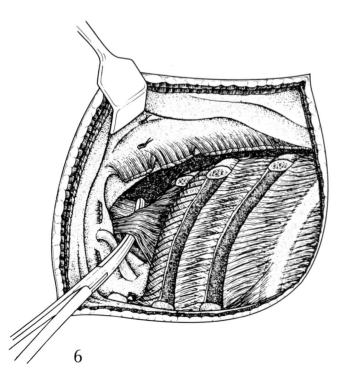

6

6

Apical mobilization

Relaxation of the upper lobe is by extrafascial apicolysis, not merely extrapleural. This is achieved by deliberately and cleanly exposing the first dorsal nerve, the subclavian artery and the innominate vein. The exposure of these structures involves division of Sibson's fascia and its three thickenings (bands of Sibelau). The first band lies superficial to the nerve, the second between the artery and the nerve and the third in front of the artery. These bands are isolated and divided and the intervening, less dense, fibrous fascia is also divided.

7

Exposure of the innominate vein

Some fibres of the scalenus anterior which insert into the pleura (scalenus pleuralis) require division in order to expose the innominate vein with the internal mammary artery running across it.

Further mobilization

The mobilization is carried out downwards separating the lung and pleura from the mediastinal structures by a process of sharp and blunt dissection until the azygos vein is reached on the right side and the aortic arch exposed on the left side.

The second and third intercostal bundles and muscles are now divided posteriorly to allow full relaxation.

After securing haemostasis, the muscles and skin are closed in layers without drainage of the space.

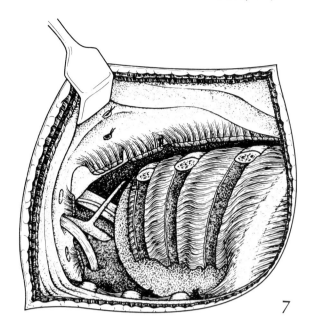

7

Complications

1. The pleura may be inadvertently torn. If noted at the time, an attempt can be made to suture the tear. Postoperative haemopneumothorax must be dealt with as necessary by aspiration or tube drainage.
2. Paradoxical movement of the freed chest wall may need support by sandbag or firm adhesive strapping for 2–3 days.
3. Atelectasis due to secretions can usually be managed by physiotherapy without bronchoscopy.
4. Excessive haemorrhage into the space may bulge into chest wall and axilla, but rarely requires reoperation.
5. Infection in the space can occur and some advocate a prophylactic antibiotic for 48 hours.
6. Scoliosis which is more than minimal should be avoided by physiotherapy.
7. Horner's syndrome is a nuisance, but at times unavoidable.

SECOND STAGE

This may be undertaken as soon as the first incision has healed cleanly and sutures have been removed; this is usually 10–14 days after the first operation. It may be delayed a further week if there is a wound or chest infection or other complication. Further delay, however, makes revision of the apicolysis difficult and risks infection of the Semb space.

The aim of the second operation is to have the scapula embedded, i.e. its tip must not lie superficial to the rib cage, nor must it ride back and forth over an unresected rib. Thus progressively shorter rib lengths are removed, and only some 10 cm of the seventh rib need be taken. The intercostal bundles are divided posteriorly to allow proper relaxation.

Occasionally a third stage may be necessary to complete the thoracoplasty.

THORACOPLASTY FOR PLEURAL SPACES

In centres where pulmonary resection is the definitive procedure for tuberculosis, thoracoplasty is reserved for chronic pleural spaces, usually following some lung resection and therefore sometimes associated with bronchopleural fistula. The thoracoplasty is adapted to the size and situation of the space. Thus, following upper lobectomy, a persistent and infected apical space may require an upper thoracoplasty; whereas after pneumonectomy, a total thoracoplasty may occasionally be indicated. Chronic empyema which is not amenable to long-term drainage or pulmonary decortication may also need thoracoplasty to obliterate an infected space.

An attempt can be made at the same operation to deal with the fistula, if necessary, by reamputation of the bronchial stump or some form of intercostal flap.

Paradoxical movement is usually no problem in these instances as the mediastinum has become sufficiently fixed by the disease process, and as many ribs as are necessary to obliterate the space may be resected at a single operation.

The object is to perform subperiosteal rib resection at least 2–3 cm beyond the edges of the space in order to ensure adequate closure. If there is a tube draining the space already, this can be left *in situ*; or if the tube lies in the area of incision, it should be relocated to an exit wound away from the incision.

Apicolysis is not indicated in these operations, but it is important to take the rib resection well postero-medially, in order to obliterate the paravertebral gutter.

Unless the pleural space to be closed clearly does not involve the apex of the thoracic cavity, it is advisable to include the first rib in all cases, though this may be a very difficult procedure.

A variety of plastic procedures has been suggested to fill the space with tissues of the chest wall, but if adequate rib resection with posterior division of the intercostal bundles has been performed, this will normally allow sufficient relaxation to obliterate the space.

Illustrations by Gillian Lee

Congenital oesophageal atresia and tracheo-oesophageal fistula

Keith D. Roberts   ChM, FRCS
Consultant Paediatric Cardiothoracic Surgeon, The Children's Hospital, Birmingham;
Senior Clinical Lecturer in Surgery, University of Birmingham, UK

Classification

Gross[1] grouped congenital oesophageal obstructions and fistulous communications with the respiratory tract into six types (*Table 1*).

Table 1 Clinical features in the various types of oesophageal abnormality

	Group A	Group B	Group C	Group D	Group E	Group F
Clinical feature						
Excess oral mucus	Always	Perhaps	Always	Perhaps	No	Perhaps
Cough and cyanosis with feeds	Always	Always	Always	Always	Perhaps	Perhaps
'Wet' bronchial tree	Usually	May be severe	Usually	May be severe	Perhaps	Perhaps
Abdominal distension	Never	Never	Frequent	Frequent	Frequent	No

Group A Oesophageal atresia without tracheo-oesophageal fistula, the upper oesophagus ending blindly, and the lower oesophagus beginning blindly with a considerable gap between the two segments.

Group B   Oesophageal atresia with a fistula between the upper pouch and the trachea, but the lower oesophagus not in communication with the respiratory tract.

Group C   Oesophageal atresia, the upper pouch being blind and the lower oesophageal segment communicating with the trachea. This is the common variety and constitutes about 90 per cent of all cases. Variation occurs between those with two portions of the oesophagus overlapping with some degree of muscular continuity to those with a considerable gap between the segments, the upper oesophagus lying in the neck and the tracheo-oesophageal fistula being connected to the trachea in the region of the right bronchus.

Group D   Oesophageal atresia with both segments communicating with the trachea by separate fistulae.

Group E   A tracheo-oesophageal fistula but without atresia (so-called 'H-fistula').

Group F   Congenital stenosis of the oesophagus.

The clinical features of congenital oesophageal atresia are primarily those of complete obstruction, namely the inability of the infant to swallow saliva. A characteristic fine frothy mucus is continually produced in the mouth, while there may be episodes of choking and cyanosis particularly if the diagnosis has not been suspected and a feed is given with 'spill-over' into the larynx. It cannot be too strongly emphasized that the diagnosis should always be suspected and made *before* any feed is given. In oesophageal atresia an important clue is the presence of maternal hydramnios in the antenatal history, this being present in well over 50 per cent of the cases. In Group C and D cases contamination of the lungs is possible not only from inhalation of infected saliva but also from regurgitation of gastric juice through the distal fistula into the bronchial tree. 'Paradoxical haematemesis' may occur[2] and the pharyngeal contents may be bile stained owing to regurgitation of alimentary contents into the trachea and so into the mouth. Respiratory obstruction with stridor may be due to a fold of mucous membrane in the trachea at the site of the fistula[3]. Occasionally air may be forced into the stomach in large volumes when the infant cries so that the abdomen is distended and tympanitic, with embarrassment of diaphragmatic movement and pulmonary ventilation. Other congenital defects (high intestinal atresia, imperforate anus, renal abnormalities and congenital cardiac defects) may be present, comprising 20 per cent in one series[4], although they are not necessarily life-threatening.

Group E cases form a special group in that the symptoms of coughing and choking with feeds and abdominal distension may not be very marked in the first few days after birth, so that only episodes of recurrent pneumonitis may lead to the suspicion of a tracheo-oesophageal communication.

Preoperative

Diagnosis

Congenital obstruction of the oesophagus is demonstrated by passage of a 10 Fr plastic radiopaque catheter (such as the Argyle feeding tube) through the mouth and into the oesophagus. In atresia it will usually be held up 10 cm from the alveolus and a radiograph will demonstrate the level of obstruction together with the presence of gas in the stomach and intestines, showing that a distal tracheo-oesophageal fistula is present. In duodenal atresia gas will not, of course, pass beyond the point of duodenal obstruction and this is an important diagnosis to make since this condition may readily be treated at the same time as the oesophageal one. There is no virtue and severe disadvantage in introducing radiopaque material such as iodized oil into the blind pouch, even if done under direct screening observation, because of the risk of 'spill-over'. Oesophagoscopy (which does not require an anaesthetic in the neonate) will confirm the diagnosis and may reveal the presence of a Group B or Group D upper fistula. A Group E abnormality (H-fistula) can be difficult to demonstrate by oesophagoscopy and/or bronchoscopy but may be facilitated by positive pressure ventilation by the anaesthetist when gas bubbles can be seen to enter the oesophagus. The most useful diagnostic aid is the use of cineradiography and the introduction of an aqueous opaque contrast medium with the child prone. This has the advantage that other conditions, such as pharyngeal or oesophageal incoordination which may mimic tracheo-oesophageal fistula, can be excluded.

Preoperative preparation

Although urgent operation is required this need not and in many cases should not, be *immediate*. Time should be allowed for the infant's temperature, often low on admission, to be restored to normal. The infant should be nursed in a humidified oxygen-enriched atmosphere in an incubator with a 10° head-down tilt, and his position changed from side to side every 30 minutes. The pharynx must be aspirated repeatedly (or continuously via a double lumen tube such as the Replogle[5] attached to low suction). Antibiotic therapy is commenced and vitamin K_1 is given by intramuscular injection in view of the normal fall in prothrombin level during the first few days of life. In the case of an H-fistula a nasogastric tube may be required to decompress a distended stomach but only rarely in other groups is a preliminary gastrostomy required for this purpose.

Choice of operation

In Groups C and D whenever possible oesophageal continuity should be restored by primary oesophageal anastomosis. If the gap between the oesophageal segments is too great for an immediate anastomosis then one of two courses can be followed. The tracheo-oesophageal fistula can be closed and a gastrostomy performed, so that growth of the upper pouch will permit a delayed anastomosis as described by Howard and Myers[6]; or the fistula can be closed and a cervical oesophagostomy done together with a gastrostomy, reconstruction of the oesophagus using colon[7] being delayed until the infant has grown to about 6 kg weight.

In Groups A and B the multiple stage plan of cervical oesophagostomy, gastrostomy and an oesophageal replacement procedure is usually employed.

Group E patients require separation of the oesophagus and trachea at the site of the fistula with repair of both structures and (in all but the highest communications which are explored through a cervical incision) this is done through a thoracotomy.

Anaesthesia

No premedication is required. An intravenous infusion of dextrose/saline is given via a percutaneous cannulation and a paediatric microset. The infant is kept on a heat-controlled water mattress and a thermistor probe is inserted into the rectum and one applied to the skin of the abdomen. ECG electrodes are applied to the limbs. Endotracheal intubation is carried out without anaesthesia; the tube is aspirated and then connected to a nitrous oxide/oxygen gas mixture with added halothane if necessary. Where there is a fistula between the distal oesophagus and trachea the infant is allowed to breathe spontaneously, to avoid the distension of the stomach resulting from positive pressure ventilation, until the intercostal space is about to be entered. At this point an intravenous relaxant is given and intermittent positive pressure ventilation commenced. It is important that the surgeon then controls the distal oesophagus *as soon as possible* to avoid anaesthetic gases passing down it into the stomach.

Primary oesophageal anastomosis

1

The incision

The infant is positioned on his left side with a rolled towel or rubber pad under the thorax towards the axilla. The skin incision is almost transverse in line with the ribs (not truly periscapular) and is positioned just below the inferior angle of the scapula extending from the lateral border of the trapezius to the nipple line. Apart from the skin itself all cutting is with surgical diathermy so that blood loss is minimal.

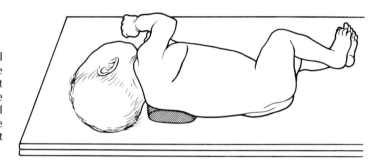

1

The transpleural approach

The periosteum on the upper border of the fifth rib is incised, and now the anaesthetist gives the intravenous relaxant. The periosteum and intercostal muscles are stripped from the rib and the thorax is entered through the fourth intercostal space, after inserting a neonatal rib spreader.

The extrapleural approach

This is more tedious. The fifth rib periosteum may be divided as in the transpleural operation but the parietal pleura is *not* opened. By careful dissection in the extrapleural plane, during which a dural elevator may be useful, sufficient space is developed to allow the insertion of a rib spreader. The extrapleural strip is carried up to the apex and posteriorly to explore the posterior mediastinum.

Choice of approach

This is largely dictated by personal preference. Thus the thoracic trained surgeon will usually opt for the transpleural route, while the general paediatric surgeon often prefers the extrapleural approach. The author prefers the transpleural operation as it gives more rapid control of the fistula and renders the anaesthetist's task much easier. Surgeons who prefer the extrapleural technique argue that the risks of oesophageal leakage are less if the pleural cavity is not contaminated; however, the extrapleural operation requires a more tedious dissection and is time consuming, while early control of leak of anaesthetic gases into the stomach is not easily attained. Anastomotic leakage is due to an ill-advised primary anastomosis under undue tension or to inadequate suturing. Provided that any leakage which occurs is managed properly, there should be no increased mortality, and this has been the case in the author's own series.

2

Control of fistula

In the transpleural operation it is often possible to bring much of the right lung out of the incision, so preventing collapse by excessive *in situ* retraction and allowing the anaesthetist to keep the lung fully inflated. An excellent view of the mediastinal pleura is obtained, and this is opened below the vena azygos arch to display the distal oesophagus. A tape is passed around the oesophagus (taking care not to injure the vagi) and gentle traction on the tape prevents further gas leak into the stomach.

In the extrapleural approach the lung and pleura are retracted forwards, and the mediastinal pleura is reflected in continuity with the parietal pleura, taking care not to rupture it. If a tear in the pleura occurs this is repaired and an intercostal tube inserted at the end of the operation. The distal oesophagus is identified and taped as above.

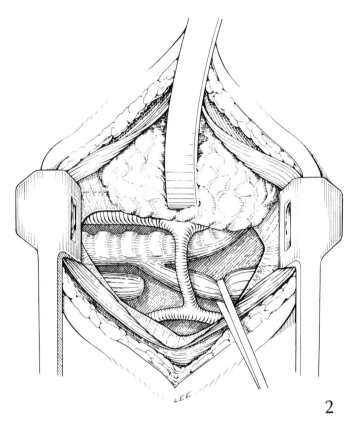

2

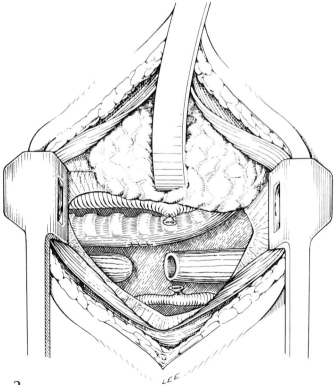

3

3

Closure of fistula

The incision in the mediastinal pleura is carried upwards to the apex of the thorax, the azygos vein being divided between ligatures. The distal oesophagus is carefully dissected with scissors to the point where it enters the membranous portion of the trachea as the tracheo-oesophageal fistula, which is then divided parallel to and close to the trachea. The lower oesophagus is allowed to lie free in the wound, while the tracheal end of the fistula is closed with interrupted 6/0 sutures on atraumatic needles (synthetic material is preferred to silk which can provoke excessive fibrous reaction).

4

Mobilization of blind upper segment

Unless very high, the blind upper segment can usually be seen as a pale pink-white bulge at the apex of the pleura lying behind the trachea. If recognition is difficult the anaesthetist can pass a plastic catheter through the mouth into the pouch.

Two 6/0 stay sutures are inserted into the lower border of the pouch, and by traction on these and careful dissection the pouch is freed. Much caution is required in separating the upper segment from the membranous portion of the trachea and care must be exercised not to injure this.

There is frequently a fibromuscular strand passing from the pouch to the prevertebral fascia and this must be divided. With full mobilization the pouch can be drawn into the thoracic cavity to a variable extent.

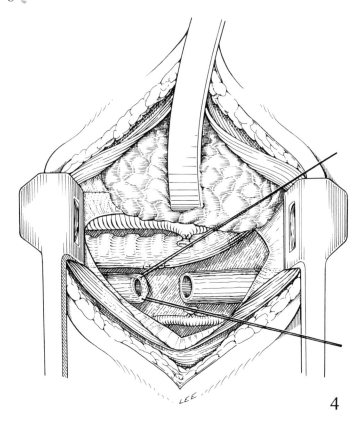

4

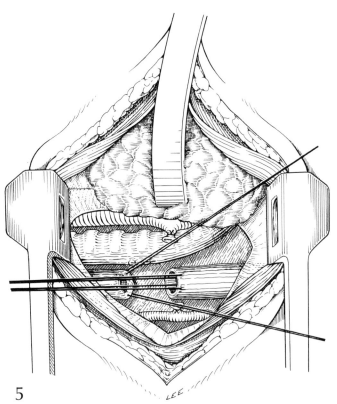

5

5

Mobilization of lower segment

The lower segment is freed from its mediastinal bed, if necessary as far as the oesophageal hiatus, segmental oesophageal arteries being coagulated and divided, until by gentle traction on two 6/0 stay sutures the upper and lower segments can be approximated without undue tension. The muscular coat of the lower segment is thin and its blood supply is easily impaired by rough handling which must be avoided.

6

Beginning the anastomosis

The blind segment is opened at its apex. A relatively *small* opening is made in view of the disparity in size between the large upper and smaller distal segments. The muscle coat of the upper pouch is thick, in contradistinction to that of the distal segment. A posterior layer of interrupted 6/0 atraumatic synthetic fibre sutures is introduced and tied, care being taken to pick up the muscle coat and mucosa of each segment. The anaesthetist now passes an 8 Fr Argyle feeding tube through the nose into the upper oesophagus, and it is guided into the distal oesophagus and so on into the stomach; the tube is left open to allow gas to escape from the stomach. The nasogastric tube is fixed firmly to the face with adhesive tape.

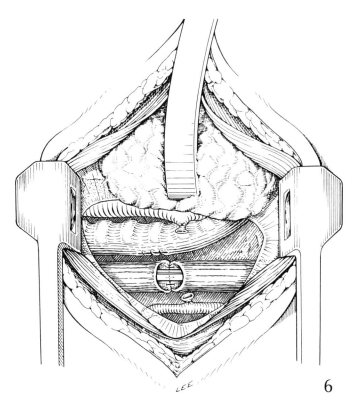

6

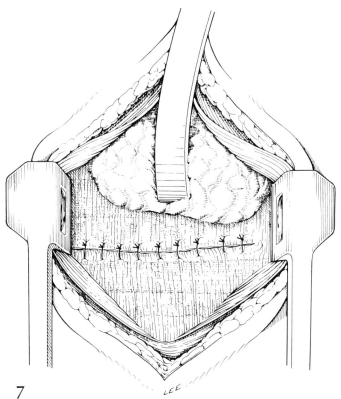

7

7

Completion of anastomosis

An anterior row of interrupted 6/0 sutures is inserted and tied over the indwelling nasogastric tube; the mediastinal pleura is then sutured over the repaired oesophagus and trachea using fine interrupted sutures.

8

Closure of chest

In the transpleural operation an intercostal drainage tube (attached to an underwater seal and gentle suction) is introduced and the lung expanded fully. With the extrapleural approach an intercostal tube is only used if the pleural cavity has inadvertently been breached, but an extrapleural drain attached to Redivac suction is left down to the posterior mediastium in the region of the anastomosis. Three non-absorbable pericostal sutures are inserted and tied. The muscle layers and fat are closed with continuous Dexon sutures and the skin by a continuous Dexon subcuticular stitch.

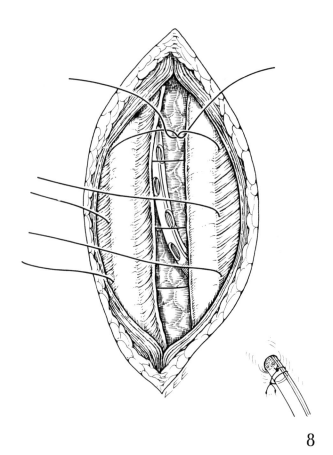

8

Delayed oesophageal anastomosis

This procedure, first described by Howard and Myers[6], may be used in Group C patients in whom immediate anastomosis is not possible because the gap between the segments is too great. The fistula is disconnected as described previously and the upper pouch mobilized. If the two segments cannot be approximated, or only brought together with undue tension with the probability of later breakdown, the distal oesophageal segment is closed with interrupted sutures and then anchored as high as possible to the prevertebral fascia. It is useful to mark this site by a metal haemostatic clip as suggested by Hamilton[8].

A gastrostomy is done for feeding purposes and the upper blind oesophagus is kept empty by continuous gentle suction on a Replogle catheter. Elongation of the upper segment may be facilitated by introducing a mercury-filled bougie twice daily, and most growth is to be expected in the first 4 weeks, with progressively smaller increments of lengthening up to 12 weeks. Some doubt has been cast on the necessity for bougienage, as

spontaneous growth of the upper segment can occur due to the swallowing reflex[9]. Reduction of the gap can be judged radiologically by measuring the distance between the end of the bougie and the metal clip. After 12 weeks, further lengthening of the upper pouch is unlikely to occur. The chest is reopened and the upper and lower oesophagus are fully mobilized. It is noteworthy that, in contradistinction to the thin-walled lower oesophagus found at the primary operation, this now has a thick muscle wall which takes sutures very easily.

The anastomosis is performed as previously described. If, however it is still not possible to bring the ends of the oesophagus together without excessive tension, the lower oesophagus must be closed and the upper oesophagus exteriorized on the side of the neck. Reconstruction is later effected by colon interposition.

Although of most use in Group C patients, success from the above technique has also been reported in Group A cases[10] although these are usually considered more suitable for a colon interposition.

Tracheo-oesophageal fistula (Group E)

Very high communications are better closed through a cervical incision, but the lower ones (including instances of recurrence of tracheo-oesophageal fistula following repair of Group C patients) are dealt with at thoracotomy.

THE CERVICAL OPERATION

9

Position of patient

The infant is placed on his back with his head to the left and a folded towel under the right shoulder. The right side is operated on to avoid risk to the thoracic duct and an incision is made 1 cm above the clavicle parallel to its medial half.

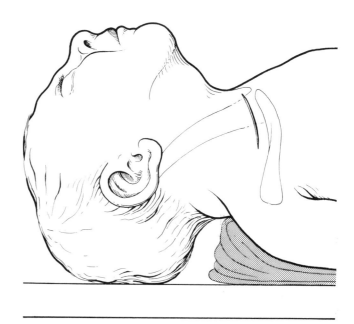

9

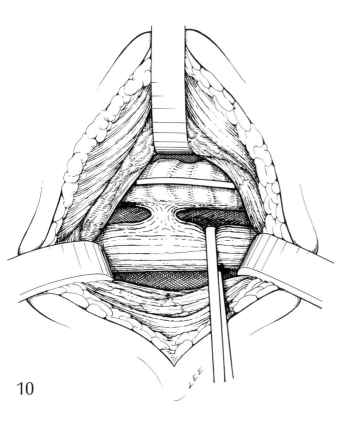

10

10

Identification of fistula

The sternal head of the sternomastoid is divided, the carotid sheath is identified and the plane behind the sheath is opened up. Dissection is carried out posterior and parallel to the trachea and care is taken to identify and preserve the right recurrent laryngeal nerve. The oesophagus is identified from its muscle fibres and a tape is passed around it below the fistula.

11

Division and closure of fistula

Traction on the tape allows the fistula to be dissected. The upper and lower limits are defined and the fistula is then divided with a knife. The tracheal end is closed first with interrupted 6/0 synthetic atraumatic sutures and then the oesophageal wound is similarly repaired taking care to pick up mucosa as well as muscle. An 8 Fr Argyle nasogastric tube is introduced for feeding purposes for the first 2–3 days and a Redivac drain is inserted through a small stab incision. The sternomastoid is repaired with interrupted Dexon sutures, the wound is then closed in layers with continuous Dexon, and a subcuticular suture is used to approximate the skin.

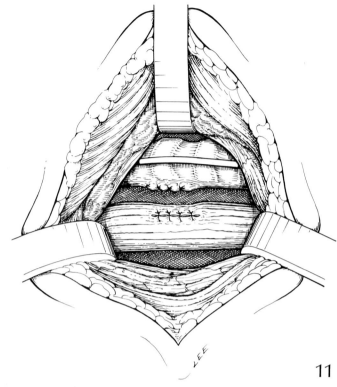

11

12

THE THORACIC OPERATION

The initial stages of this are the same as for primary oesophageal anastomosis for oesophageal atresia.

12

Identification of fistula

After opening the chest the oesophagus is taped below the fistula, as in the primary oesophageal atresia repair operation, in order to control leak of anaesthetic gases into the stomach. The azygos vein is doubly ligated and divided, and the upper part of the oesophagus is also encircled by a tape.

13

Closure of fistula

By traction on the tapes and cautious dissection with scissors the oesophagus above and below the fistula is freed from the trachea to the upper and lower margins of the fistula. This is then incised with a knife parallel to the trachea, and the tracheal end is closed with interrupted 6/0 atraumatic synthetic sutures. The oesophagus is closed similarly, taking care to include both mucosa and muscular coats. An 8 Fr Argyle nasogastric tube is introduced and left *in situ* for 2–3 days. The repair is covered with mediastinal pleura and the chest closure is as detailed for primary anastomosis.

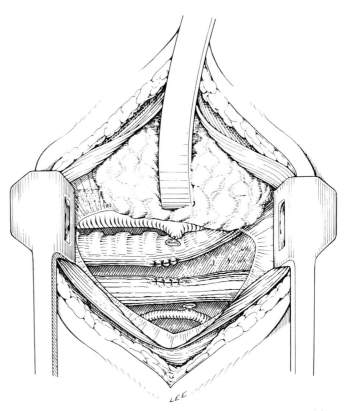

13

Oesophageal replacement with colon

In Group A patients, in those Group C cases in whom it is decided not to proceed to primary or delayed oesophageal anastomosis, or in failed delayed anastomosis, it is necessary to ensure that the baby will not die of inhalation pneumonia, and that feeding can be carried out pending the reconstruction. Drainage of the blind upper oesophagus is achieved by cervical oesophagostomy, the pouch being exteriorized and opened just to the left of the midline above the suprasternal notch. The exposure for this is similar to that described in the cervical operation for Group E tracheo-oesophageal fistula, except that the operation is done on the left side of the neck. A Stamm gastrostomy is done through a small left transverse upper abdominal incision. The gastrostomy tube is brought through a separate stab incision in the abdominal wall above the laparotomy wound.

In Group A patients it is not necessary to open the chest but this will have already been done in Group C patients in whom, in any case, it is necessary to disconnect the tracheo-oesophageal fistula and close both the tracheal and oesophageal ends.

It is important in such patients to preserve the mechanism of feeding and swallowing in response to hunger, so that food should be given by mouth at the same time as gastrostomy feeds and allowed to discharge through the cervical oesophagostomy into a dressing.

Transverse colon is preferred in the intrapleural (left mediastinal) position, rather than in the retrosternal site. Retrosternal colon has to be anastomosed to the stomach and it is impossible to control reflux, so that a 'reflux colitis' can occur, with the possibility of peptic ulceration. In the intrapleural operation the cardio-oesophageal sphincter mechanism is preserved.

Prior to operation low-residue gastrostomy feeds are given, such as Vivonex. The bowel may be prepared, if desired, with a preoperative course of succinylsulphathiazole and neomycin, but it is more important to administer systemic metronidazole. Enemas are unnecessary.

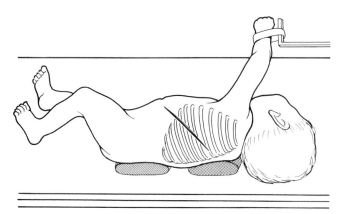

14

14

The incision

The baby is positioned on his right side with a slight backward inclination and a pad is placed under the right loin. The left arm is placed so that, with a pad under the shoulder and the head turned to the right, the left cervical oesophagostomy is accessible. Drapes are applied to leave an area exposed for an abdominothoracic incision, the suprasternal and left cervical regions are also left exposed. The abdomen and chest are opened through an abdominothoracic incision passing below the gastrostomy stoma (the tube having been removed prior to operation), across the costal margin and into the eighth intercostal space. The diaphragm is incised radially in the line of the incision but not across the lateral pillar of the right crus. Alternatively, the abdomen can be entered by incising the diaphragm along its periphery about 1 cm from the costal attachment. A transverse incision is made in the neck below the oesophageal stoma and the sternal head of the sternomastoid is divided.

15

Mobilization of colon

The lienorenal ligament is divided so that the spleen, tail of the pancreas and stomach can be retracted medially, exposing the kidney and suprarenal gland. The transverse colon is seen at the lower limit of the wound and the gastrocolic omentum is divided. The mediastinal pleura over the lower oesophagus is divided; the oesophagus is freed from its bed taking care to avoid injury to the vagi. It is convenient to pass a tape (not shown) around the oesophagus so that it can be drawn towards the surgeon when the anastomosis is performed.

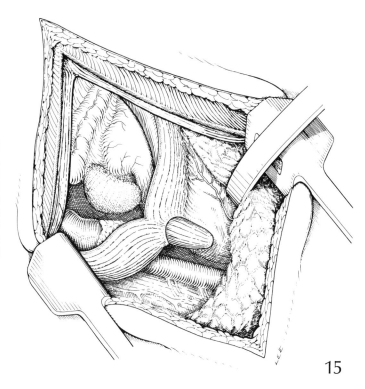

15

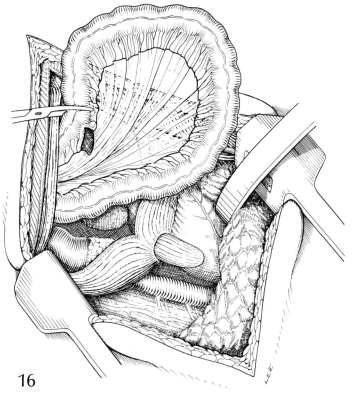

16

16

Preparation of pedicled colon segment

The middle colic artery is ligated close to its origin and divided, taking care not to imperil the lumen at the bifurcation. Before dividing the colon a careful estimate is made of the length required to bridge the gap between the lower oesophagus and the neck (see chapter on 'Colon replacement of the oesophagus', pp. 355–369). If necessary the right colic artery must be divided. The transverse colon is now supplied by the ascending branch of the left colic artery. The colon is divided in the region of the flexures. A tunnel is made from the apex of the pleura to the cervical incision, lying medial and anterior to the subclavian artery; care is taken to avoid injury to the subclavian vein and obstruction of the airway. It is convenient to pass a nylon tape through the tunnel in order to facilitate positioning of the colon.

17

Positioning of colon

Continuity of the colon is restored by end-to-end anastomosis in two layers using interrupted 6/0 synthetic atraumatic sutures. The proximal end of the pedicled colon is ligated and attached to the nylon tape. If the abdomen has been entered by peripheral detachment of the diaphragm, a suitable small incision must be made in the diaphragm lateral to the right crus and oesophageal hiatus. The pedicled colon is then carefully drawn behind the hilum of the lung until it appears in the neck. The pedicle *must* lie without tension in the space behind the displaced spleen and anterior to the kidney. The colon segment will be found to be too long distally and redundant colon is carefully excised, preserving the left colic artery, so that an anastomosis without tension can be made to the distal oesophagus.

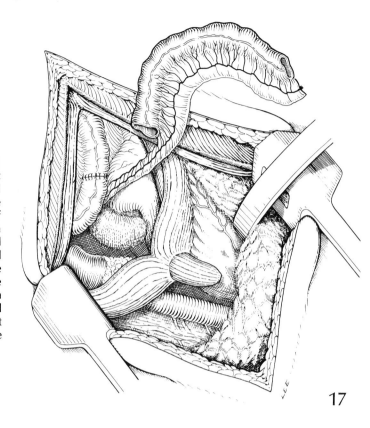

17

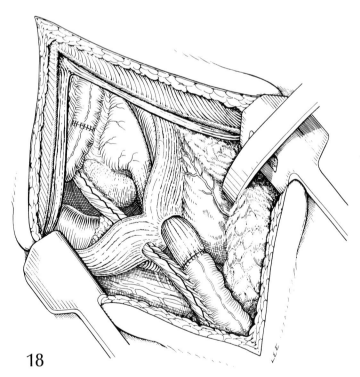

18

18

Distal oesophagocolic anastomosis

After trimming back the redundant colon an oblique incision is made in the distal oesophageal segment, which can conveniently be drawn towards the operator by an encircling tape (not shown). A one-layer anastomosis of interrupted 6/0 synthetic atraumatic sutures is made between the end of the colon and the oesophagus, care again being taken not to imperil the blood flow in the pedicle.

19

Closure of the wound

The diaphragm is carefully closed with interrupted sutures in front of the pedicle so as not to compromise its blood flow; the closure is carried forwards to the costal margin and so on to the transversus abdominis/internal oblique/ peritoneum layer. Two strong through-and-through sutures are passed through the divided costal margin and repaired diaphgram to be tied when the thoracic part of the incision is closed; this step is important in order to ensure that the diaphragm is securely attached at this point. In the case of peripheral detachment of the diaphragm this is then reconstituted by a single layer of interrupted non-absorbable sutures. Pericostal sutures are used to approximate the ribs and the wound is closed in layers, leaving an intercostal pleural drain inserted via a stab incision and attached to underwater seal drainage with gentle suction. The gastrostomy tube is then reinserted.

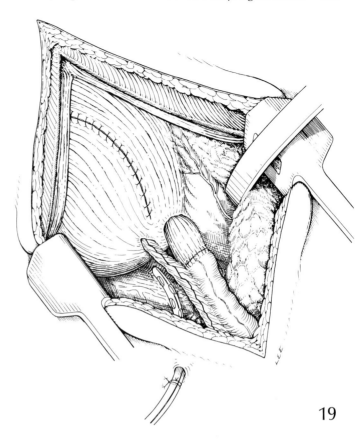

19

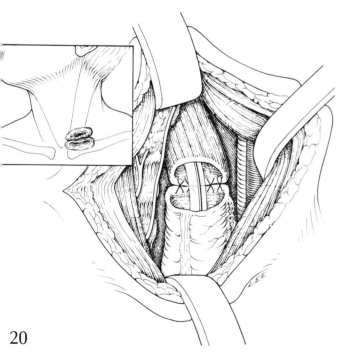

20

20

The cervical anastomosis

This may be done immediately or may be deferred for 1–2 weeks, which has the advantages that the viability of the colon is established without doubt, and peristaltic activity will have returned to it. If the delayed anastomosis is decided upon, the ligature attaching the colonic segment to the nylon tape is removed and the colon is anchored to the skin by interrupted sutures. When the anastomosis is done the oesophagus and colon are dissected free of any scar tissue so that after trimming back they lie together without tension. A posterior layer of interrupted 6/0 synthetic atraumatic suture is inserted and tied and a 10 Fr Replogle tube is passed through the nose into the oesophagus and across the anastomosis into the colon. The anterior layer is completed and the wound is closed leaving a small corrugated or Redivac drain down to the anastomosis.

Infants of low birth weight

Infants of under 1.5 kg weight present particular problems, and require meticulous preoperative, intraoperative and postoperative care if a successful outcome is to be achieved. Aspiration pneumonitis is a fatal hazard, and, if it is to be prevented, early endotracheal intubation with repeated endotracheal suction may be necessary. Transport from the referring maternity unit must be in a neonatal portable incubator and the infant should be wrapped in aluminium foil to reduce loss of body heat. He must be accompanied by an anaesthetist or paediatrician expert in neonatal intubation and resuscitation. On admission to the neonatal surgical unit the baby is transferred to a preheated incubator and the endotracheal tube is connected to warmed and humidified air, oxygen enriched if necessary, with due precautions to prevent pulmonary or ocular damage from oxygen toxicity. The operation is conducted in an operating theatre at about 28°C ambient temperature and the infant is largely swaddled in sterile Gamgee tissue with a panel cut out through which the incision can be made. The core temperature is measured by a thermocouple placed over the liver (this is preferable to the use of a rectal probe which may be insulated by meconium), and the skin temperature by a probe taped to the dorsum of the foot.

Postoperatively, these infants are preferably treated by artificial ventilation with a suitable neonatal mechanical respirator, from which the infant will eventually be weaned by a period of constant airway pressure. Suitable circuits are easily devised[11]. Gastric feeding is delayed and parenteral alimentation is provided, via a central venous catheter inserted percutaneously, for the first 7–14 days postoperatively.

Rickham[12] considers that today death of babies with oesophageal malformations is usually due to associated anomalies, particularly those of the heart and brain, and that with proper care the majority of low birth weight infants should survive.

Postoperative care

Infants who have had oesophageal anastomotic operations or repair of tracheo-oesophageal fistula are nursed in an incubator in a moist atmosphere which is oxygen-enriched if necessary. Antibiotic therapy will be needed for the first few days, particularly if aspiration pneumonitis has been present preoperatively. Lobar or lung collapse will require endotracheal intubation with suction and possibly bronchial lavage. Intercostal drainage is removed when chest radiographs show full lung expansion with no pleural fluid or air – usually in 24–48 hours. Nasogastric tube feeds are allowed after 48 hours, prior to which intravenous fluid is given and, in the case of an oesophageal anastomosis, radiological examination using a swallow of aqueous contrast medium is carried out on the seventh day in order to see if oral feeds may be commenced, supplemented at first by tube feeds.

Following oesophageal anastomosis with excessive tension the two most probable complications are leakage and stricture formation. An oesophagopleural leak is initially managed by intercostal drainage, with nasogastric or gastrostomy feeding, or parenteral nutrition. If not excessive and the lung is kept expanded, the leak will usually heal. A life-threatening huge leak will require a salvage procedure of ligation of the distal oesophagus, exteriorization of the proximal oesophagus in the neck, and a feeding gastrostomy. Continuity is restored later by a colon interposition.

Stricture formation almost always responds to intermittent dilatation, but in the early stages difficulties with oral feeding may necessitate a gastrostomy.

In the case of staged colon replacement it is important to maintain the swallowing reflex by giving food by mouth while the infant is awaiting reconstruction. The infant does not require hospitalization during the waiting time as the mother can be taught to give the gastrostomy feeds. Stenosis of the oesophageal stoma in the neck may need periodic dilatation.

After the positioning of the colonic segment in colon reconstruction the gastrostomy tube should be drained and intravenous fluids given until postoperative ileus has recovered and stools are being passed, when gastrostomy feeds can be resumed. The intercostal tube can usually be removed after 48 hrs.

When the cervical anastomosis has been completed, the Replogle tube is kept on gentle suction to prevent distension of the colonic segment due to air swallowing. The neck drain is removed after 3 days, and, provided there is no anastomotic leak in the neck, the Replogle tube can be removed on the fourth day and oral feeds commenced in small amounts, supplemented by gastrostomy feeds. The gastrostomy tube is retained until oral feeding is well established, when it is removed and the sinus allowed to close.

Late complications

The late complications of anastomotic procedures for oesophageal atresia, whether primary or delayed, include the following.

Anastomotic stricture

This usually responds to intermittent oesophageal dilatation, and in the young infant the mother can be trained to do this using a plastic Jaques type catheter. A tight stenosis will necessitate dilatation using oesophagoscopic visualization, while in any event this is required in older patients who will not tolerate bougienage without anaesthesia.

Recurrence of tracheo-oesophageal fistula

This is fortunately a rare complication which is due to the formation of a small mediastinal abscess caused by a tiny anastomotic leak, with eventual partial breakdown of the tracheal suture line. The symptoms are those of repeated respiratory infections perhaps with episodes of coughing and choking with food, usually liquid. Treatment requires operative separation of the oesophagus and trachea and repair of both. A pleural flap can be placed between the two structures to prevent further recurrence.

Incoordination of swallowing

Occasionally children for years after operation may have episodes of dysphagia and impaction of food debris despite the absence of anatomical obstruction. Cine-oesophagograms and oesophageal manometric measurements reveal the presence of disordered peristalsis in the lower oesophagus, that is, distal to the anastomosis. This results in to-and-fro movement of radiopaque material, some of which passes into the stomach, while some may regurgitate into the upper oesophagus and into the pharynx. Fortunately, most children in the course of time are able to accommodate the problem.

Gastro-oesophageal reflux

There seems to be a significant proportion of patients with Group C repair who develop gastro-oesophageal reflux in the months or even years after operation. Early cases may present with recurrent acute aspiration pneumonitis, but late presentation is usually as a result of reflux oesophagitis. It has been suggested that the condition is due to some shortening of the oesophagus with opening up of the gastro-oesophageal angle[13]. If conservative positional management in the young infant fails to relieve the condition, then an operative antireflux procedure must be considered, though the problem of selection for surgery of patients who may also have a motility disorder is difficult[14].

In the case of reconstruction of the oesophagus by colon interposition late complications include dilatation of the colon, kinking and stasis in the conduit which inevitably has somewhat sluggish peristalsis[15]. The author has also observed anastomotic stricture always at the cervical end and usually due to inadequate dissection and mobilization at the time of the initial anastomosis; stricture at the distal colo-oesophageal anastomosis has not been seen in his series.

References

1. Gross, R. E. The surgery of infancy and childhood: its principles and techniques. Philadelphia and London: Saunders, 1953

2. Lecutier, E. R. Paradoxical haematemesis in oesophageal atresia. British Medical Journal 1955; 1: 647

3. Franklin, R. H., Graham, A. J. P. Atresia of the oesophagus with an abnormal tracheal fold. Thorax 1953; 8: 102–103

4. Roberts, K. D. Congenital oesophageal atresia and tracheo-oesophageal fistula: a review of 36 patients. Thorax 1958; 13: 116–129

5. Replogle, R. L. Esophageal atresia: plastic sump catheter for drainage of the proximal pouch. Surgery 1963; 54: 296–297

6. Howard, R., Myers, N. A. Esophageal atresia: a technique for elongating the upper pouch. Surgery 1965; 58: 725–727

7. Waterston, D. J. Colonic replacement of oesophagus (intrathoracic). Surgical Clinics of North America 1967; 44: 1441–1447

8. Hamilton, J. P. Esophageal atresia: technical points in the staged procedures leading to oesophageal anastomosis. Journal of Pediatric Surgery 1966; 1: 253–255

9. Puri, P., Blake, N., O'Donnell, B., Guiney, E. J. Delay primary anastomosis following spontaneous growth of esophageal segments in esophageal atresia. Journal of Pediatric Surgery 1981; 16: 180–183

10. Hays, D. M., Woolley, M. M., Snyder, W. H. Esophageal atresia and tracheo-oesophageal fistula: management of the uncommon types. Journal of Pediatric Surgery 1966; 1: 240–252

11. Roberts, K. D., Edwards, J. M. Paediatric intensive care: a manual for resident medical officers and senior nurses, 2nd ed. Oxford: Blackwell, 1975

12. Rickham, P. P. Infants with eosophageal atresia weighing under three pounds. Journal of Pediatric Surgery 1981; 16: 595–598

13. Ashcraft, K. W., Goodwin, C., Amoury, R. A., Holder, T. M. Early recognition and aggressive treatment of gastro-oesophageal reflux following repair of oesophageal atresia. Journal of Pediatric Surgery 1977; 12: 317–321

14. Parker, A. F., Christie, D. L., Cahill, J. L. Incidence and significance of gastro-oesophageal reflux following repair of eosophageal atresia and tracheo-eosophageal fistula and the need for anti-reflux procedures. Journal of Pediatric Surgery 1979; 14: 5–8

15. Louhimo, J., Pasila, M., Visakopri, J. K. Late gastrointestinal complications in patients with colonic replacement of the eosophagus. Journal of Pediatric Surgery 1969; 4: 663–673

Illustrations by Susan W. Evans

Surgical treatment of achalasia of the cardia

Diffuse oesophageal spasm ('corkscrew oesophagus') and periphrenic diverticulum

A. W. Jowett FRCS
Consultant Thoracic Surgeon, The Royal Hospital, Wolverhampton, UK

ACHALASIA OF THE CARDIA

Preoperative

Diagnosis

Though barium swallow examination usually confirms clinical suspicion, manometric tests should be performed to demonstrate the motility disorder; these are essential in mild or early cases.

Oesophagoscopy should be carried out to exclude a carcinoma, either one involving the cardia and mimicking the X-ray appearance of achalasia or one which has already developed in the dilated oesophagus above. In all but the mildest cases the oesophagus contains a large volume of secretions and decomposing food. Rigid rather than fibreoptic endoscopy allows this to be cleared with large-bore suction. Washing out is often necessary. Anaesthetic induction should be in the semi-sitting position to reduce overspill risks, and, for the same reason, the cuff of the endotracheal tube should be inflated except at the moment of introduction of the rigid oesophagoscope. The oesophageal mucosa is often inflamed. The cardia is usually further from the incisor teeth than normal for the patient's size. However, if long enough, the oesophagoscope can usually be passed into the stomach without encountering much resistance or requiring dilatation, especially if a small bougie is used to indicate the forward direction to be followed.

Indications

Surgery is indicated in all cases except when the general condition and especially when respiratory function is poor and cannot be adequately improved. In these, daily self-bouginage using a Hurst mercury bougie may be considered. Older endoscopic procedures aimed at rupturing the circular muscle at the cardia, using instruments such as Plummer's hydrostatic bag or the Henning dilator, cannot be recommended. Newer instruments for forceful dilatation which can be introduced using a fibreoptic instrument without general anaesthesia have still not been fully assessed but may prove to have a place in a few high-risk patients.

Heller's myotomy is, however, the treatment for all uncomplicated cases but must always be accompanied by a definitive hiatus hernia repair to prevent the risk of subsequent complications from gastro-oesophageal reflux. In cases with gross megaoesophagus or where, for some other reason, a previous Heller's operation has failed, partial or total excision of the thoracic oesophagus should be considered. Direct anastomosis between the dilated oesophagus and the fundus of the stomach must never be contemplated as this must always result in severe reflux.

HELLER'S MYOTOMY

The operation consists of complete division of the circular muscle at the oesophagogastric junction.

The length of this division must always be adequate. Below, it should extend for a short distance onto the stomach, and above, it should be continued until no more hypertrophied muscle is encountered. In cases which show little muscle hypertrophy, the myotomy should extend for at least 7 cm up the oesophagus.

A thoracic, thoracoabdominal or entirely abdominal approach can be used. For the majority of cases, the operator should select the approach normally preferred for repair of the hiatus. However, the exposure obtained by thoracotomy is the most satisfactory and always allows upward extension of the myotomy if necessary. In the rare case of achalasia associated with an elevated cardia the thoracic approach is essential.

Preoperative preparation

Even in cases with little oesophageal dilatation, careful clinical and radiological assessment should be made to estimate the degree of 'overspill pneumonitis'. When the oesophagus is large and oesophagoscopy reveals much debris, this should be cleared completely, washing out if necessary. Following this, the patient should be allowed a fluid diet only and must not be allowed to sleep flat. Physiotherapy and appropriate antibiotic treatment may be required for some time before the pneumonitis is adequately controlled.

The operation

Care should again be exercised during the anaesthetic induction. Oesophagoscopy is performed to clean the oesophagus thoroughly.

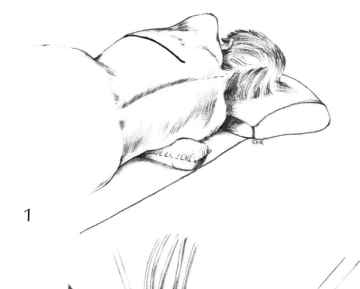

1

For the thoracic approach, the patient is allowed to roll about 15° forwards from a true lateral position. This allows good exposure from a higher and therefore less painful thoracotomy. A sandbag is placed under the lower ribs.

2

Exposure of lower end of the oesophagus

The thorax has been opened by stripping the periosteum from the upper border of the left seventh rib. The pleura over the lower oesophagus is incised vertically and carefully dissected to form flaps for subsequent reconstitution.

3

Mobilization of oesophagus, cardia and upper stomach

Dissecting with care to avoid the adjacent right pleura, the oesophagus is lifted out of its bed and a tape passed round it. Further dissection around the hiatal margin allows the cardia and some stomach to be pulled up into view. Any fat in this area is carefully removed and the vessels always present just below the cardia are identified, ligated and divided to allow access in the line of the proposed myotomy.

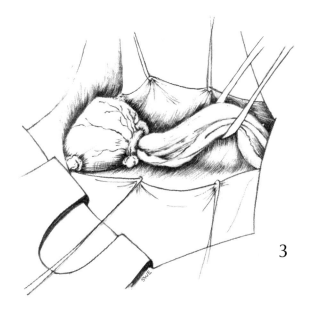

3

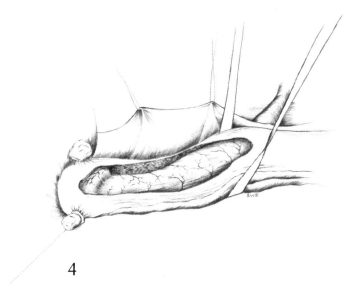

4

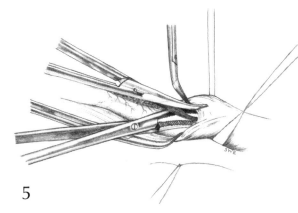

5

4 & 5

Division of the muscle

The incision along the line of the oesophagus, avoiding the vagal nerves, should be started some distance above the oesophagogastric junction. It is deepened until the mucosa is exposed. The submucosal venous plexus is a guide to this plane. At this stage diathermy must be avoided because of the risk of mucosal damage. Once identified, this plane is followed downwards across the junction onto stomach for a short distance. Here, at the oesophagogastric junction, the risk of opening the mucosa is greatest. The incision is then extended upwards on the oesophagus until the circular muscle no longer appears hypertrophied. Unless circular muscle hypertrophy is obviously extending higher than this, upward myotomy can be stopped at the level of the inferior pulmonary vein.

Holding up the cut muscle edges with forceps, a third pair of forceps can be used to extend the plane between the mucosa and the circular muscle and this facilitates safe muscle division. The use of scissors rather than a knife decreases the risk of mucosal damage.

It is unwise to have an oesophageal tube *in situ* during the myotomy as this may also increase the risk of opening the mucosa. However, a tube gently introduced at this stage by the anaesthetist will demonstrate the finest fibres of any residual circular muscle requiring division. Accidental perforation of the mucosa is immediately obvious and should be carefully repaired using fine interrupted sutures, and the postoperative regimen will require modification.

HIATUS HERNIA REPAIR

A formal hiatus hernia procedure will guard against reflux complications and does not appear to impede oesophageal emptying. The thoracic approach for Heller's myotomy described allows a Belsey type of operation (see chapter on 'Thoracic repair of hiatus hernia', pp. 286–291) to be performed which has the additional possibility of placing the cardia well below the hiatus. This helps to correct the often sigmoid deformity of the usually elongated oesophagus which will further assist oesophageal emptying. However, because the myotomy lays bare the mucosa on the front of the oesophagus, only the medial and lateral pairs of mattress sutures can be inserted.

Reconstitution of the pleura

The pleural flaps are approximated with interrupted sutures. A single intercostal tube is inserted and the sandbag removed before closure of the chest.

Postoperative care

Prevention of chest complications

Because of chronic lung damage from overspill, special care needs to be taken. Certainly if it was considered necessary during the preoperative preparation, appropriate antibiotic cover should be continued after surgery. The intercostal tube can usually be removed on the day following operation.

Resumption of feeding

Oral fluids can normally be started on the day following operation. However, if the mucosa has been damaged and repaired, antibiotics should be given, the intercostal tube should be kept in for longer and oral intake delayed until mucosal integrity has been checked radiographically on the fifth to seventh day.

Follow-up

Though swallowing is greatly improved after Heller's myotomy it must be remembered that achalasia is a disease which affects more of the oesophagus than just the cardia. Oesophageal motility remains abnormal and a megaoesophagus does not return to normal size.

Also, it appears that an adequate Heller's operation does not overcome the predisposition of achalasia patients to develop oesophageal carcinoma later. Even with diligent and extended follow-up a carcinoma developing in a megaoesophagus is almost always inoperable by the time symptoms suggest investigation.

DIFFUSE OESOPHAGEAL SPASM ('Corkscrew oesophagus')

Diagnosis

Barium swallow examination suggests the condition and frequently also demonstrates the presence of a hiatus hernia with gastro-oesophageal reflux. Manometric studies in a specialist unit and other oesophageal function studies are essential before considering surgical intervention.

Surgical treatment

This should be considered only when the symptoms are very severe and do not respond to a strict medical hiatus hernia regimen. Some cases may benefit from repair of the hiatus hernia. In others an extended Heller's myotomy is indicated. The upward extent of muscle division is indicated by the manometric test findings. The technique is similar to that described for the standard myotomy and, again, an efficient repair of the hiatus must be carried out.

PERIPHRENIC DIVERTICULUM

Should the symptoms from a periphrenic diverticulum of the oesophagus indicate the need for surgical intervention, simple excision of the diverticulum alone is liable to be followed by breakdown of the suture line. A Heller's myotomy at the cardia should always be carried out to prevent this complication.

Further reading

Harley, H. R. S. Achalasia of the Cardia. Bristol: John Wright, 1978

Oesophagoscopy

K. Michael Pagliero FRCS
Consultant Thoracic Surgeon, Royal Devon and Exeter Hospital;
Clinical Tutor, Exeter University Postgraduate Medical School, Exeter, Devon, UK

Indications

Diagnostic

Oesophagoscopy is used to identify and grade the severity of mucosal lesions such as tumour, peptic oesophagitis, leucoplakia, moniliasis and lye oesophagitis, and to obtain specimens for biopsy. It is further used to observe oesophageal motility and lower oesophageal sphincter tone, assess gastro-oesophageal competence and identify any extrinsic compression by mediastinal tumour, enlarged lymph nodes or aberrant blood vessels. Finally, it will reveal structural abnormalities such as diverticula, hiatal hernia, dilatation, stricture or perforation.

Therapeutic

Its therapeutic applications include: removal of foreign bodies; bougienage of strictures; intubation for carcinoma; balloon dilatation for achalasia; injection of sclerosants for oesophageal varices; cauterization of fistula; vaporization of tumours by laser beam; and intracavity irradiation of cancer.

Preoperative

1

Special preparation for oesophagoscopy

Barium swallow is advised especially if it is anticipated that the oesophagoscope will not pass beyond the lesion and to exclude a pharyngeal diverticulum which may be damaged if not suspected. Chest X-rays (posteroanterior and lateral) should be available for postoperative comparison, and if the rigid oesophagoscope is to be used in elderly people or others with suspected osteoarthritis, X-rays of the cervical spine are also required.

Oesophageal wash-outs and a clear fluid diet are indicated in patients with obstructive lesions. In achalasia, for example, the usual period of restriction of eating and drinking (4 hours) is insufficient to guarantee an empty oesophagus and evacuation may be necessary before induction of anaesthesia.

The need for concomitant examination of the larynx, bronchial tree, stomach or duodenum should be assessed preoperatively. Attention should be paid to dental hygiene, and any loose teeth extracted.

Equipment

A rigid oesophagoscope or flexible fibreoptic gastroscope may be used. The rigid instrument is superior for examining lesions close to the cricopharyngeal sphincter; removal of foreign bodies; obtaining large biopsy specimens; and cautery of oesophageal fistula.

The flexible instrument gives a better field of view and greater accuracy of biopsy, and is superior for examination of the stomach and duodenum, and of the oesophagogastric junction from below. It is also superior for negotiating spinal deformities and/or narrow strictures, and is the instrument of choice when general anaesthesia is contraindicated. Finally, it is superior for photography.

The instruments are complementary and, ideally, both should be available. In the author's opinion, however, the indications for rigid oesophagoscopy are extremely limited.

2

Rigid oesophagoscope

The Negus pattern is recommended with proximal lighting. A fibrelight is desirable but low voltage is acceptable. A variety of sizes is available and it should be remembered that in order to see the entire length of the adult male oesophagus the instruments must be longer than 40 cm; its diameter should not exceed 20 mm in the adult male and 16 mm in the adult female. Scaled-down instruments are available for children. Higher lesions are better viewed with a shorter instrument.

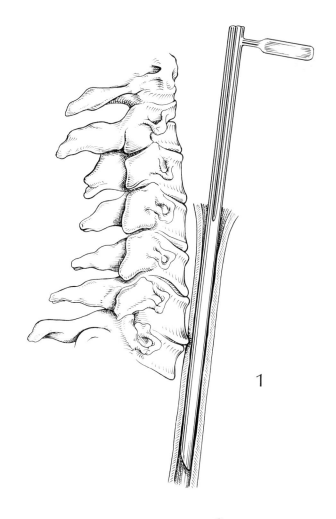

1

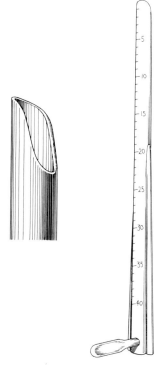

2

3

The sucker and biopsy forceps (a Brock angled bronchus biopsy forceps or a Souttars cup forceps is recommended) must be longer than the oesophagoscope. A sucker with a side hole is preferred to avoid trapping the mucosa. Both a fine-bore sucker for accurate atraumatic suction and a large-bore sucker for solid retained food matter should be available.

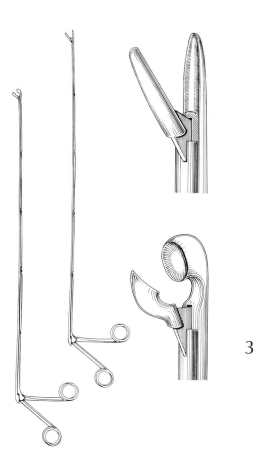

3

4a & b

A set of graduated bougies (*see Illustration 21*) is required for dilatation. Hurst mercury-loaded bougies may also be used (*a*). These are flexible and depend more on the weight of the mercury when used vertically than on the pressure that can be transmitted by hand. A set of graduated Chevalier Jackson gum elastic bougies mounted on rigid wire stems (*b*) is useful for assessment of an obstruction and dilatation under direct vision.

4a

4b

Flexible gastroscope

5

A forward-viewing instrument gives the best view of the oesophagus. Retroflexion and rotation of the instrument allows full examination of the lower oesophageal sphincter, cardia, stomach, pylorus and duodenum, and any fluid obstructing the view can be aspirated via the suction channel. A separate channel permits passage of biopsy forceps, cytology brush or guide wire. A water jet clears the lens. A camera attachment allows photography.

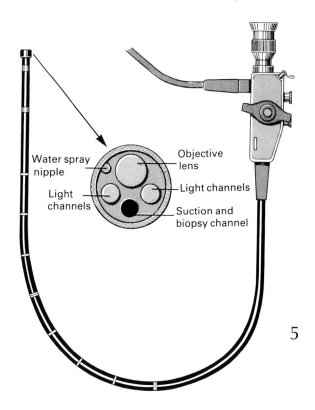

Water spray nipple

Objective lens

Light channels

Light channels

Suction and biopsy channel

5

6 & 7

In addition to simple biopsy forceps, there are biopsy forceps with a central spike for lesions difficult to grasp. A cytology brush is also available to obtain material for microscopic examination.

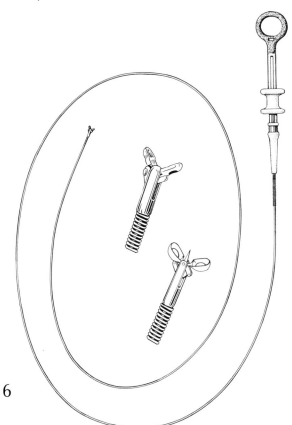

6

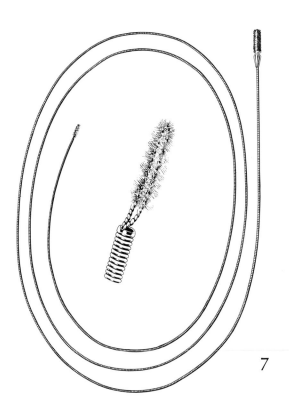

7

8, 9 & 10

A guide wire is passed under direct vision through the strictures and dilatation can be achieved by graded olivary dilators or graded inflatable balloon dilators.

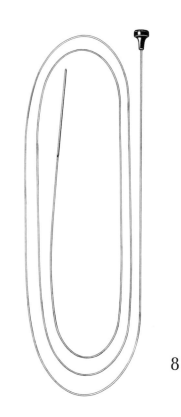

8

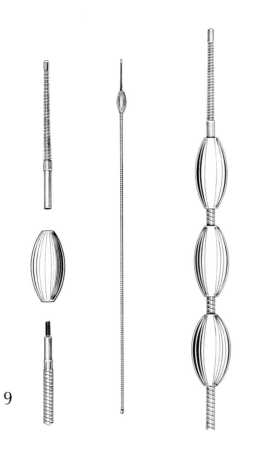

9

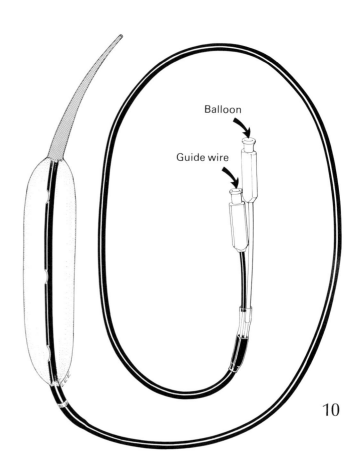

Balloon

Guide wire

10

The operations

RIGID OESOPHAGOSCOPY

Anaesthesia

General anaesthesia is recommended, with muscle relaxant and the use of an endotracheal tube large enough to accommodate the fibreoptic bronchoscope if this investigation is also anticipated. In cases where it is suspected that the oesophagus is not completely empty (recent intake of food or fluids, hiatus hernia, achalasia, foreign body, stricture or neoplasm), copius reflux of oesophageal contents to the pharynx at the time of induction can be prevented by pressing the cricothyroid against the spine and maintaining pressure until the endotracheal tube is in place and its cuff inflated.

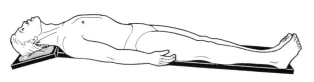

11

Position of patient

The patient is placed on the operating table, with the head resting – stabilized on a grommet – on an extension piece capable of flexing and extending the neck.

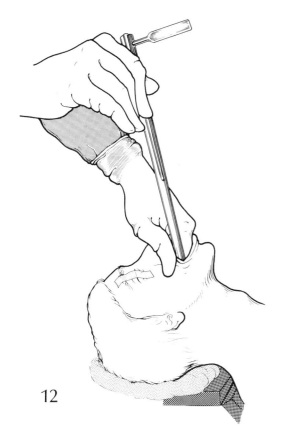

12

Insertion of rigid oesophagoscope

Using the thumb as a fulcrum to avoid damage to the upper jaw, the well-lubricated distal end of the instrument is used to lift the tongue forward without damaging the lips or teeth. Under direct vision the cricopharyngeal inlet is located with the head flexed. The beak of the instrument is introduced through the inlet without force, gently elevating the larynx. If this is difficult, insertion may be facilitated by prior passage of a large Mercury bougie (50 Fr) or by passing the oesophagoscope over a bougie (35 Fr), using it as a guide. However, in this latter recourse the bougie obstructs the view, increasing the risk of mucosal damage. Only minimal force should therefore be applied and the advancing oesophagoscope must not be allowed to advance the bougie, otherwise the bougie tip itself may cause damage.

As the instrument is gently advanced the neck is extended to maintain alignment with the oesophagus and reduce the risk of injury by compression of the posterior oesophageal wall against vertebral osteophytes.

13

The position of lesions should be recorded in centimetres from a standard reference point, customarily the upper incisor teeth, as indicated on the instrument.

Examination

Taking advantage of the anaesthetic and muscle relaxation, the abdomen is palpated carefully for other pathology, especially enlarged liver and gastric neoplasm.

The oesophagus is then examined for any contents such as saliva, retained food or barium which should not ordinarily be present in the unobstructed organ. Its calibre and any rigidity, extrinsic compression or distortion of the wall are noted, as well as any mucosal abnormalities. It is important to proceed cautiously and expeditiously before trauma by the instrument or biopsy forceps causes bleeding which could interfere with the examination.

The stricture lumen is usually visible. If it is difficult to locate, previously ingested thread, with the upper end strapped to the face, may be found to have negotiated it. Alternatively, insufflation of a puff of air may localize a pinhole stricture as it bubbles back through it. The puff of air has the additional advantage that it may distend the oesophagus distal to the obstruction, thus reducing the risk of perforation beyond the stricture.

14

Biopsy

An adequate specimen should be obtained by accurate placement of the forceps. It is important to avoid large bites, especially from normal mucosa, that may cause perforation. If there is no bleeding from the biopsy site the specimen may be necrotic and unsuitable for histological examination. A further specimen should be obtained – and several specimens are recommended. Mucosal biopsy is not recommended if oesophago-myotomy is planned. If biopsy examination is desired subsequent myotomy should be delayed for 2 or 3 weeks to allow complete mucosal healing.

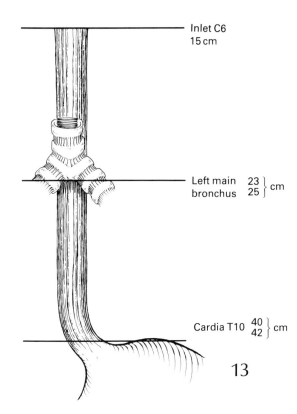

Inlet C6 15 cm

Left main bronchus 23 / 25 } cm

Cardia T10 40 / 42 } cm

13

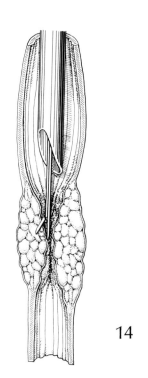

14

Therapeutic procedures

Removal of foreign bodies

If the object is opaque, its position should be checked radiologically immediately before the procedure since it may have moved and be capable of being passed without the need for intervention. Oesophagotomy may be required in cases of failure to extract the object. The object is grasped with suitable biopsy forceps and dislodged if impacted, if necessary by rotating or advancing it before withdrawal. If the object is wider than the lumen of the oesophagoscope the oesophagoscope is withdrawn together with the forceps, firmly grasping and lodging the foreign body in the mouth of the oesophagoscope. Undue traction on spiky objects may cause oesophageal injury and it may be more prudent to perform oesophagotomy.

Dilatation of strictures

15

Dilatation is achieved by sequential passage of graduated bougies under direct vision until an optimum lumen is achieved or the resistance to dilatation is such that injury is feared. Some mucosal bleeding is common but should not normally discourage further bougienage. Maximal dilatation is not advised in cases of proven or suspected carcinoma.

16a & b

There is an ever present hazard of perforation, rupture of the stricture or creation of a false passage.
   Study of the anatomy beyond the stricture on barium swallow is advised to guard against more distal injury beyond the field of view. Dilatation beyond the internal diameter of the oesophagoscope (usually about 38 Fr) may be achieved by withdrawing the oesophagoscope and introducing graduated Maloney bougies as described below. Dilatation with the oesophagoscope is not recommended.

Cauterization

Persistent small oesophageal fistulae may be cauterized with 20 per cent sodium hydroxide applied on a pledget. Care must be taken not to oversaturate the pledget and risk damage to normal mucosa. Any excess is then neutralized with 30 per cent acetic acid.

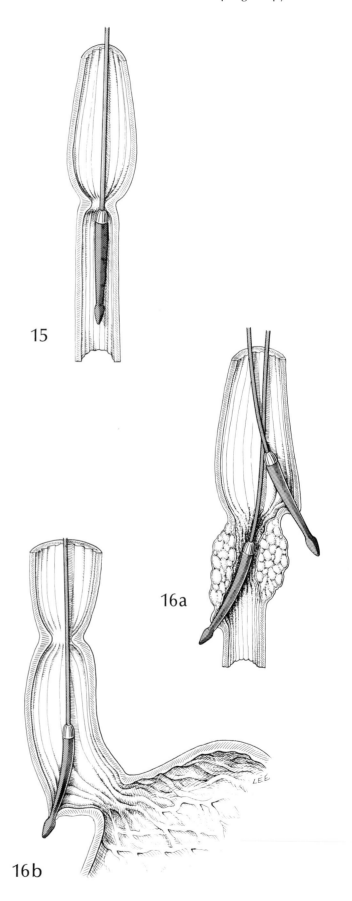

15

16a

16b

FIBREOPTIC OESOPHAGOSCOPY

This may be performed under general anaesthesia with the patient supine, or under local anaesthesia with intravenous sedation in the lateral position. Under general anaesthesia, insertion is facilitated by gentle elevation of the larynx with a laryngoscope; the instrument is passed if necessary under direct vision. Occasionally, excessive cricopharyngeal tone resists the passage of the endoscope. This can be overcome by dilatation of the cricopharyngeal sphincter with Maloney mercury bougies. The guard previously threaded on the oesophagoscope should be placed between the upper and lower teeth.

If using local anaesthesia sedation, the patient is asked to swallow as the oesophagoscope is gently but firmly advanced. In this case the guard is placed between the teeth before passage of the endoscope.

17a–e

Examination

By gently advancing the gastroscope and distending the organ with air, the contents and calibre of the oesophagus are observed, as well as any distortion and mucosal abnormalities such as carcinoma or oesophagitis. The abdomen is examined frequently to avoid overdistension, especially in obstructing lesions, which may make evacuation by suction difficult. Fluid interfering with the view may be cleared by lavage from the water jet. Care must be taken to avoid trauma to lesions which could bleed and thus interfere with the examination. The tone of the lower oesophageal sphincter and its relation to the diaphragmatic impression are noted from above. The position of the squamocolumnar epithelial junction is identified and, if required, confirmed by biopsy. The cardia is examined from below by retroflexing the oesophagoscope, looking for gastric herniation and lower oesophageal sphincter competence on gently distending the stomach with air. Any other pathology in the stomach, pylorus and duodenum that may coexist with oesophageal pathology should be noted at the same time. There may be bile in the stomach or oesophagus.

Biopsy

A specimen is obtained, by taking care to place the forceps accurately. There is little danger of perforation with these forceps but in view of their small size several samples should be taken. Bleeding from the biopsy site assures a viable rather than necrotic specimen. Specimens for cytological examination are obtained with the flexible brush under direct vision. Satellite lesions may be made more obvious by staining the mucosa with Toluidine Blue; mucosal distortion may indicate a submucosal tumour.

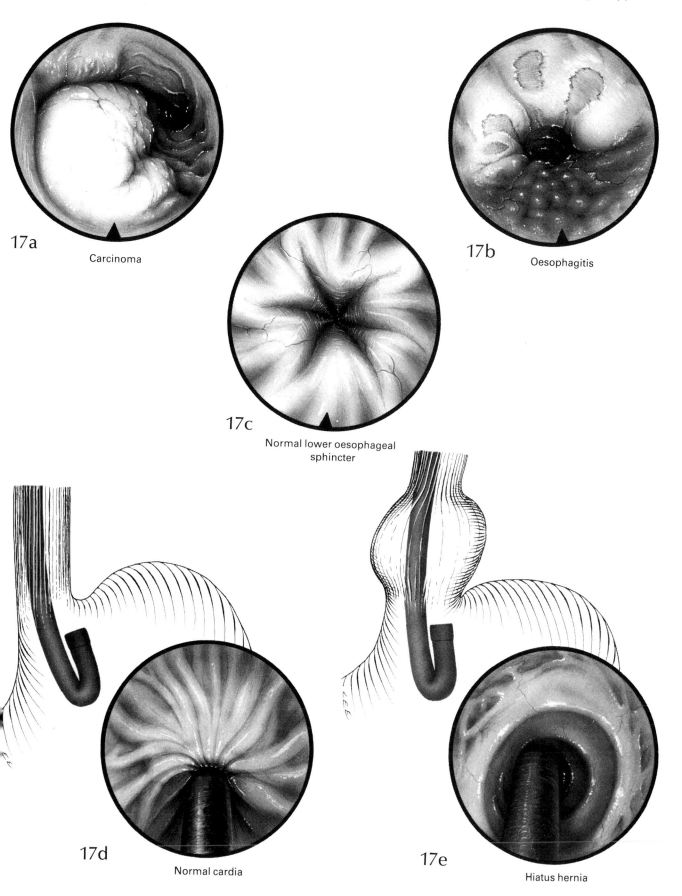

17a
Carcinoma

17b
Oesophagitis

17c
Normal lower oesophageal
sphincter

17d
Normal cardia

17e
Hiatus hernia

Therapeutic procedures

Dilatation of strictures

18

An Eder Puestow guide wire is inserted through the stricture under direct vision and then advanced into the stomach under X-ray control. Care must be taken to avoid a large loop in the stomach as this could knot itself. In order to avoid pushing the guide wire through the oesophageal or gastric wall, the position of the guide wire within the gastric lumen, as outlined by the gastric air bubble, should be carefully observed under X-ray control. If the gastroscope can be pushed past the stricture, it is advanced into the stomach together with the guide wire, which is kept in place as the gastroscope is withdrawn.

19 & 20

Dilatation is achieved by sequential passage of graduated Eder Puestow olivary bougies (range 21–58 Fr) over the guide wire, checking its position radiologically to ensure that it has not become displaced above the stricture. Gentle tension is applied to the wire to prevent kinking especially while negotiating the cricopharyngeal sphincter.

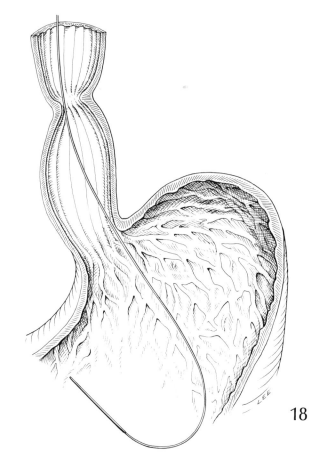

18

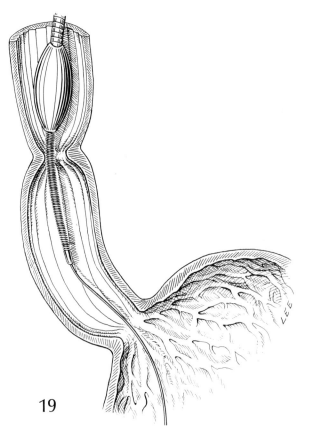

19

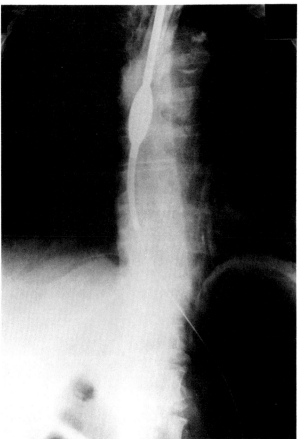

20

21, 22 & 23

In less severe strictures and severe strictures that have been dilated by the Eder Puestow system to about 30 Fr, it is recommended that dilatation be continued with mercury-filled graduated Maloney bougies which are less rigid and prevent unduly forceful dilatation. Used under X-ray control, failure of the highly flexible tip to negotiate the stricture can be readily identified before inappropriate pressure is applied. Injury is extremely rare. Once optimal dilatation has been achieved, often between 50 and 60 Fr, the final bougie may be left in place for a while to gain maximum benefit.

Occasionally a stricture may resist the forward pressure of a bougie or may be so eccentric that forward pressure is impossible to apply. In these cases dilatation may be achieved by a balloon dilator (*see Illustration 10*) that can be positioned within the stricture over a guide wire.

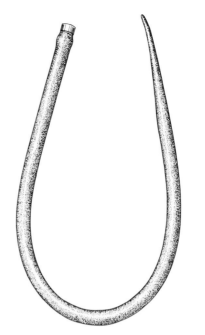

21

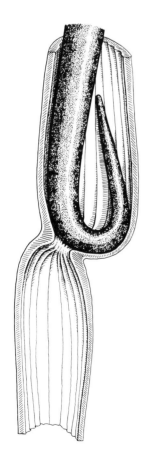

22

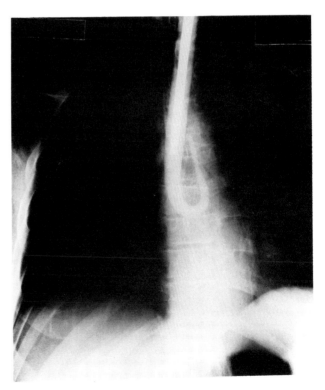

23

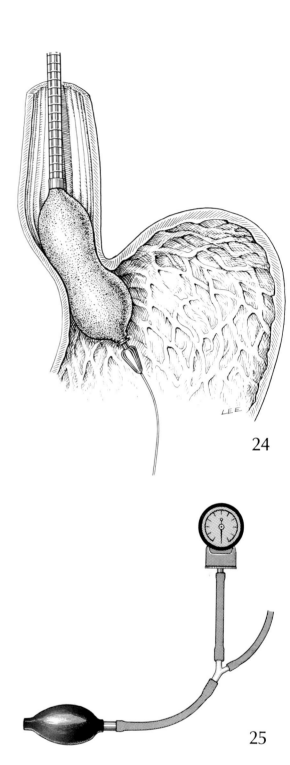

24

25

24 & 25

Balloon dilatation for achalasia

This may be used to forcibly rupture the inner circular muscle fibres of the lower oesophageal sphincter in achalasia of the oesophagus. A guide wire is placed in the stomach as described above. The balloon is passed over the wire and sited to straddle the lower oesophageal sphincter. The bag is then inflated with air to a pressure of 250 mmHg for a period of 3 minutes, checking radiologically that inflation does not dislocate the balloon upwards into the oesophagus or downwards into the stomach. Endoscopic examination after dilatation is recommended to exclude mishap. If a perforation has occurred, examination should be brief to avoid overdissection of tissue planes by injected air. Such an event may be suspected if surgical emphysema presents in the neck.

26, 27 & 28

Injection of sclerosant[1]

Sclerosant such as ethanolamine oleate may be injected
directly into oesophageal varices through either the
fibreoptic or the rigid oesophagoscope under direct
vision. Immediately after each 2–5 ml injection the varix
should be compressed to encourage retention of sclerosant for about 5 minutes. Using the fibreoptic endoscope
through a Williams tube, a varix can be made to pout into
the lumen. After injection the tube is rotated to compress
the varix. Some prefer perivariceal to intraluminal injection. The correct siting of such injections may be
confirmed by adding radio-opaque or fluorescent mate-
rials to the sclerosant.

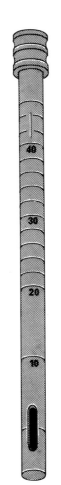

26

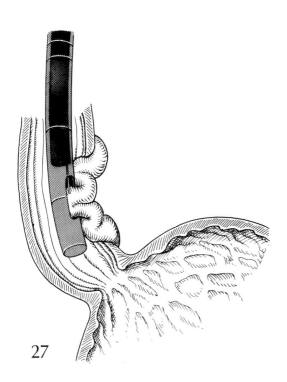

27

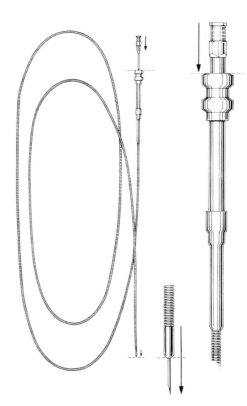

28

Laser photocoagulation

It has recently been shown that laser beams can be used to photocoagulate bleeding vessels and to vaporize solid lesions. The merits and constraints of the different systems are presently under review.

29, 30 & 31

Intracavity irradiation[2]

Intracavity irradiation for oesophageal cancer has recently been introduced and is indergoing review. An applicator containing radio opaque marker pellets is passed into the oesophagus over a guide wire, having first established endoscopically and by fluoroscopy the upper and lower extent of the tumour. It may be necessary to dilate the tumour first, to the diameter of the endoscope, to allow inspection. The applicator is then introduced over the guide wire in such a way that its subsequent radiation field will embrace the tumour. This portion is maintained by fixation to a face mask and the guide wire is withdrawn. The patient is then transferred to a special room screened for radiation. Here the marker pellets are removed and Caesium-137 pellets substituted for a period of about 1 hour to achieve a dosage of 1250cGy.

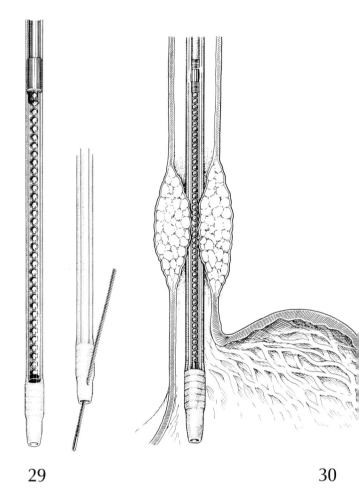

29   30

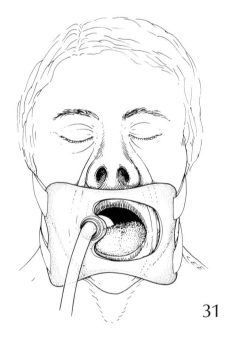

31

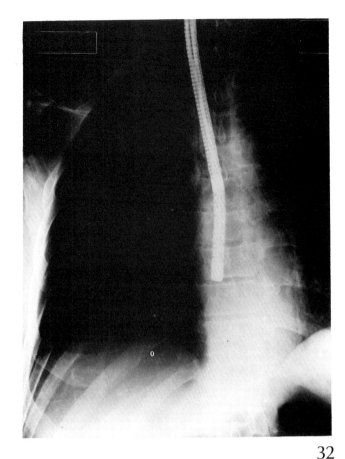

32

Insertion of indwelling tube by pulsion

This is for palliation in carcinoma and rarely in benign obstruction. The lesion is dilated to 45 Fr gauge using Eder Puestow bougies under X-ray control (see chapter on 'Pulsation intubation of the oesophagus', pp. 370–373). Injury is not uncommon in friable malignant lesions but perforation usually heals, responding to the defunctioning role of the indwelling tube. One can, therefore afford to be a little more enthusiastic with the dilatation than in cases where an indwelling tube is not contemplated.

32 & 33

X-ray

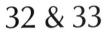

The level and length of the obstruction should be defined in relation to other mediastinal structures so that the radio-opaque tube can be correctly positioned. The position of the oesophagoscope tip on X-ray screening indicates the site of the lesion.

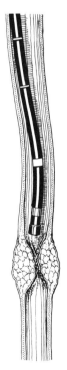

33

34

Tubes of varying diameter and length are available. A large diameter is recommended whenever possible for maximum relief of symptoms and to minimize the risk of blockage. A short tube is recommended to permit the lower oesophageal sphincter to function normally below it. If the tube has to traverse the lower oesophageal sphincter a longer tube will discourage gastro-oesophageal reflux.

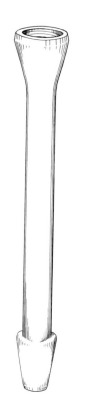

34

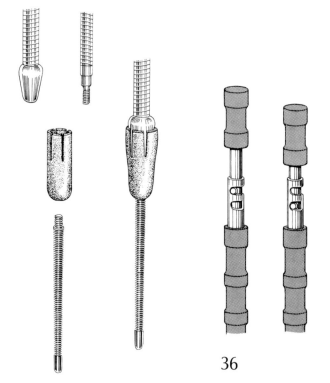

35

36

35 & 36

A Nottingham introducer appropriate to the diameter of the tube is chosen, and its fixing and release mechanism is checked before use. The tube and introducer are then passed on to the guide wire.

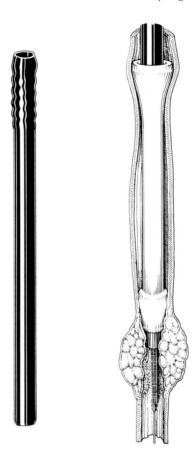

37

The ram rod is placed in the cup and advanced with the apparatus until the tube is correctly sited through the lesion. The introducer is then released and withdrawn, maintaining the tube position with the ram rod which is then also withdrawn. Successful positioning should be confirmed by X-ray screening and further endoscopy.

37

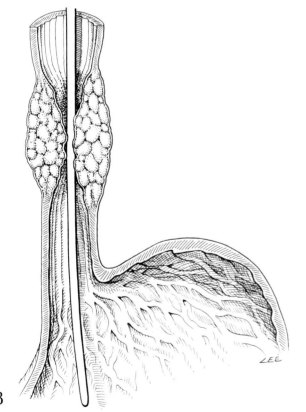

38

Traction insertion of indwelling tube

Failure to insert a tube by pulsion should be anticipated and both the patient and theatre staff should be prepared for this event. The procedure is carried out under general anaesthesia and requires two surgeons: one to make the upper midline abdominal incision, the other to perform rigid oesophagoscopy.

38

Under direct vision a pilot bougie is passed through the stricture into the stomach where its position is confirmed by palpation.

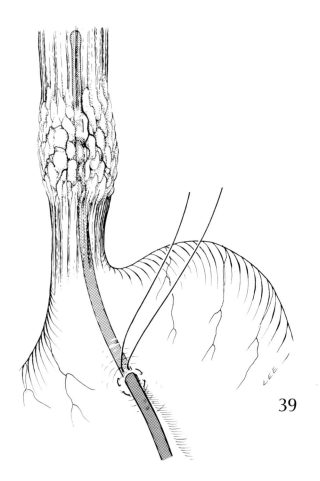

39

If passage is impossible, a gastrostomy is performed and an 18 Fr gum elastic bougie passed upwards towards the oesophagoscope.

39

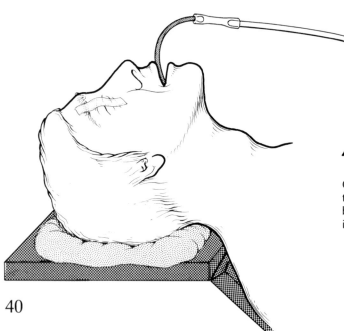

40

Once through the stricture, the bougie is passed upwards to the mouth where it can be connected to the pilot bougie with a short length of 16 Fr tubing. The pilot bougie is drawn into the stomach.

40

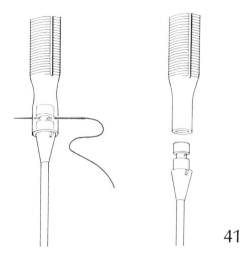

41

A Celestin tube is sutured to the pilot bougie.

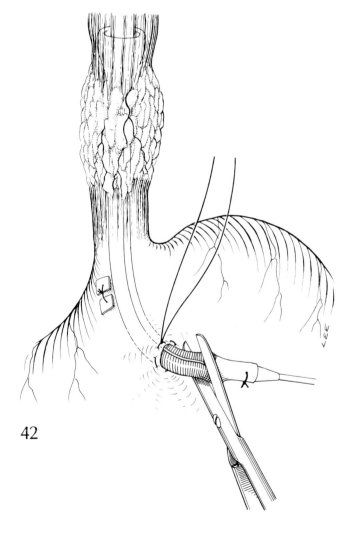

42

With gentle traction below and pulsion by the oesophago-scope or Maloney bougie, the tube is passed through the stricture until its cup is felt and measured to be sitting above it.

The tube is fixed to the lesser curve of stomach with a Teflon buttressed '0'-thread suture encircling a strand of the nylon spiral in the wall of the tube without encroaching on the lumen. Excess tube is cut off with a rounded bevel towards the cavity of the stomach.

43

The gastrotomy is closed in two layers. Complete sterility in this operation is impossible; however, by carefully avoiding too much contamination and using peritoneal lavage and perioperative antibiotics, the risk of infection can be minimized.

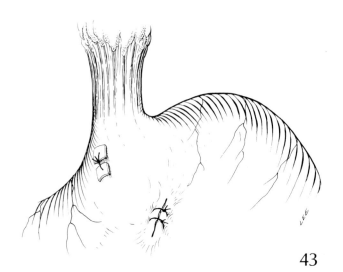

43

Postoperative care

Specific complications of oesophageal endoscopy are bleeding and perforation. Basic haemodynamic parameters should be recorded regularly. A history of postoperative pain as opposed to the customary discomfort indicates leakage of air and other contents into the neck, mediastinum, pleura or peritoneal cavity and, if suspected, straight X-rays or X-ray contrast studies may be used for confirmation and localization. Oral fluids need only be restricted until the effects of general and local anaesthesia have subsided or if perforation is anticipated or suspected.

References

1. Terblanche, J. Sclerosant injection of oesophageal varices. In Operative Surgery, 4th ed, Alimentary Tract and Abdominal Wall. Vol. 2. Butterworths: London. 1983: 528–534

2. Rowland, C. G., Paliero, K. M. Intracavity irradiation in palliation of carcinoma of oesophagus and cardia. Lancet 1985; ii: 981–983

Perforation of the oesophagus

W. F. Kerr FRCS(Ed)
Formerly Consultant Thoracic Surgeon, Norfolk and Norwich Hospital, Norwich, UK

Introduction

Perforation or rupture of the oesophagus happens most often during endoscopy or endoscopic instrumentation. Other causes are comparatively rare and include the so-called 'spontaneous' or 'emetogenic' ruptures (the Boerhaave* syndrome), simple and malignant ulceration, impaction of swallowed foreign bodies, operations in the vicinity of the oesophagus and penetrating wounds of the neck and, less often, the chest. Dehiscence of anastomoses and acquired oesophagotracheal fistulae are not included.

The principal considerations which govern the management of a case are:

1. whether the perforation is intramural (incomplete)[1] or transmural (complete);

and, if transmural,

2. its location and extent;
3. its age – in hours; and
4. whether there is pre-existing local disease, obstruction distal to the perforation being most important[2].

The overall figure for mortality is approximately 30 per cent in specialized units[3, 4, 5] and 50 per cent in the general wards of a teaching hospital[6]. As mortality and morbidity rates rise steeply the longer the institution of appropriate treatment is delayed, the key to success is a complete and anatomically precise diagnosis within 12, or at the most, 24 h. The possibility of an oesophageal perforation therefore needs to be kept in mind, particularly after endoscopy, and the mere suspicion that one may have occurred is indication enough for immediate investigation.

* Hermann Boerhaave (1668–1738) – Dutch physician

Diagnosis

Clinical

Instrumental injury not recognized at the endoscopy is unlikely to be suspected before the anaesthetic or sedative has worn off. The leading symptom is severe and constant pain which is aggravated by attempts to swallow. Irrespective of the level of the perforation the pain may be referred to the throat, the chest or the upper abdomen and in many cases is worst in the back. Pleuritic pain and dyspnoea are somewhat less frequent complaints that tend to be too readily attributed to aspiration pneumonitis or spontaneous pneumothorax. Vomiting fresh or altered blood directs attention to the upper alimentary tract but the quantity is seldom sufficient to explain the degree of shock that is a feature of many cases and is particularly impressive in the Boerhaave syndrome, often misdiagnosed as an 'acute abdomen', a myocardial infarct or an aortic dissection. Surgical emphysema in the neck is a positive though inconstant sign that ought to be looked for routinely after oesophagoscopy and gastroscopy.

1

Radiological

Perforation of the oesophagus may be deduced from plain films of the chest and abdomen and a lateral view of the neck, but normal appearances do not exclude it. Gas shadows in the soft tissues of the neck and mediastinum are significant as is rapidly accumulating pleural fluid with or without pneumothorax.

2

The one indispensable investigation is a radiopaque swallow, *carried out as an emergency procedure* and if possible attended by the surgeon. Except in a very small proportion of cases expert screening demonstrates the site of a perforation, its relationship to a pre-existing lesion if there is one and the extent of involvement of neighbouring tissues. Thin barium is best for the *initial* examination[7] as it gives the sharpest definition and does no harm if it spills into the airways, whereas water-soluble contrast media such as Gastrografin and Dionosil may be so diluted by fluid in the mediastinum or pleural cavity that an indubitable perforation is not outlined. An added disadvantage of Gastrografin is the severe irritation it causes if aspirated into the trachea.

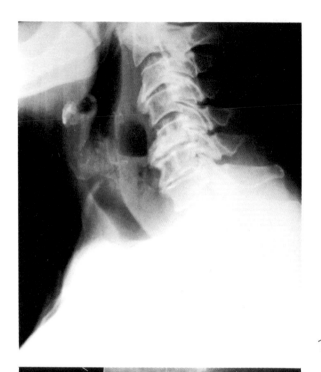

1

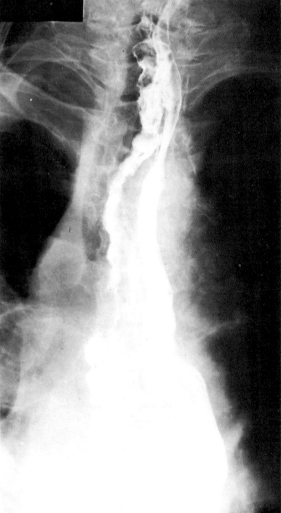

2

Treatment

3a & b

Intramural rupture: instrumental (*a*) or spontaneous (*b*)

The radiographic appearances are diagnostic and oesophagoscopy is not necessary. Treatment is conservative whatever the level. Oral feeding is stopped and nutrition maintained through a nasogastric tube or parenterally. A broad-spectrum antibiotic is given for aerobic micro-organisms and metronidazole for anaerobes. When pain subsides, usually in 3 or 4 days, oral feeding is cautiously reintroduced. Progress is checked with weekly barium or Gastrografin swallows; most cases heal completely within 2 or 3 weeks but a few take much longer.

Transmural perforation of the cervical oesophagus

When the laceration is minor such as occurs when the oesophagus is caught between a rigid instrument and vertebral osteophytes (see *Illustration 1*), treatment is conservative as for an intramural perforation. If an abscess forms, it is drained externally through an incision along the anterior border of the sternomastoid muscle.

Some surgeons advocate the same treatment for more extensive injuries of the cervical oesophagus but it is safer to operate immediately. Free external drainage of the false passage should be ensured and, if practicable, the defect in the mucous membrane is sutured, but a perforated pharyngeal pouch must be excised and cricopharyngeal myotomy performed (see volume on *Nose and Throat*, p. 248). A false passage that enters a pleural cavity requires the insertion of well placed chest drains by thoracotomy if intercostal intubation is contraindicated or does not immediately result in complete re-expansion of the lung.

Transmural perforation of the thoracic oesophagus

In dealing with this most dangerous of all oesophageal injuries, the prime object is to save the patient's life; except when necessary for the relief of obstruction, a definitive operation for associated disease is a secondary consideration to be contemplated only when circumstances are entirely favourable. A successful outcome depends largely on gaining and keeping control of infection in the mediastinum, pleural cavity and lungs; therefore the source must be eliminated by closing, resecting or excluding the perforation, and thoroughly effective drainage must be provided to permit and maintain full expansion of both lungs. Half-hearted measures will not suffice.

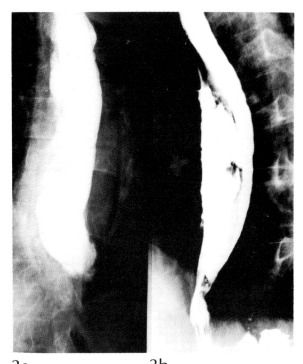

3a   3b

Figure 3b is reproduced by courtesy of the Publishers of 'Thorax'[1]

Preoperative

Preparation

Resuscitation of a shocked patient is started immediately and antibiotics effective against anaerobic and aerobic micro-organisms are given to all suspected cases without waiting for confirmation of the diagnosis. If fluid or air in a pleural cavity is causing respiratory embarrassment, a 28 Fr, or larger, intercostal tube is inserted under local anaesthesia while preparations are being made for surgery. However, one should not expect or await much improvement as opening the chest and evacuating the irritant and infective material from the pleural cavity and mediastinum is the only really effective countermeasure.

Anaesthesia

A double-lumen tube that allows the lung on the operation side to be collapsed is a great help but the preliminary oesophagoscopy is easier if the operation is started with an endotracheal tube.

Operation for intrathoracic perforation (instrumental or spontaneous) of an unobstructed oesophagus

Oesophagoscopy

A rigid oesophagoscope and a 4–6 mm diameter suction tube are used to aspirate the fluid, stained with altered blood, that wells back through the laceration and up from the stomach. (Quite apart from the inadequacy of its suction channel, a fibreoptic oesophagoscope blows air through the perforation and makes matters worse.) The position, direction and extent of the tear(s) and the presence or absence of other lesions should be confirmed. The stomach is then emptied with a 36 or 39 Fr stomach tube, which is left in position until the end of the operation.

4

After the anaesthetist has substituted an endobronchial tube for the endotracheal one, the chest is opened, the side and level of the incision depending on the radiological and oesophagoscopic findings. All fluid and debris are evacuated from the pleural cavity.

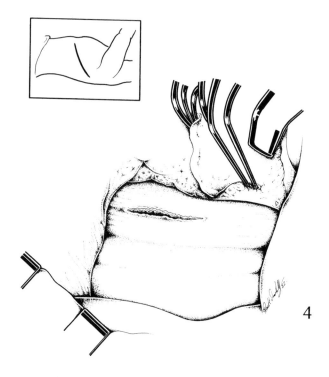

4

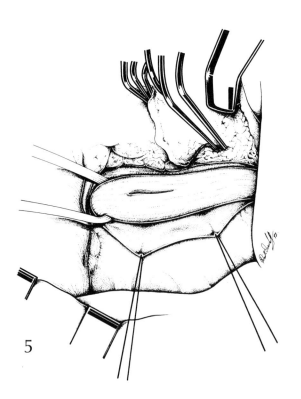

5

5

Taking care to preserve the attachment of the mediastinal pleura posteriorly, the mediastinum is opened widely – from the diaphragm to the arch of the aorta on the left, to the azygos vein or higher on the right. The oesophagus is mobilized and a tape is passed round it to display the perforation. If the perforation cannot be found, the oesophagus is submerged in normal saline solution while the anaesthetist blows air or oxygen into it.

6

The rent in the muscular coat is enlarged upwards and downwards until the limits of the defect in the mucosal layer have been positively identified.

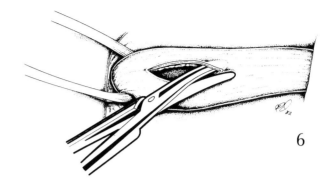

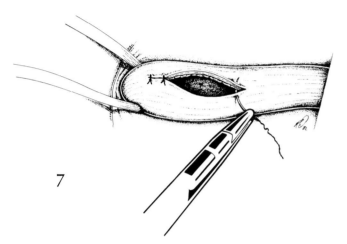

7

The oesophagus is repaired with a single layer of interrupted non-absorbable sutures, e.g. 2/0 (3 metric) Prolene, making sure that each stitch includes both muscle and mucosa.

8

The closure is reinforced by stripping a large flap of pleura from the posterolateral chest wall, leaving it hinged on the aorta and stitching it to the muscular coat of the oesophagus all round the sutured perforation.

A hinged flap of thick and inflamed pleura may be used as a patch to seal perforations that come so late to surgery that the edges of the oesophagus cannot be drawn together[8]. In such cases, oesophageal mucous membrane is included in stitches placed a good 1 cm away from the margins of the defect. If pleura is not available or seems unsatisfactory, a hinged flap of pericardium makes a good alternative[9].

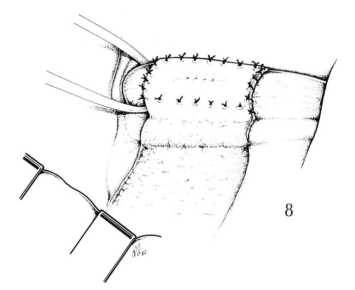

9

The stomach tube is removed and a nasogastric tube advanced through the nose until its tip lies a little above the repaired segment. The inside of the rib cage is then abraided with dry gauze to encourage rapid adhesion of the lung and thus localization of the empyema should a leak develop. Any remaining fibrinous plaques are peeled off the lung (easier after it has been reinflated). The chest is drained with two tubes, preferably Silastic, size 36 Fr or larger. One is placed in the paravertebral gutter with a side-hole opposite the repaired perforation, the other anteriorly; the ends of both should reach the apex of the pleural cavity. The chest is then closed.

With the patient supine, a draining gastrostomy for protection of the lower oesophagus and a separate jejunostomy for feeding are made (see Alimentary Tract, Volume 1, p. 22). Double-lumen tubes such as the Burns-Menzies do not always function satisfactorily. Alternatively, nasogastric suction may be employed to protect the repair from reflux of gastric juice while nutrition is maintained by intravenous feeding.

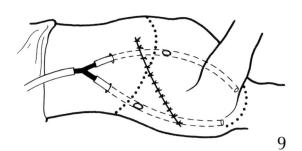

9

Postoperative management

1. The patient is nursed in an intensive therapy unit for the first 24–48 h. Advantage should be taken of all available supportive measures including intermittent positive pressure ventilation – this not only compensates for failing respiration but, by assisting full expansion of the lungs, tends to prevent the development of empyema and bronchopneumonia which are the complications mainly responsible for the high mortality rate. Frequent and skilled physiotherapy is most important but unless attention is given to adequate relief of pain, its benefits are lost. Antibiotics in high dosage are continued for at least 5 days.
2. The oesophageal tube is connected to a continuous suction pump and the gastric secretions are allowed to drain by gravity into a collecting bag. The gastrostomy tube is intended to protect the oesophagus from reflux of gastric juice and accidental obstruction must be guarded against.
3. Ranitidine or cimetidine is given intravenously for 2 weeks.

4. A close check is kept on electrolyte and fluid balances and if the haemoglobin level falls below 12.0 g/dl it is raised by blood transfusion.
5. Jejunostomy feeds are started when bowel sounds return, usually on the second or third day.
6. A barium or Gastrografin swallow is requested on the 12th day and if it shows the repair intact, the chest drains and the nasal and gastrostomy tubes are removed and oral feeding commenced.

   If dehiscence has occurred, the drains are left until the lung is firmly adherent to the parietes and the fistulous track is well localized. The anterior tube is then removed and the posterior tube changed to a shorter one with its internal end opposite the disruption. The oesophageal and gastrostomy tubes are also removed and the patient is encouraged to drink and eat; a proportion of the intake will be lost through the pleural drain but spontaneous closure of the fistula will not be hindered and the jejunostomy is still available for supplementary feeds.

Alternative procedures

THE THAL OPERATION[10]

In this procedure the intact gastric fundus is used as a patch for the oesophagus when the edges of the tear are too friable to hold stitches. This involves opening and perhaps contaminating the peritoneal cavity and, as with any operation that leaves stomach in the chest, there is a calculated risk of complications in the long term.

10

The hiatus is dissected and, if necessary, enlarged by incising the diaphragm forwards in the midline. The vagus nerves are identified and preserved. The fundus is mobilized by ligating and dividing the short gastric vessels.

11

The seromuscular coats of the stomach are sutured to the oesophagus about 1 cm away from the edges of the defect, including the oesophageal mucous membrane in the stitches, and a partial fundoplication to counteract gastro-oesophageal reflux is added.

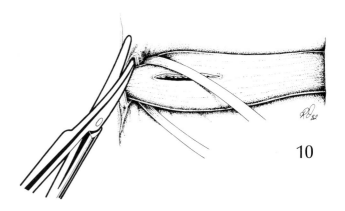

10

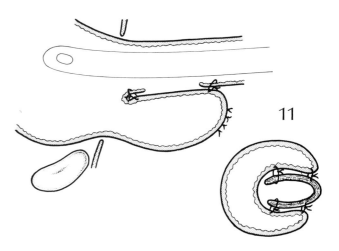

11

FUNDOPLICATION

This has been used with success to buttress a lower oesophageal suture line when surgery has been delayed[11]. Before repairing the oesophagus the fundus is mobilized as in the Thal procedure, and no attempt is made to reduce the hiatal hernia so formed.

12

EXCLUSION OF RUPTURED SEGMENT[4]

When extreme debility or gross sepsis as a result of late diagnosis or failure of a previous operation for perforation threatens to overwhelm the patient, exclusion of the ruptured segment constitutes the last line of defence. The oesophagus is ligated with nylon tape above and below the perforation and the drainage of the chest is augmented to clear any residual pockets of infection. The lungs are protected with an oesophagostomy-in-continuity in the neck and the patient is fed through a gastrostomy until his condition is good enough to permit reconstruction.

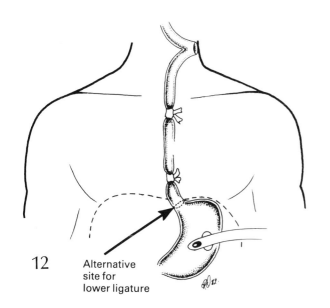

12   Alternative
site for
lower ligature

Operations for perforation of an obstructed oesophagus

An instrumental perforation is usually located at or just above the site of obstruction. It is essential that the obstruction be relieved[2] and a number of options are available. The choice depends on the disease and the general condition of the patient.

ACHALASIA

The perforation is repaired and an adequate cardiomyotomy performed (see chapter on 'Surgical treatment of achalasia of the cardia', pp. 252–255). This is not easy but not impossible if a right-sided approach to the perforation is indicated.

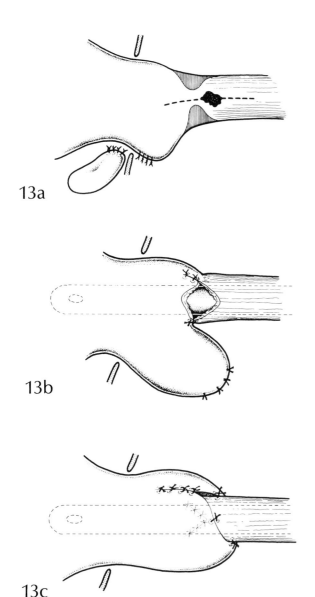

13a

13b

13c

BENIGN STRICTURE ASSOCIATED WITH A HIATAL HERNIA

If, exceptionally, *the stricture has been or can be satisfactorily dilated* (to size 40 Fr at least) treatment is as for an unobstructed oesophagus but, with the fundus of the stomach already displaced into the chest, fundoplication (see above) is preferred to a pleural flap for covering the suture line. Then, provided that the perforation is so recent that infection has not had time to become established, the hernia is reduced and repaired.

When *adequate relief of obstruction cannot be obtained by dilatation* and the condition of the patient is reasonably good, the stricture is resected together with the perforation. The cardia is closed and the fundus of the stomach anastomosed to healthy oesophagus[2]. This comparatively quick and easy operation does not involve opening the peritoneal cavity and it preserves the whole of the stomach for restoration to the abdomen when reconstruction is less hazardous.

13a, b & c

For a *frail patient with an intractable stricture*, a modified Milstein oesophagoplasty[12] may be applicable even if the perforation is into the right pleural cavity[13]. One should check that the cardia and fundus of the stomach can comfortably be raised to a level well above the perforation; if necessary the peritoneal sac is opened and the short gastric vessels divided. The perforation is incorporated in an incision reaching a good 2 cm above the stricture and an equal distance below it. This incision is closed transversely over a 36–39 Fr stomach tube, *bringing the distal end up* to meet the proximal which is relatively fixed. There must be no tension whatsoever on the suture line which when finished will be >-shaped. The oesophagoplasty is supported with a 360° fundoplication and the chest closed without attempting to reduce the hiatal hernia.

MALIGNANT OBSTRUCTION

Carcinoma suitable for radical treatment

The lesion is formally resected together with the perforation and, provided conditions are favourable, continuity is restored immediately by oesophagogastrostomy (see chapter on 'Operations for carcinoma of the thoracic oesophagus and cardia', pp. 326–342). Otherwise the patient is left with a terminal oesophagostomy in the neck and a gastrostomy, and reconstruction is carried out when the prospects for healing of anastomoses are better.

Inoperable carcinoma

Heroic measures are out of place and no surgical procedure is indicated other than drainage of the pleural cavity and oesophageal intubation for relief of dysphagia. The occasional successful result of treatment of the very frail by intubation[9, 14] should not tempt one to use it routinely for good-risk cases; only non-intervention has a higher mortality rate (but see chapter on 'Pulsion intubation of the oesophagus', pp. 370–373).

References

1. Kerr, W. F. Spontaneous intramural rupture and intramural haematoma of the oesophagus. Thorax 1980; 35: 890–897

2. Kerr, W. F. Emergency oesophagectomy. Thorax 1968; 23: 204–209

3. Sandrasagra, F. A., English, T. A. H., Milstein, B. B. The management and prognosis of oesophageal perforation. British Journal of Surgery 1978; 65: 629–632

4. Skinner, D. B., Little, A. G., DeMeester, T. R. Management of esophageal perforation. American Journal of Surgery 1980; 139: 760–764

5. Michel, L., Grillo, H. C., Malt, R. A. Operative and nonoperative management of esophageal perforations. Annals of Surgery 1981; 194: 57–63

6. Banks, J. G., Bancewicz, J. Perforation of the oesophagus: experience in a general hospital. British Journal of Surgery 1981; 68: 580–584

7. Appleton, D. S., Sandrasagra, F. A., Flower, C. D. R. Perforated oesophagus: review of twenty-eight consecutive cases. Clinical Radiology 1979; 30: 493–497

8. Grillo, H. C., Wilkins, E. W. Esophageal repair following late diagnosis of intrathoracic perforation. Annals of Thoracic Surgery 1975; 20: 387–399

9. Keen, G. The surgical management of old esophageal perforations. Journal of Thoracic and Cardiovascular Surgery 1968; 56: 603–606

10. Thal, A. P. A unified approach to surgical problems of the esophagogastric junction. Annals of Surgery 1968; 168: 542–550

11. Finley, R. J., Pearson, F. G., Weisel, R. D., Todd, T. R., Ilves, R., Cooper, J. The management of nonmalignant intrathoracic esophageal perforations. Annals of Thoracic Surgery 1980; 30: 575–583

12. Milstein, B. B. An operation for the treatment of intractable peptic stricture of the esophagus. Israel Journal of Medical Sciences 1975; 11: 281–286

13. Cooper, D. K. C. Management of oesophageal perforation associated with benign stricture and hiatus hernia by oesophagoplasty and fundoplication. Thorax 1981; 36: 541–542

14. Sandrasagra, F. A., English, T. A. H., Milstein, B. B. Esophageal intubation in the management of perforated esophagus with stricture. Annals of Thoracic Surgery 1978; 25: 399–401

Illustrations by Christopher Tyrrell

Thoracic repair of hiatus hernia

G. Keen MS, FRCS
Consultant Cardiothoracic Surgeon,
United Bristol Hospitals and Frenchay Hospital, Bristol, UK

Introduction

There are two distinct varieties of hiatus hernia, each with characteristic anatomical features and pathological consequences. By far the commoner (Type I), the so-called sliding hiatus hernia, is associated with failure of the barriers to gastro-oesophagitis and stricture formation. A variant of this group is the syndrome of patulous cardia, in which a hernia is absent but the florid picture of gastro-oesophageal reflux and its consequences may be seen.

The second distinct group (Type II), that of para-oesophageal hiatus hernia (sometimes called rolling hiatus hernia) is not usually associated with gastro-oesophageal reflux. The intrathoracic portion of the stomach is prone to congestion and chronic bleeding, and patients with this condition frequently present with severe anaemia. Such a hernia is liable to incarceration, volvulus and acute dilatation within the chest. The last complication may follow a trivial injury or illness and has caused fatal respiratory embarrassment in one elderly patient with a fractured fibula.

Rarely, the two distinct types of hernia may co-exist (mixed Type I and Type II). It is with the surgical treatment of the Type I hernia that this chapter is concerned.

Preoperative

Aims of surgery

1. The correction of gastro-oesophageal reflux.
2. Preservation of the ability to belch or vomit when necessary.
3. Maintenance of normal swallowing mechanisms.

Anatomical and physiological barriers to gastro-oesophageal reflux

1. The pinchcock effect of contraction of the crura of the diaphragm is undoubtedly contributory although this is an over-simplification of what is a complex mechanism.
2. A lower oesophageal sphincter can be demonstrated manometrically and the point of transition between the negative intraoesophageal pressure above and the positive pressure below is described as the pressure inversion point. This sphincter is a complicated and dynamic structure which responds to physical and humoral stimuli and provides part of the barrier to the reflux of gastric contents.
3. The antireflux effect of the oblique entry of the oesophagus into the stomach has probably been over-emphasized. Certainly, many patients with severe reflux have a normal angle of entry of the oesophagus and in others with an apparently wide angle no reflux can be demonstrated.
4. An adequate length of intra-abdominal oesophagus is considered to play a major part in the prevention of gastro-oesophageal reflux. The positive intra-abdominal pressure flattens this segment against the supporting crura which prevents suction of gastric contents into the chest during inspiration or during changes in posture.

An adequate surgical operation seeks to correct or modify these mechanisms although it is unlikely that any surgical procedure can influence the function of the physiological lower oesophageal sphincter.

Preoperative assessment

The repair of radiological hiatus hernia in the absence of specific symptoms related to this condition is not advised. Postoperative persistence of symptoms related to undiagnosed and untreated disease elsewhere serves only to discredit the surgical treatment of hiatus hernia.

In addition to eliciting the specific symptoms of gastro-oesophageal reflux, which are aggravated by postural changes and sometimes complicated by dysphagia, oesophagoscopy is required in all patients. This should be conducted using the conventional oesophagoscope or the fibreoptic instrument under local or general anaesthesia. Should general anaesthesia be used, it is important to maintain normal respiration in the patient to ensure that the negative pressure phase of respiration is maintained during which gastro-oesophageal reflux may be observed and the cardia examined under relatively normal conditions. Oesophagoscopy will furthermore ensure the accurate assessment of oesophagitis and biopsy may be undertaken. Barium studies should be carefully scrutinized, for in addition to the condition under discussion careful assessment of the stomach and duodenum is necessary. Evidence of hold-up at the pylorus, whether by spasm, ulcer or fibrosis, will indicate the need for pyloroplasty in addition to hiatal hernia repair. Manometric studies, although elegant, are not readily available in most centres.

Indications for transthoracic repair

The controversy concerning the choice of transthoracic or abdominal repair of hiatus hernia will subside as the specific indications for each become clear. As it becomes more universally recognized that gastro-oesophageal reflux can be controlled by specific local procedures, the wide variety of transabdominal manoeuvres and quaint gastric operations for the management of gastro-oesophageal reflux will be restricted to few situations. Although simple hiatus hernia is often repaired from below, either as a definitive procedure or during the course of another abdominal operation, care should be taken to avoid an inadequate repair offered as an afterthought with poorly defined indications. There is no doubt that in patients with oesophagitis, oedema and fibrosis, the consequent shortening of the lower oesophagus will prevent adequate mobilization from below and such an operation is unlikely to produce an effective reduction and repair without tension. Furthermore, mediastinal adhesions frequently require accurate sharp dissection under direct vision which is unobtainable via the abdominal route. Inadequate reduction under tension is inevitably followed by recurrence of symptoms. It is claimed that the transabdominal approach is justified during other operations such as cholecystectomy or pyloroplasty but it is under these conditions that repair of the difficult hiatus hernia will fail. On the other hand, pyloroplasty is readily undertaken during transthoracic hiatus hernial repair when the operative exposure is extended into the left upper quadrant of the abdomen.

The operation

1

Position of patient

The patient is placed in the right lateral position with 45° backward rotation. This enables the thoracic incision to be extended, should this prove necessary, across the costal margin and into the upper abdomen.

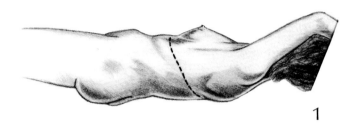

1

The incision

The left chest is opened through the bed of the left sixth rib. Rib resection or rib division is usually unnecessary. The exposure enables adequate mobilization of the oesophagus to be undertaken and gives an excellent view of the cardia and subdiaphragmatic structures. Furthermore, this incision is readily extended across the costal margin to enter the upper abdomen, such extension being required when pyloroplasty is undertaken, or should reduction of the hernia prove impossible and resection be necessary.

The left lung is retracted upwards and forwards by an assistant and the diaphragm is retracted downwards. The oesophagus, cardia and diaphragm are thus exposed.

2

The lateral pulmonary ligament is divided and the oesophagus is dissected from its bed, ligating and dividing the aortic branches to the oesophagus as high as the aortic arch. The oesophagus is dissected with the left vagus nerve, which is readily palpated posteriorly, and the oesophagus is encircled by a rubber sling.

The pleura at the junction between the oesophagus and cardia is incised circumferentially and by gentle traction on the rubber sling the hernia is drawn into the chest. Incision of the phreno-oesophageal ligament, the extraperitoneal fat and the lesser sac of the peritoneum anteriorly enables the cardia to be freed in its entirety apart from musculovascular connections posteriorly. The latter contain arterial branches to the lower oesophagus from the inferior phrenic and left gastric arteries which must be carefully divided and tied.

Following complete mobilization of the lower oesophagus and cardia, a trial of reduction is then undertaken by reducing the cardia into the abdomen as far as possible. In the majority of instances, this is readily accomplished but in patients with chronic and severe oesophagitis, or oesophageal fibrosis, shortening of the oesophagus may be so marked that reduction is impossible despite adequate mobilization. This situation must be recognized, for attempting hernial repair in these circumstances will result

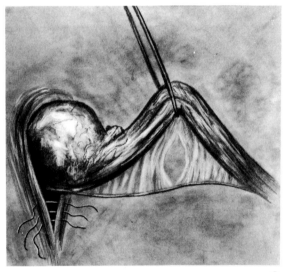

2

in the persistence of symptoms and possible formation of strictures. In these patients, resection of the lower oesophagus with short segment colon interposition should be undertaken. Oesophagogastrectomy is employed as a last resort in patients in whom colonic interposition is not possible for anatomical reasons and in the elderly, for the exchange of a natural hiatus hernia for a man-made hiatus hernia is followed in many cases by stricture formation some years postoperatively. Oesophagogastrectomy is an operation best reserved as a palliative procedure in carcinoma and is to be avoided in patients with benign conditions.

3

When it is clear that satisfactory reduction is possible, the operation is continued. The pad of fat which occupies the angle between the oesophagus and gastric fundus must be carefully removed, preserving the right vagus nerve which runs close to the stomach and oesophagus in this situation.

The gastro-oesophageal hiatus usually requires narrowing and the sutures for this procedure are placed at this stage of the operation but are not tied. Traction on the oesophageal sling holds the stomach and lower oesophagus forwards, and exposes the crura. Three or four linen sutures are placed and held by artery forceps, and these are to be tied later (see *Illustrations 2* and *3*).

Sutures are now placed at the cardia. The aim of these is twofold: to restore the acute angle of entry of the oesophagus into the stomach (see cut away in *Illustration 5*); and to ensure the reduction into the abdomen of an adequate length (5 cm) of intra-abdominal oesophagus.

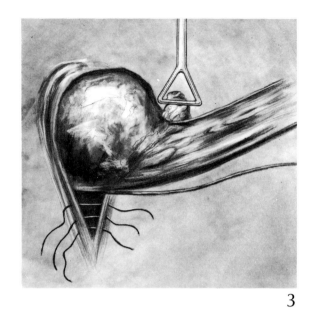

3

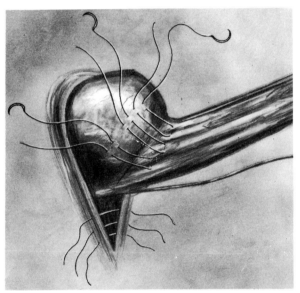

4

4, 5 & 6

First layer

Mattress sutures are taken from the stomach to the oesophagus. These linen thread sutures pick up and secure the stomach wall 2 cm below the cardia and the oesophagus at the cardia. Although the bites should not be too superficial, care must be taken to avoid penetrating the full thickness of the oesophagus. Usually three or four such sutures are required and when these are tied the stomach embraces the lower oesophagus. Encircling the oesophagus with the stomach should be resisted for this has been shown to interfere with the mechanism of belching and may cause dysphagia. The ideal result is achieved by wrapping the oesophagus with the stomach over three-quarters of a circle (270°).

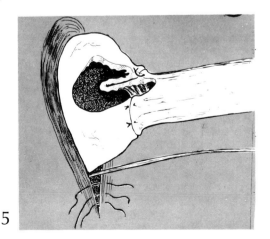

5

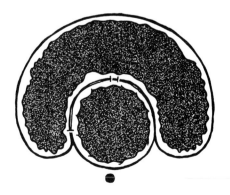

6

Second layer

7

The second layer of sutures enters the lower oesophagus and stomach and attaches this to the underside of the diaphragm 4 cm away from the hiatus which ensures reduction and fixation of the hernia. The diaphragmatic sutures are inserted with the aid of a spoon introduced through the hiatus from above (Belsey). This spoon ensures the safe passage of the sutures through the diaphragm whilst subdiaphragmatic structures are safely displaced. Again, three or four sutures are placed, entering the diaphragm from above, the stomach 3 cm below the first row, and then the oesophagus, returning to the stomach and emerging again through the diaphragm.

Gentle traction on this row of sutures reduces the hernia and when these sutures are tied, fixation is complete. Adequate mobilization of the oesophagus and preparation of the cardia will result in a tension-free reduction and in these circumstances the oesophagus will be lax and freely movable. Should the oesophagus be as tight as a bow string the scene is set for postoperative recurrence and further mobilization of the oesophagus is necessary.

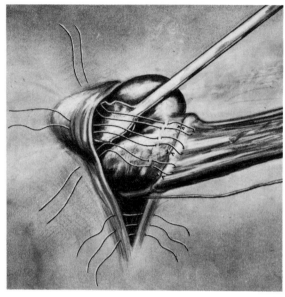

7

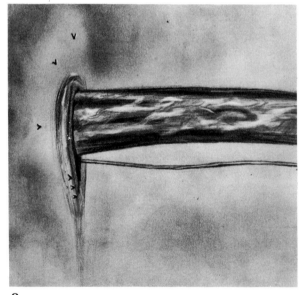

8

8

The previously placed crural stitches are now tied, commencing with the most posterior. Tight closure of the hiatus should be avoided, as food needs to pass through the oesophagus. The sutures should be tied in order until the hiatus posterior to the oesophagus will take the first digit of the surgeon's forefinger and will have the feel of an anal sphincter.

The chest is closed with drainage. The passage of a nasogastric tube is unnecessary. Indeed, the presence of such a tube in the presence of oesophagitis may predispose to ulceration and stricture formation.

It is usually possible to remove the intercostal drainage tube on the first postoperative day, following which the patient is mobilized. Fluids by mouth are allowed after 24 h if bowel sounds are present, gradually progressing to free fluids and a light diet over the subsequent 2 days.

Postoperative results

A barium swallow after a correctly performed operation should demonstrate the intra-abdominal segment of oesophagus. If this is not seen it is likely that the antireflux repair has been unsuccessful. However, in the majority of patients a 4 cm segment of intra-abdominal oesophagus will be restored. In these patients an early postoperative acid reflux test or 24 h pH monitoring will demonstrate the repair to be highly effective. Pressure studies will also demonstrate a considerable rise in pressure of the distal high pressure zone[1]. In 1972 Orringer, Skinner and Belsey[2] undertook a 10 year follow-up study on 892 patients who had undergone transthoracic repair of hiatus hernia by this technique between the years 1955 and 1965. Follow-up was complete in 86 per cent of cases and 94 per cent were followed for more than 3 years. The operative mortality was 1 per cent and the overall recurrence rate was 11 per cent. The recurrence rate in patients followed from 3 to 10 years was 12 per cent, and 7 per cent in patients followed for more than 10 years; 84 per cent of patients had excellent or good results from operation at their last follow-up evaluation and it was found that most clinical recurrences occurred within 5 years of the operation.

The operation is readily taught to resident staff but this investigation clearly demonstrated that improved long-term results were associated, as is to be expected, with that group of operations undertaken by experienced surgeons. It was found that the recurrence rates for the consultant and trainees were 5.9 per cent and 14.6 per cent respectively. The type of hiatus hernia and the degree of oesophagitis in the absence of shortening did not significantly influence results. However, this operation failed in 45 per cent (9 of 20) of patients with severe oesophagitis and stricture and the recurrence rate in children (20 per cent) was twice that in adults.

The management of the 98 patients in this series who had very unsatisfactory surgical results was medical in 32 and surgical in 45; 21 of these patients either required no treatment or declined treatment; 24 of 33 patients who had a second transthoracic repair and 8 of 9 patients who required stricture resection had good or excellent results, an overall success rate of 75 per cent.

The long-term evaluation of this operation for the treatment of hiatus hernia has demonstrated the value of this procedure in treating gastro-oesophageal reflux and its complications but emphasizes that to obtain consistently good results it is necessary for the surgeon to be experienced in the procedure.

Acknowledgement

The opinions and operation described here are based on the philosophy and teaching of R. H. Belsey at Frenchay Hospital, to whom the author is indebted.

References

1. Demeester, T. R., Johnson, L. F., Joseph, G. J., Toscano, M. S., Hall, A. W., Skinner, D. B. Patterns of gastro-oesophageal reflux in health and disease. Annals of Surgery 1976, 184: 459–470

2. Orringer, M. B., Skinner, D. B., Belsey, R. H. R. Long-term results of the Mark IV operation for hiatal hernia and analyses of recurrences and their treatment. Journal of Thoracic and Cardiovascular Surgery 1972; 63: 25–33

Further reading

Fyke, F. E., Code, C. F., Schlegel, J. F. The gastroesophageal sphincter in healthy human beings. Gastroenterologia 1956; 86: 135–150

Hiebert, C. A., Belsey, R. Incompetency of the gastric cardia without radiologic evidence of hiatal hernia. The diagnosis and management of 71 cases. Journal of Thoracic and Cardiovascular Surgery 1961; 42: 352–362

Johnson, L. F., Demeester, T. R. Twenty-four hour pH monitoring of the distal oesophagus: a quantitative measure of gastroesophageal reflux. American Journal of Gastroenterology 1974; 62: 325–332

Skinner, D. B. Hiatal hernia. In: Keen, G., ed. Operative surgery and management. Bristol: John Wright & Sons, 1981

Skinner, D. B., Belsey, R. H. R. Surgical management of oesophageal reflux and hiatus hernia: long-term results with 13 000 patients. Journal of Thoracic and Cardiovascular Surgery 1967; 53: 33–54

Skinner, D. B., Booth, D. J. Assessment of distal esophageal function in patients with hiatal hernia and/or gastroesophageal reflux. Annals of Surgery 1970; 172: 627–637

Illustrations by Charles Wood

Surgical management of hiatus hernia and complications of gastro-oesophageal reflux

Lucius D. Hill MD
Head, Section of General, Thoracoesophageal and Vascular Surgery,
Virginia Mason Medical Center, Seattle, Washington, USA

Colin O. H. Russell FRACS
Prince Henry's Hospital, Melbourne, Australia

Nicolas Velasco MD
Virginia Mason Medical Center, Seattle, Washington, USA

Kjell Thor MD, PhD
Associate Professor of Surgery, Karolinska Institute,
Ersta Hospital, Stockholm, Sweden

Introduction

Once considered a rarity, gastro-oesophageal reflux, with or without a hiatus hernia, is now recognized as the most common clinical abnormality of the upper gastrointestinal tract.

Since the symptoms of the disease may vary, indication for surgery must be clearly defined in relation to the patient's overall physical well-being, otherwise a large number of needless operations will be performed and this type of surgery will have a bad reputation.

With the development of precise methods of gastro-oesophageal pH and manometric measurements, our understanding of the pathophysiology of hiatus hernia has been enhanced, enabling us to define strict indications as well as a coherent rationale for corrective surgery. The surgeon has been challenged by gastroenterologists who state that the intrinsic defect in hiatus hernia with reflux cannot be changed. These workers state that the underlying abnormality in hiatus hernia is an abnormal gastro-oesophageal sphincter which is incompetent and does not respond to neural or humoral stimulation, thus permitting reflux. Reflux is presumed to lead to spasm and shortening of the oesophagus which pulls the gastro-oesophageal junction cephalad, creating the common sliding hiatus hernia. However, by careful manometric and pH measurements, before, during and after surgery, the surgeon can demonstrate that the sphincter is not abnormal and that when it is placed in its subdiaphragmatic position, both normal anatomy and function can be restored.

Preoperative

Indications

The corrective procedure is not to be undertaken lightly and strict indications for surgery must be observed. Bleeding oesophagitis, oesophageal ulceration and oesophageal stricture as the result of reflux are unequivocal indications for surgery. The patient with uncomplicated reflux oesophagitis should be evaluated in the usual manner after which a trial of intensive medical therapy under the direction of an interested physician or gastroenterologist is warranted. Symptomatic control and objective improvement in oesophagitis can often be obtained. However, it has been clearly shown[1], with careful measurement of lower oesophageal sphincter pressure and reflux, that after 1 year of continued medical treatment there was no change in the underlying disease. Overflow of gastric contents in the tracheobronchial tree is an important and often overlooked indication for surgery. Repeated nocturnal overflow can be elicited by careful history in 20–30 per cent of patients with reflux and can lead to severe chronic obstructive pulmonary disease and even to lung abscess.

In addition to the reflux problems already listed, a small group of patients require surgery to correct pressure symptoms and cardiorespiratory embarrassment secondary to organ displacement. Incarceration and subsequent ulceration or bleeding can occur in large hiatus hernias as well as in paraoesophageal hernias. Another group of patients has an incompetent gastro-oesophageal junction with reflux without demonstrable hiatus hernia.

In our own series, 9 per cent of patients required abdominal surgery for other indications including cholelithiasis, peptic ulcer disease and diverticulitis. In these, a careful preoperative history revealed reflux symptoms, and preoperative pressure manometry and reflux determinations were performed. With confirmation of significant reflux, an effective antireflux procedure was performed as part of the necessary surgical treatment.

Preoperative evaluation

The usual careful history and physical examination is performed with attention focused on the problems already listed. The standard contrast X-ray evaluation follows with emphasis on observation of free and induced reflux. Endoscopic evaluation of patients with reflux oesophagitis is mandatory, especially if surgery is considered. It is also important to rule out oesophageal cancer or other diseases in the stomach and duodenum. At endoscopy, hiatal hernia can be observed with erythema, friability, erosions, exudates, ulceration, stricture, or columnar-lined oesophagus (Barrett's oesophagus). If endoscopy with biopsy is used together with careful evaluation of symptoms and barium study, one can establish the correct diagnosis in most cases.

In our laboratory, pre- and postoperative measurement of lower oesophageal sphincter pressure (LOSP) and simultaneous pH began in 1956 and we have examined 16 000 patients with a variety of oesophageal disorders by this method. It has been found that an LOSP of less than 9 mmHg generally indicates incompetence whereas a pressure of 30 mmHg or greater indicates a hypertensive sphincter. Swallow waves are observed with a triple lumen manometric tube and motility abnormalities are noted. After a standard acid load has been administered through a stomach tube, the pH electrode is utilized to determine the presence of spontaneous reflux in upright and supine positions. Induced reflux is then sought by standard manoeuvres. This simple and safe technique not only can detect the presence of reflux more accurately than X-ray examination but also give the surgeon a clear indication of the level of the lower oesophageal sphincter pressure. With this kind of objective data, the surgeon can then demonstrate whether or not the underlying abnormality has been altered by surgical manoeuvres.

Another method with high sensitivity and specificity is ambulatory 24-hour pH monitoring. The collected data is analysed by computer which gives us all the relevant data in print and graphically within minutes. Other methods such as the Bernstein test, the standard acid reflux test, the acid clearing test are used but in our hands clinical history with physical examination, endoscopy with biopsy, and pressure measurements with ambulatory 24-hour pH measurements provide the surgeon with the information needed for operation.

Radionuclide transit (RT) is currently being employed at the Virginia Mason Medical Center, Seattle as a preoperative screening test for oesophageal dysfunction. In a recent study 10 normal volunteers and 30 subjects with dysphagia not related to mechanical obstruction were studied by this technique. RT studies detected a higher incidence of oesophageal motor abnormality than manometry or radiology in the dysphagia group. In addition, a definitive description of the functional problem was possible in most cases. RT is a safe non-invasive test and suitable as a screening test for oesophageal motor disorders[2].

Rationale for surgery

The primary objectives of surgical repair of hiatus hernia are the prevention of recurrence and the elimination of gastro-oesophageal reflux by a procedure that can be performed with technical ease and low morbidity and mortality. In order to fulfill these objectives, the surgeon must understand the normal anatomy of the gastro-oesophageal junction. Cadaver dissections have demonstrated that the oesophagus is anchored primarily posteriorly to the preaortic fascia by a dense plate of fibroelastic tissue. Anteriorly, its attachments to the oesophageal hiatus are loose, allowing the diaphragm to move freely in relationship to the oesophagus during its respiratory excursions. It is this loose anterior attachment which allows the sphincter to open and close in response to deglutition. Attenuation or lengthening of the posterior phreno-oesophageal plate allows the sphincter mechanism to slide cephalad in the posterior mediastinum. This visceral displacement of the oesophageal hiatus leads to reflux.

With these anatomical relationships in mind, the median arcuate posterior gastropexy was designed. This procedure, in conjunction with intraoperative manometry, can precisely calibrate the lower oesophageal sphincter mechanism and ensure consistent and lasting results.

The operation

1

A left paramedian incision is made beginning high up in the notch between the xiphoid and left costal margin. If the costal margin is narrow or the xiphoid is large, exposure is enhanced by removal of the xiphoid. The upper hand retractor is used to improve exposure of the upper abdominal contents.

The abdomen is thoroughly explored with careful attention to palpation and invagination of the pylorus as any obstruction here may, if not corrected, compromise the repair. The left triangular ligament is then divided, allowing the left lobe of the liver to be reflected out of the operative field to the patient's right. This uncovers the phreno-oesophageal membrane and the oesophageal hiatus.

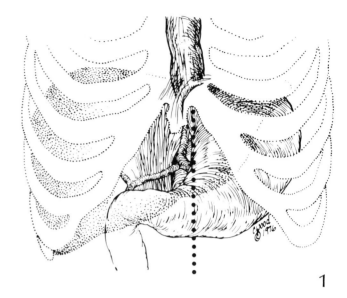

2

At this point, before disturbing the pathological anatomy, a measurement of the lower oesophageal sphincter pressure is obtained with the aid of a calibrated manometric tube attached to the usual plastic nasogastric tube. This tube, which is placed preoperatively, contains a side hole 12 cm from the tip and is connected to a unit which contains a constant-flow infusion pump, a pressure transducer and a graphic recorder. With the surgeon monitoring the position of the tube, the side hole is slowly passed across the gastro-oesophageal junction while the tube position and corresponding pressure is recorded. Three measurements are taken of the lower oesophageal sphincter pressure and the mean recorded is a prerepair sphincter pressure.

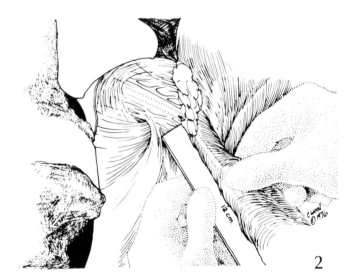

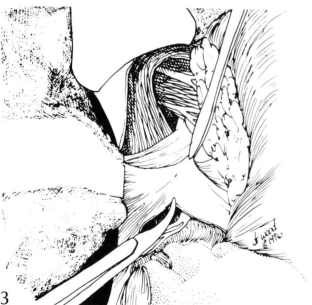

3

The phreno-oesophageal membrane and the peritoneum of the lesser sac are divided. This manoeuvre exposes the underlying preaortic fascia as well as the attenuated posterior phreno-oesophageal bundle.

4

The phreno-oesophageal membrane attaching the greater curvature to the diaphragm is then divided. Great care should be taken to divide the peritoneum on the diaphragm in order to preserve the phreno-oesophageal bundles. The stomach is further mobilized by ligating one or two short gastric vessels. Rarely, the spleen may be densely adherent to the greater curvature and may require removal to provide adequate mobilization, but the spleen should be preserved if at all possible. The stomach may now be rotated to facilitate exposure of the attenuated posterior phreno-oesophageal attachments. These may now be divided and the oesophagus mobilized by blunt and sharp dissection.

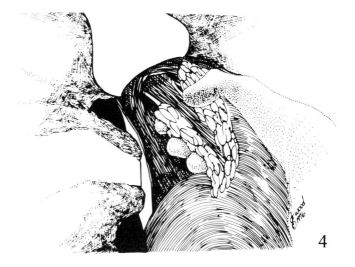

4

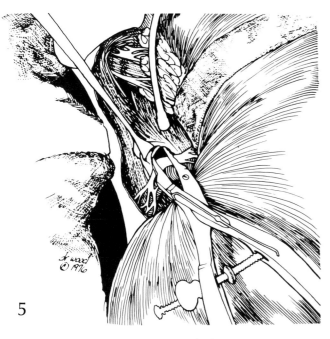

5

5

The stomach is then retracted to the patient's left, exposing the preaortic fascia. The aorta, coeliac axis and overlying coeliac nerve plexus are identified by palpation. By depressing these structures posteriorly, the surgeon can readily palpate the overlying band of dense fibres comprising the median arcuate ligament. This ligament is then defined by dissecting away the surrounding fibroareolar tissue and the coeliac ganglion is retracted caudally; the midline plane is developed. A diaphragmatic artery usually arises from each side of the coeliac axis and travels cephalad to its respective crus. Care must be taken to stay in the midline and to avoid vigorous dissection as avulsion of one of the branches will lead to troublesome bleeding. If encountered, haemorrhage may be controlled by pressure or careful arterial suture techniques to avoid compromising the lumen of the coeliac trunk.

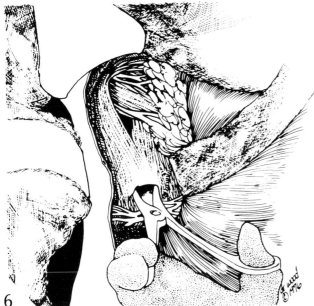

6

6

The median arcuate ligament is then elevated from the coeliac axis and a Goodell cervical dilator is placed beneath it and passed cephalad. No resistance to the passage of this instrument is encountered if the instrument is in the correct plane. If resistance is encountered, further dissection to identify the coeliac artery and the median arcuate ligament is essential.

7

The crura of the oesophageal hiatus are then loosely approximated by heavy mattress sutures taken widely so that fascia propria and peritoneum are included to lend strength to the closure. These sutures must be tied gently so that a finger can be easily placed alongside the oesophagus and the oesophageal hiatus. A tight hiatal closure neither aids in preventing recurrence nor does it help to eliminate reflux and may contribute to postoperative dysphagia.

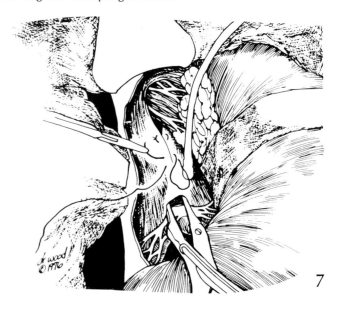

7

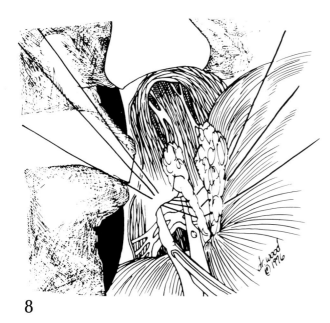

8

8

Four or more sutures are then placed which serve both to imbricate the phreno-oesophageal bundle and to anchor the gastro-oesophageal junction. These are passed deeply through the anterior and posterior phreno-oesophageal bundles while keeping the vagal trunks under direct vision to avoid including them. The sutures are then passed through the median arcuate ligament and preaortic fascia.

The most cephalad of these is referred to as the key suture as the tension applied to this suture is mainly responsible for proper calibration of the lower oesophageal sphincter pressure. A suture cephalad to the key suture is usually placed simply to imbricate further or to bring together the phreno-oesophageal bundle and support the lower oesophageal sphincter.

9

The initial imbricating suture and the key suture are then tied with two slip knots to allow adjustment. The lower oesophageal sphincter pressure is then measured by passing the side hole of the pressure tube across the gastro-oesophageal junction. The distance from the tip of the tube to the side hole is 12 cm and is carefully measured with the use of a ruler. If the mean pressure is between 50 and 55 mmHg the imbricating and key suture are secured by placing further ties in the suture, the remaining sutures are tied and the final measurement is obtained. If the lower oesophageal sphincter pressure is less than 50 mmHg, the key suture and imbricating suture are tightened, and if necessary an additional imbricating suture is taken, including more of the seromuscular layer of the wall of the stomach. If the lower oesophageal sphincter pressure is over 58 mmHg, the key suture is loosened slightly. A mean intraoperative lower oesophageal sphincter pressure of 50–55 mmHg is ideal and post repair will yield a postoperative pressure of 20–25 mmHg.

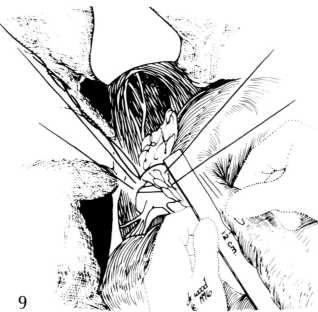

9

10

Upon completion of the repair the introitus of the oesophagus can easily be palpated along the nasogastric tube and should admit a fingertip. The flap valve arrangement can also be palpated.

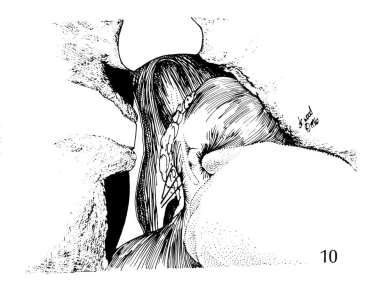

10

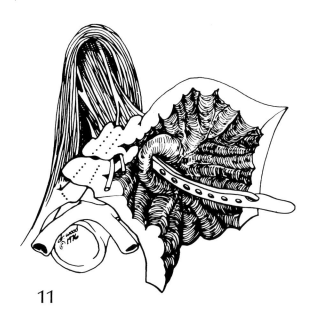

11

11

This cutaway diagram demonstrates the anatomy of the complete repair. The flap valve that has been reconstructed is shown as if viewed through a gastrotomy. From this, it can be seen that increase in intragastric pressure will serve to close the flap valve and raise the oesophageal sphincter pressure which will assist in correction of reflux.

Recurrent hernia

The experience at this institution, with various types of recurrent hernia, involves 209 referred patients. Some of these patients have had as many as five previous operations, both transthoracic and transabdominal. In these, the takedown of the previous operations may be exceedingly difficult. Rarely a thoracoabdominal approach using a counterincision in the chest may be required. After the takedown of the previous repair, we have been successful in all but two patients in performing the median arcuate gastropexy. In only two patients, in whom the distal oesophagus had actually been destroyed by perforation or by a Heller-type procedure, the imbrication of the introitus of the oesophagus was done in the thorax. Whenever possible, it is felt important to fix the oesophagus in its normal subdiaphragmatic position. Recent studies on patients who have had Nissen procedures and been referred for repair of recurrent hernias, have shown that these patients without normal fixation of the oesophagus below the diaphragm have a serious motility disorder because the musculature of the oesophagus is not attached distally. Poorly coordinated swallow waves similar to those seen in the small bowel propel portions of the oesophageal contents in both cephalad and caudad directions simultaneously. Once the oesophagus is returned to its normal subdiaphragmatic position, this motility disturbance is corrected. The results with the median arcuate posterior gastropexy in recurrent hernia have been good in 88 per cent of cases.

In a recent study done in Seattle, 25 failed Nissen operations were reported and a method of classifying the type of failure presented[3]. Manometric studies documented disordered motor activity in 10 of these patients with return to normal activity after rerepair. With these difficult patients, intraoperative manometrics allowed a satisfactory antireflux barrier to be created with posterior gastropexy. Good to excellent results were achieved in 22 of 24 patients.

The mortality rate and failure rate in repair of recurrent hernias is understandably higher than in primary hernias, indicating that the optimum time to correct the hiatus hernia is at the first operation.

Oesophageal stricture

In the presence of reflux strictures, even with penetrating ulcers and transmural involvement, we have been able by careful manometric determination to locate the sphincter distal to the level of the stricture. In our experience, the strictures occur at the squamocolumnar junction. By careful freeing of the oesophagus by blunt and sharp dissection we have been able to bring the sphincter down to its normal location below the diaphragm in all 177 patients. Shortening of the oesophagus has not been apparent.

With the correction of reflux, strictures with penetrating ulcers and transmural involvement have cleared within 2–3 months. These patients often require one to two dilatations postoperatively but with complete correction of reflux the oesophagus demonstrates a remarkable healing capacity and the strictures have cleared to the point that the patient is able to swallow all solid food. When the surgeon is faced with a purely reflux stricture, a simplified approach is to be recommended rather than an oesophageal resection with its increased mortality and morbidity.

Results

With the use of intraoperative manometrics in 514 patients, there are only 6 patients with symptomatic reflux in the 308 patients operated upon for primary hiatus hernia. An intraoperative pressure of only 30 mmHg was accepted in one of these patients as she was among the first done by this technique. With an intraoperative pressure of 45–55 mmHg there have been 4 recurrences of hernia or reflux. Reflux was corrected in all but 14 patients in this group. Of these 14 patients with reflux documented on postoperative pH and pressure study, 6 were primary hiatal hernias and they remain only mildly symptomatic. Of 84 patients with stricture and 107 patients with recurrent hiatus hernia, there are 8 patients with some degree of continued reflux (1 a recurrent hiatus hernia, 3 patients with stricture and 4 with recurrent hiatus hernias with stricture). This study indicates that sphincter competence was restored in this group of patients, thus confirming the work of Lipshutz et al.[4] which showed that an antireflux procedure can restore the resting lower oesophageal sphincter pressure and the ability of the sphincter to respond to neural and humoral stimuli.

References

1. Behar, J., Sheahan, D. G., Biancani, P., Spiro, H. M., Storer, E. H. Medical and surgical management of reflux esophagitis: a 38 month report on a prospective clinical trial. New England Journal of Medicine 1975; 293: 263–268

2. Russell, C. O. H., Hill, L. D., Holmes, E. R., Hull, D. A., Gannon, R. Pope, C. E., Radionuclide transit: a sensitive screening test for esophageal dysfunction. Gastroenterology 1981; 80: 887–892

3. Hill, L. D., Ilves, R., Stevenson, J. K., Pearson, J. M. Reoperation for disruption and recurrence after Nissen fundoplication. Archives of Surgery 1979; 114: 542–548

4. Lipshutz, W. H., Eckert, R. J., Gaskins, R. D., Blanton, D. E., Lukash, W. M., Normal lower esophageal sphincter function after surgical treatment of gastroesophageal reflux. New England Journal of Medicine 1974; 291: 1107–1110

Illustrations by P. Somerset

Nissen's fundoplication

A. H. K. Deiraniya FRCS
Consultant Cardiothoracic Surgeon, Wythenshawe Hospital, Manchester, UK

Introduction

Recognition of the role played by reflux in the causation of symptoms and pathological changes in patients with sliding hiatus hernia diverted attention away from the anatomical aspects of surgical repair of the hernia and emphasized the primary importance of the antireflux component of the operation.

Nissen's fundoplication[1,2] is most effective in abolishing reflux at the gastro-oesophageal junction, irrespective of whether it is carried out above or below the diaphragm. The success of intrathoracic fundoplication in controlling reflux undermined the long-held surgical belief that the presence of an intra-abdominal segment of the oesophagus was essential to gastro-oesophageal competence.

It is now well established that the vast majority of peptic strictures of the oesophagus can be managed successfully without the necessity for oesophageal resection and replacement once reflux at the gastro-oesophageal junction is abolished. Fundoplication alone, or in combination with a Collis gastroplasty[3], is now frequently used in the management of patients with peptic strictures of the oesophagus. A stricture that is easily dilatable endoscopically or retrogradely at operation will resolve in the vast majority of cases with fundoplication alone. Fibrous strictures associated with a short oesophagus require the addition of a Collis gastroplasty as in the combined Collis-Belsey operation pioneered by Pearson (*see* volume on *Cardiothoracic Surgery*, 3rd ed., p. 439), or preferably by the combined Collis-Nissen fundoplication. Fundoplication plays a dual role in the combined operation: it prevents reflux and provides added cover to potential sites of leakage.

The likelihood of reflux oesophagitis and its sequelae developing in patients following local resection of the oesophagus and gastro-oesophageal anastomosis or Heller's myotomy is considerably reduced by the addition of fundoplication.

Extensive mobilization of the oesophagus under direct vision allows the reduction of the cardia below the diaphragm in the vast majority of patients with sliding hiatus hernia and reflux. However, there remain a small number of patients in whom reduction is impossible owing to gross shortening of the oesophagus. The technical simplicity and reliability of the intrathoracic Nissen wrap in controlling reflux in this small group of patients led to its use by surgeons as an alternative to the more major operation of resection and/or replacement. However, in some patients the intrathoracic fundoplication is liable to the potentially lethal complication of rupture into the pleural cavity, pericardium or bronchial tree. Accordingly, intrathoracic fundoplication should be reserved for elderly and frail patients with severe reflux symptoms in whom the cardia cannot be placed below the diaphragm. A gastroplasty and intra-abdominal fundoplication is recommended for the remaining patients in that group.

History of operation

The first fundoplication was performed by Nissen in 1936[1] as an added protection against leakage from an oesophagogastric suture line in the course of a limited oesophageal resection for benign disease in a young man. The lower oesophagus was implanted into the anterior wall of the stomach, in the same fashion as the rubber tube is implanted in a Witzel's gastrostomy. The patient was noted to be free from reflux symptoms 16 years later, an observation which led Nissen to recognize the crucial role played by the gastric wrap-round in reflux control. In 1955 he added fundoplication to anterior gastropexy (Nissen I), then his operation of choice for sliding hiatus hernia. Shortly afterwards the combined operation was superseded by fundoplication alone (Nissen II)[2]. The operation soon gained widespread acceptance in Europe and America. Nissen performed the operation through a left subcostal incision and stated the aims of the operation as the elimination of the hernia, reduction of the cardia below the diaphragm, reconstruction of the oesophagogastric angle and the re-establishment of a valvular mechanism at the cardia.

Preoperative

Preoperative investigations

A thorough evaluation of the clinical and laboratory data as well as the results of radiological and endoscopic examination is essential for accurate diagnosis and management. The importance of ascertaining that symptoms are not due to other conditions cannot be overstated. The presence of associated diseases of the gall bladder, stomach or duodenum should be remembered and their contribution to the overall clinical picture assessed. Barium examination of the oesophagus, stomach and duodenum is routine in all cases and gives essential information concerning oesophageal motility and length and the reducibility or fixation of the hiatus hernia as well as its type. Furthermore, radiological studies will reveal the presence and location of a stricture and demonstrate the presence of gross gastro-oesophageal reflux and any associated lesions in the stomach or duodenum. A preoperative oesophagoscopy is mandatory as it will reveal the extent and severity of oesophagitis and allow dilatation and biopsy of stricture, as well as biopsy of any other suspicious area of oesophageal mucosa. Routine biopsy of grossly 'inflamed' oesophageal mucosa occasionally reveals unsuspected neoplasia and is recommended.

Indications for operation

The chief indication for operative treatment is the presence of severe symptoms of reflux unresponsive to medical treatment. Other indications for operative intervention are severe oesophagitis at oesophagoscopy, dysphagia due to stricture formation, bleeding, whether acute or chronic, and aspiration pneumonitis. All patients with paraoesophageal hiatus hernia who are acceptable operative risks should be advised to undergo operation in view of the unacceptably high risk of major complications associated with this type of hernia. The operation is inappropriate in patients with oesophageal motility disorders.

The operation

The operation can be performed using either an abdominal or transthoracic approach. The abdominal route may have some merit in patients with coexistent abdominal pathology. The thoracic approach is indicated in obese patients, in recurrent herniation, in patients with panoesophagitis and oesophageal shortening and where a suspicion of malignancy exists. Extensive oesophageal mobilization can be performed under direct vision using the thoracic approach, thus making it possible in the vast majority of patients to replace the gastro-oesophageal junction below the diaphragm without undue tension. Our preferred approach to be described later is thoraco-abdominal. This provides good access to both the chest and the upper abdomen, making it possible to carry out lower oesophageal and upper gastric resection with considerable ease. However, access to the duodenum and gall bladder through this incision is limited and can be improved by extending the incision across the costal margin into the left upper quadrant of the abdomen.

Anaesthesia

After induction, a double-lumen endotracheal tube is introduced. While the patient is still in the supine position a 40–50 Fr Maloney dilator is introduced into the upper oesophagus. The patient is then placed in the lateral decubitus position.

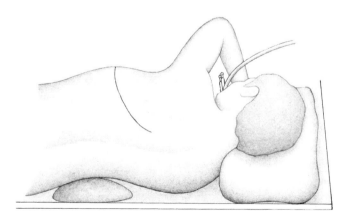

1

The incision

A standard posterolateral thoracotomy incision is made along the line of the eighth rib. The periosteum is incised with a fine diathermy needle from the sacrospinalis muscle at the back to the cartilage in front. The periosteum is stripped off the upper border using a curved raspatory and a small segment of the back end of the rib under the sacrospinalis muscle is removed with a costotome. The pleural cavity is entered by incising the rib bed. A Finochietto chest spreader is inserted and gradually opened to provide wide exposure. The anaesthetist is asked to deflate the left lung.

1

Mobilization of the oesophagus and hernia and diaphragmatic incision

2

The inferior pulmonary ligament is divided until the inferior pulmonary vein comes into view. The lung is retracted forwards and upwards. The posteromedial pleura overlying the oesophagus is incised. The oesophagus, with the vagus nerves attached to its wall, is encircled with a nylon tape and elevated from its bed by gentle traction. The lower oesophagus is mobilized upwards and downwards, dividing the oesophageal arterial branches between ligatures and carefully preserving the vagus nerves. The extent of the oesophageal mobilization necessary to effect reduction without tension depends on the presence or absence of perioesophagitis and the size of the hiatal hernia. Mobilization up to the level of the aortic arch is likely to be necessary in the presence of perioesophagitis and a large hernia. The oesophagus is mobilized downwards to the hernia or phreno-oesophageal ligament if no hernia is present. At the diaphragmatic level the crural fibres of the hiatal margin are displayed. The diaphragm is incised circumferentially through the muscular part, about 5 cm from its costal attachment, for a distance of 15 cm. The incision lies anterior to the phrenic nerve as it enters the diaphragm and extends backwards to well beyond the lateral extent of the spleen. It is important not to divide the diaphragm too close to the chest wall as it will make subsequent closure difficult. This type of incision preserves the nerve supply to the diaphragm and gives excellent access to the upper abdomen.

Two fingers of the left hand are passed through the incision in the diaphragm up through the hiatus to act as a guide while the phreno-oesophageal ligament and peri-

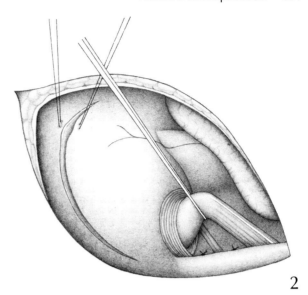

2

toneal reflection in front and on each side of the hernia are divided. Complete freeing of the cardia is achieved by division of the remaining connections posteriorly between clamps, as these contain significant arterial branches of the phrenic and gastric arteries. The fat pad overlying the gastro-oesophageal junction is completely removed as far laterally as the vagus nerves. The nylon tape round the oesophagus is passed through the hiatus into the abdomen.

3

Exposure of hiatal region and oesophagus from abdomen

The left triangular ligament is divided, taking care not to injure the inferior phrenic vein. The left lobe of the liver is retracted to the right. The upper part of the gastrohepatic omentum is divided between ligatures. This will bring into view the caudate lobe of the liver and, lying alongside it on the left, the right limb of the right crus of the diaphragm. The proximity of the inferior vena cava to this structure must be remembered. It lies immediately posterolateral to the right margin of the hiatus and can be injured if excessively deep bites are taken in the right limb of the crus.

The widened hiatus can now be narrowed using interrupted No. 1 silk sutures on a 45 mm atraumatic needle, taking generous, full-thickness bites of both margins of the hiatus and including the peritoneum. Before these sutures are tied the Maloney bougie, which had been previously introduced into the upper oesophagus, is passed into the stomach and the sutures tied sufficiently tightly to approximate the crura. Excessive tension while tying these sutures will result in strangulation of the crural muscle and cutting out of sutures. The reconstructed hiatus should have enough room to accommodate the oesophagus, with the indwelling bougie, and the tip of the index finger; otherwise, troublesome postoperative dysphagia may occur.

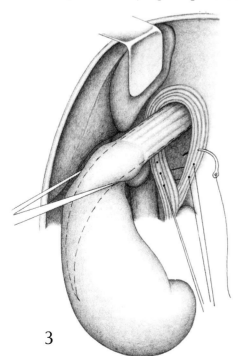

3

4

Fundoplication: stage 1

The fundus and the upper third of the greater curvature are completely mobilized by division of the vasa brevia, taking special care not to injure the spleen or to include any of the stomach wall in the ligatures. Any adhesions to the posterior wall of the proximal half of the stomach should be divided. After mobilization is complete the fundus is pushed, from the patient's left to right, behind and around the posterior wall of the terminal oesophagus until the edge of the fundal fold appears on the right side of the oesophagus. The edge of the fold is held in this position with Duval tissue forceps. Further gentle traction on the Duval forceps, aided by pushing with the surgeon's right hand, ensures that a good fold of fundus lies to the right of the oesophagus. At the conclusion of this manoeuvre there should be two stomach pouches, one on either side of the oesophagus.

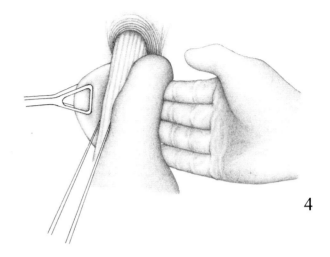

4

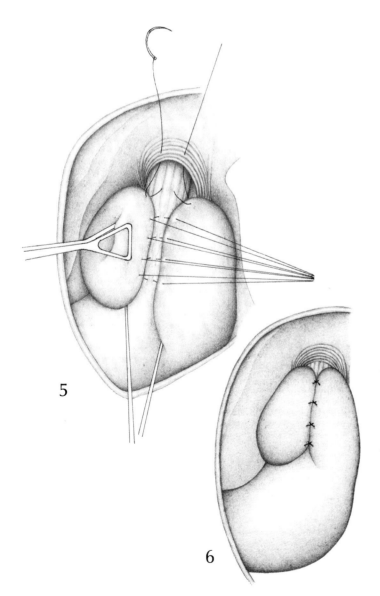

5

6

5 & 6

Fundoplication: stage 2

The pouches are brought together in front of the oesophagus by four or five interrupted 2/0 silk sutures, inserted at 1 cm intervals. The sutures pick up the seromuscular layer of the stomach pouch on either side and the muscle layer of the oesophagus in the middle. Extra care is taken to avoid penetration into the lumen of the oesophagus or stomach. (Fatalities have followed careless placement of these sutures.) All the sutures are put in before they are tied. The first and uppermost suture is a mattressed suture which passes first through the hiatal margins, then through one side of the stomach, the oesophagus, the other side of the fundus and then back through the hiatus. When all sutures have been placed they are tightened, while a finger is placed beneath the fundal cuff thus formed and alongside the oesophagus with its indwelling bougie to ensure that the calibre of the oesophageal lumen and space for expansion during swallowing is not compromised. Should the fundal wrap prove to be tight, the sutures are repositioned; otherwise they are tied with a bougie in position. Too tight a fundoplication will produce dysphagia and too lax a wrap will not restore competence. The Maloney bougie is now removed.

7

Closure of the diaphragm

Meticulous closure of the diaphragm is essential to prevent herniation. The diaphragm is closed with interrupted, figure-of-eight, silk sutures, placed so that every stitch takes up, in addition to muscle, the peritoneum and the diaphragmatic pleura. The chest is closed, leaving a basal drainage tube connected to an underwater seal.

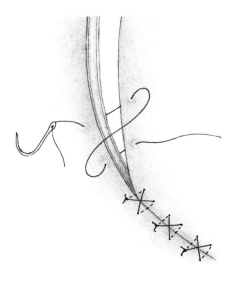

7

Postoperative care

Physiotherapy, instituted preoperatively, is continued in the postoperative period to prevent pulmonary atelectasis from sputum retention. The chest tube is usually removed within 24 hours, after a chest film has confirmed satisfactory expansion of the lungs. We have found the use of a nasogastric tube unnecessary. Fluids are commenced on the return of peristalsis, usually within 48 hours. In the early postoperative phase carbonated drinks are discouraged as they may produce gastric distension. The oral intake is progressively increased and patients are usually able to tolerate a normal diet within a week of operation. Transient dysphagia due to oedema at the cardia is encountered in a few patients. Venous thrombosis and pulmonary embolism pose a constant threat to patients after hiatus hernia repair, particularly if a concomitant splenectomy is necessitated by inadvertent injury of the spleen. Prophylactic measures, including early ambulation and minidose heparin anticoagulation, are advisable.

References

1. Nissen, R. Die Transpleurale Resektion der Kardia. Deutsche Zeitschrift für Chirurgie 1937; 249: 311–316

2. Nissen, R., Rossetti, M. Surgery of the cardia ventriculi. Ciba Symposium 1963; 11: 195–223

3. Orringer, M. B., Sloan, H. Combined Collis-Nissen reconstruction of the oesophagogastric junction. Annals of Thoracic Surgery 1978; 25: 16–21

Further reading

Mansour, K. A., Burton, H. G., Miller, J. I., Hatcher, C. R. Complications of intra-thoracic Nissen fundoplication. Annals of Thoracic Surgery 1981; 32: 173–178

Nicholson, D. A., Nohl-Oser, H. C. Hiatus hernia. a comparison between two methods of fundoplication by evaluation of the long-term results. Journal of Thoracic and Cardiovascular Surgery 1976; 72: 938–943

Rossetti, M. Allgöwer, M. Fundoplication for treatment of hiatal hernia. Progress in Surgery 1973; 12: 1–21

Reflux oesophagitis treated by gastroplasty

F. G. Pearson MD, FRCS(C), FACS
Professor of Surgery, University of Toronto;
Surgeon-in-Chief, Toronto General Hospital, Toronto, Ontario, Canada

History

The technique of gastroplasty was designed by Collis[1] in Great Britain and first reported in 1957. The operation is used in patients with acquired short oesophagus due to reflux oesophagitis, in whom a standard or simple antireflux repair may be inadequate. We subsequently described a modification of Collis' gastroplasty[2] using a transthoracic rather than thoracoabdominal approach, and partial fundoplication rather than Collis' own technique of repair. Still further modifications, such as the 'uncut gastroplasty'[3] and gastroplasty combined with complete fundoplication[4,5], have since been reported.

Preoperative

Indications

The commonest indication for the addition of gastroplasty is severe peptic oesophagitis with transmural inflammatory changes in the distal oesophagus leading to acquired shortening and frequently, although not always, associated stricture. In such patients, standard techniques of hiatal hernia repair may fail because the oesophagogastric junction cannot be restored to its intra-abdominal position without undue tension.

Assessment of acquired shortening

In cases of acquired shortening, the barium swallow will demonstrate an irreducible hernia when the patient is in the upright position. Preoperative oesophagoscopy, using the flexible instrument, is essential and will determine the level of the squamo-columnar interface, esophagogastric junction and diaphragmatic hiatus with reasonable accuracy. Some estimates of the presence and extent of shortening can be made from the level of the junction in relation to the diaphragmatic hiatus. An acquired columnar-lined segment of oesophagus is always an indication of prior ulcerative oesophagitis and is inevitably associated with some degree of shortening. Confluent peptic ulceration of the squamous epithelium and stricture are usually associated with panmural inflammation and shortening.

Dilatation of stricture

Most peptic strictures can be adequately dilated before operation. To restore normal swallowing, it is usually necessary to dilate the stricture with bougies of 50 Fr diameter or greater. In most cases, this can be accomplished with indirect dilatation using the taper-tipped, mercury-weighted Maloney bougies. However, severe strictures may initially require more forceful dilatation with Puestow or Savary dilators, or rigid oesophagoscopy with direct bouginage.

The operation

1

Exposure is obtained via a left posterolateral thoracotomy through the sixth intercostal space. The incision is carried well forward, to within a few centimetres of the diaphragmatic attachment at the anterior end of this interspace, in order to provide optimal access for dissection at the level of the diaphragmatic hiatus and for application of the GIA stapler for construction of the gastric tube.

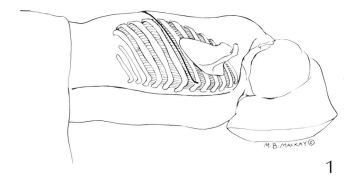

1

2

With the left hemithorax open, the inferior pulmonary ligament is divided and the left lung retracted antero-superiorly to expose the posterior mediastinum. Use of a double-lumen endotracheal tube or left endobronchial blocker permits collapse of the left lung, which facilitates exposure.

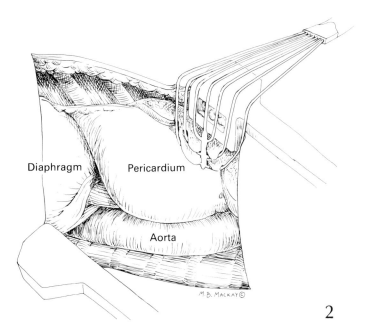

2

3

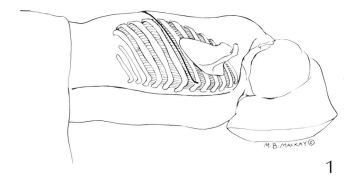

3

The mediastinal pleura is incised and the oesophagus mobilized circumferentially from the level of the diaphragmatic hiatus to the pulmonary hilum above the level of the inferior pulmonary vein. At the outset of this mobilization, both vagus nerves (LVN and RVN) are identified. They are carried with the mobilized oesophagus and carefully preserved throughout the remainder of the operation. Elevation of the oesophagus from its mediastinal bed exposes the pleura covering the right lung. The diaphragmatic reflection of the right pleura is often close to the posterior margin of the oesophageal hiatus and can be displaced by blunt dissection in order to avoid entry into the right pleural space.

4

The margins of the oesophageal hiatus are circumferentially freed by sharp dissection, the greater peritoneal sac is opened anteriorly and, the lesser sac posteriorly, and the upper part of the gastrohepatic omentum is divided. This dissection allows the cardia and fundus of the stomach to be elevated freely into the left hemithorax. Adequate mobilization of the greater curvature side of the stomach does not require division of any short gastric vessels.

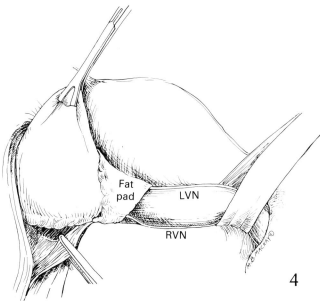

4

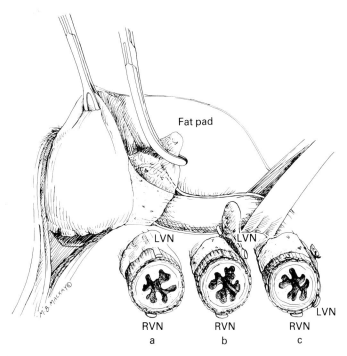

5

5

There is always a collection of fat lying between the upper and lower limbs of the phreno-oesophageal membrane which envelops the oesophagogstric junction (a). This fat pad is meticulously dissected from most of the circumference of the oesophagogastric junction. With this dissection, the left vagus nerve (LVN) is lifted free from the muscular wall of the oesophagus and carried with the fat pad (b). The fatty tissue is cleared away from the entire anterior surface of the oesophagogastric junction and adjacent upper part of the lesser curvature. The dissection is tedious and requires coagulation or ligation of many small penetrating vessels similar to the technique of highly selective vagotomy. The gastric tube can then be constructed through an area of stomach which is free of any fatty covering. This dissection results in displacement of the left vagus nerve to a more posterior location (c) close to the right vagus nerve (RVN).

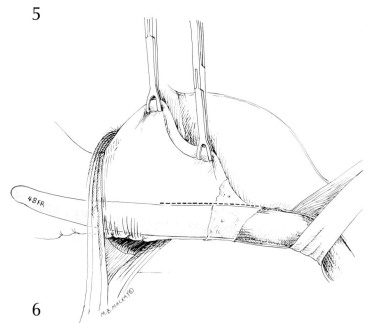

6

6

A 48 Fr Maloney bougie is then passed via the mouth through the oesophagus and well into the stomach beyond. The interrupted line indicates the proposed line of division of the gastric wall in order to create a gastric tube in continuity with the distal oesophagus.

7

The stomach is now divided with the GIA stapler. Alternatively, it may be divided between two obtuse-angled clamps. The length of gastric tube to be created depends on the degree of acquired shortening. A 5 cm long gastric tube is sufficient in the majority of cases and can be accomplished with a single application of the GIA stapler. Traction is exerted on the greater curvature side of the gastric fundus before closing the jaws of the stapler in order to ensure that the gastric tube closely approximates the diameter of the indwelling 48 Fr bougie throughout its length. The length and diameter of the newly created gastric tube significantly affect the antireflux properties of the repair: the smaller the tube diameter, the higher the intraluminal pressure created. These effects on pressure have been studied by both intra- and postoperative manometry[7].

The GIA stapler may prove awkward to apply through this sixth left interspace exposure, and precise application is most easily accomplished when the oesophagus and the oesophagogastric junction are firmly elevated from the mediastinal bed by traction on the stomach and the Penrose drain which encircles the mobilized thoracic oesophagus.

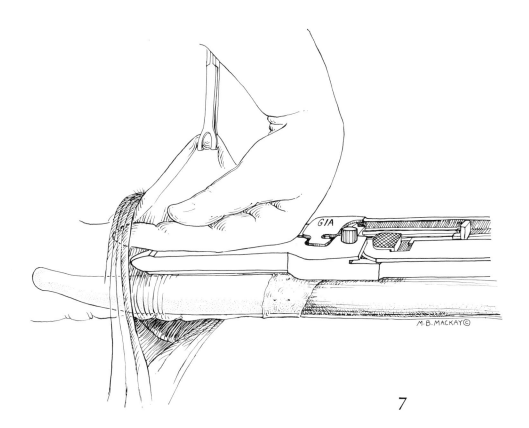

7

8

The GIA stapler drives a double row of staggered staples on each side of the divided gastric wall. The oesophageal side of the newly formed gastric tube is reinforced with a running suture of 3/0 chromic catgut. This staple line is not invaginated, since invagination might further decrease the diameter of the gastric tube.

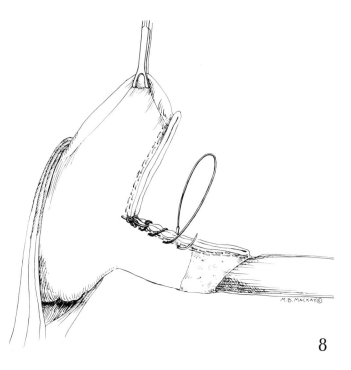

8

9

The gastric side of the staple line is invaginated with a running suture of 3/0 chromic catgut. This will obliterate the 'dog ear' of stomach (arrow) which is created at the gastric end of this staple line.

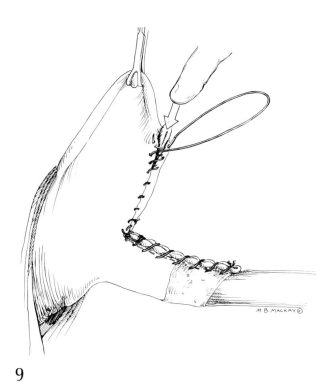

9

10

Interrupted sutures of No. 1 silk are then placed through the crural margins of the hiatus, but are not tied at this stage of the operation. The sutures in the right limb of the crus are more widely spaced than those in the left limb. The most anterior of these crural sutures should include the edge of a stout tendonous diaphragmatic band which is present in this anterior part of the right limb.

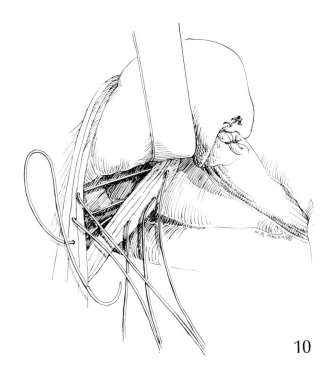

10

11

Using 3/0 silk sutures and double-ended needles, the fundoplication is now begun. This will partially wrap the distal 4–5 cm of the gastric tube with the adjacent gastric fundus. In the illustration, the first of three tiers of fundoplicating sutures has been placed. Three horizontal mattress sutures are used for each tier and the sutures are placed so as to produce a 270° fundoplication.

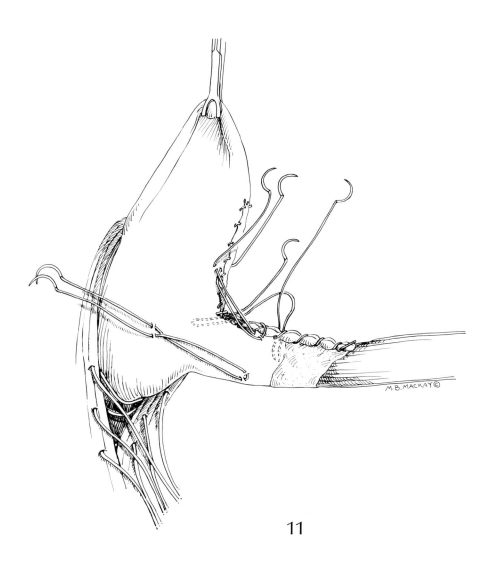

11

12a, b & c

The three stages of fundoplication are shown. The first tier of sutures has been placed but not tied (a). The first tier has been tied and the second tier has been placed but not tied (b). The first two tiers are tied, and the third and final tier of three sutures has been placed (c). The distance between tiers is 1.5–2 cm.

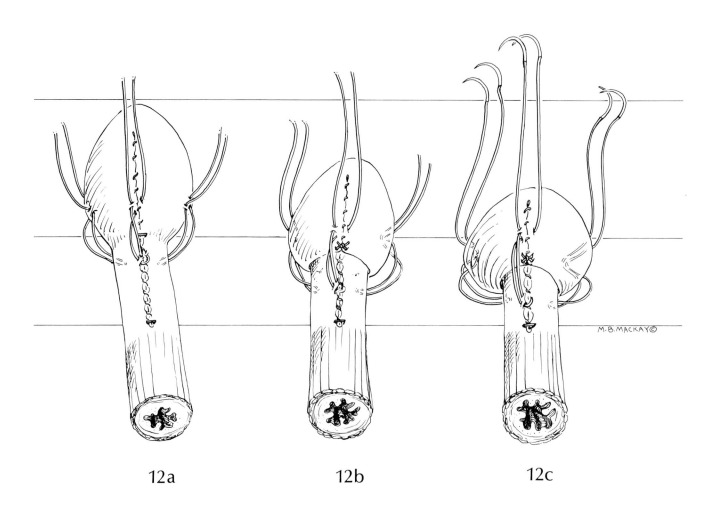

12a   12b   12c

13

This projection of the fundoplication shows the final tier of three fundoplicating sutures placed in the wall of the gastric tube and in the adjacent gastric fundus.

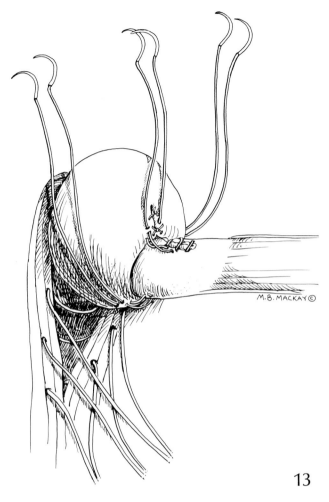

13

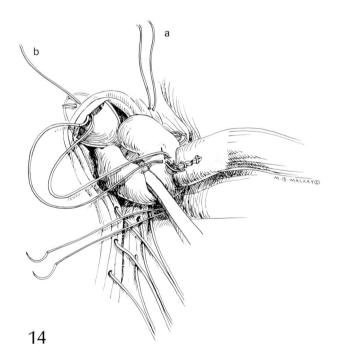

14

14

A spoon is placed in the anterior opening of the hiatus to facilitate passage of the last tier of fundoplicating sutures. These sutures are directed through the hiatus and then brought back up through the diaphragmatic margin from the abdominal to the thoracic side. In this illustration, both ends of the fundoplicating suture on the right side have been passed in this fashion but not tied. This suture is passed through the diaphragm just to the right of the anterior 'apex' of the hiatus (a). The middle suture is in the process of being placed just to the left of the 'apex' of the hiatus (b). These three sutures are spaced apart in the diaphragmatic margin by the same distances that separate them on the circumference of the gastric tube or oesophageal wall.

15

The gastric tube and fundoplication have been reduced in the abdomen and the last tier of three fundoplicating sutures has been tied. Between 4 and 5 cm of gastric tube or 'neo-oesophagus' now lie in the intra-abdominal position and are secured to the abdominal side of the diaphragmatic hiatus without tension on the intrathoracic oesophagus or the antireflux repair.

The No. 1 silk sutures in the posterior crura are then tied to reduce the size of the diaphragmatic hiatus.

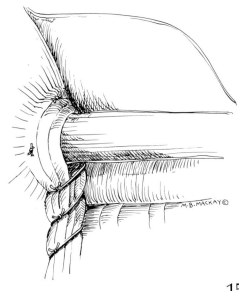

15

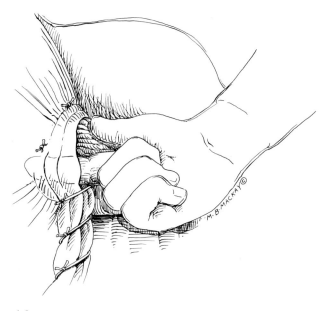

16

16

The diaphragmatic hiatus is closed relatively loosely. It should be easy to slip the index finger through the narrowed hiatus behind and alongside the oesophagus and gastric tube. The incision is then closed and the left pleural space vented with a single No. 28 intercostal drain.

Postoperative care

Prophylactic antibiotics are given. A suitable cephalosporin (e.g. cephazolin 1 g) is administered intravenously at the time of anaesthetic induction and a second dose is given in the recovery room 4 hours later. The intercostal tube is attached to suction drainage and can usually be removed after 24 hours. Nasogastric suction is not necessary – ileus is a very rare complication of this transthoracic repair. Clear fluids are given within 24–48 h of operation, with rapid advancement to a solid diet if this is well tolerated. Most patients are taking a relatively normal diet and can be discharged after 7 days.

Postoperative dilatation

The need for postoperative dilatation is variable and depends on the severity of the stricture. Short, mild strictures are easily dilated by the single passage of a 50 Fr Maloney bougie before operation and rarely require further treatment after repair. Postoperative dilatation is, however, necessary in many patients with moderate degrees of stricture, and in all patients with severe strictures. Such dilatation is best done by indirect bouginage with Maloney bougies in the outpatient clinic using topical anaesthesia which may be supplemented by intravenous diazepam. In the most severe cases, intermittent postoperative dilatation may be necessary for up to 1 year, by which time the healing process in the oesophageal wall is complete and scar contracture has ceased. The techniques of dilatation have been described in detail by Pearson[8].

Results

Between 1964 and 1984 at Toronto General Hospital, 424 patients were managed by this modification of Collis' gastroplasty and partial fundoplication. The indications for operation were: short oesophagus and peptic stricture (201 cases), oesophagitis and shortening without stricture (97 cases), re-do cases without gross oesophagitis or stricture (64 cases), and massive sliding hernia (intrathoracic stomach) without gross oesophagitis or stricture (62 cases).

Two patients died during the first 30 days after operation (0.5 per cent). There were six transient leaks from the region of the gastroplasty and repair, and four of these six leaks occurred in re-do cases. The remaining postoperative complications, e.g. atelectasis and pneumonia, wound infection, cardiac arrythmia, were similar in frequency and severity to those anticipated after a standard hiatal repair.

Most (90 per cent) of these 424 patients have undergone follow-up within the last available year and 265 have been followed for more than 5 years. Good to excellent results were obtained in 93 per cent of the 214 patients with peptic stricture and/or oesophagitis and shortening but without an associated primary motor disorder or previous antireflux surgery. The results were less favourable for re-do cases. Nevertheless, 80 per cent of the 118 patients who had had one or more prior antireflux operations had a good to excellent result. The results were least satisfactory in the group of 37 patients with oesophagitis and stricture associated with an underlying primary motor disorder (scleroderma 16, achalasia 14, diffuse spasm 7). Only half of these patients (19 of 37) had a good or excellent result. In most cases, the fair and poor results were evident within the first few years after operation. There was no significant further deterioration in those followed for more than 5 years.

References

1. Collis, J. L. An operation for hiatus hernia with short esophagus. Journal of Thoracic and Cardiovascular Surgery 1957; 34: 768–778

2. Pearson, F. G., Langer, B., Henderson, R. D. Gastroplasty and Belsey hiatus hernia repair. Journal of Thoracic and Cardiovascular Surgery 1971; 61: 50–63

3. Langer, B. Modified gastroplasty: a simple operation for reflux esophagitis with moderate degrees of shortening. Canadian Journal of Surgery 1973; 16: 84–91

4. Henderson, R. D. Reflux control following gastroplasty. Annals of Thoracic Surgery 1977; 24: 206–214

5. Orringer, M. B., Sloan, H. Complications and failings of combined Collis-Belsey operation. Journal of Thoracic and Cardiovascular Surgery 1977; 74: 726–735

6. Pearson, F. G., Cooper, J. D., Ilves, R., Todd, T. R., Jamieson, W. R. E. Massive hiatal hernia with incarceration: a report of 53 cases. Annals of Thoracic Surgery 1983; 35: 45–51

7. Cooper, J. D., Gill, S. S., Nelems, J. M., Pearson, F. G. Intraoperative and postoperative esophageal manometric findings with Collis gastroplasty and Belsey hiatal hernia repair for gastroesophageal reflux. Journal of Thoracic and Cardiovascular Surgery 1977; 74: 744–751

8. Pearson, F. G. Surgical management of acquired short esophagus with dilatable peptic stricture. World Journal of Surgery 1977; 1: 463–473

Reflux oesophagitis with stricture: alternative methods of management

W. Spencer Payne MD
Consultant, Section of Thoracic, Cardiovascular, Vascular and General Surgery, Mayo Clinic and Mayo Foundation;
James C. Masson Professor of Surgery, Mayo Medical School, Rochester, Minnesota, USA

Introduction

The sensitivity of oesophageal mucosa to the corrosive effects of certain digestive secretions has been implicated in the genesis of almost all the complications of gastro-oesophageal reflux. Gastro-oesophageal incompetence permits the free reflux of acid peptic secretions from the stomach to the oesophagus. The oesophageal consequences of this reflux are directly related to the noxious effects of these secretions on the oesophagus and to the tissue response to chemical injury. Desquamation, erosion, ulceration, inflammation, pain, bleeding, motility disturbances, oesophageal shortening, and stricture formation, as well as columnar epithelial lining of the lower oesophagus (Barrett's oesophagus), are the recognized consequences of such injury. Complications occur in varying intensity from patient to patient, and the pathological processes are often reversible once physical contact between corrosive secretions and oesophagus is eliminated.

The following two surgical techniques currently provide the chief means of control of the complications of gastro-oesophageal reflux.

1. Surgical restoration of gastro-oesophageal competence.
2. Surgical alteration of the quality of secretions present in the stomach, so that the secretions are no longer corrosive to the oesophagus when they reflux.

In the management of benign strictures of the oesophagus due to gastro-oesophageal reflux, rehabilitation of oesophageal function entails, in addition, restoration of oesophageal lumen size or patency. The majority of such benign strictures readily respond to simple dilatation by the passage of sounds or bougies of appropriately graduated sizes. Subsequent stabilization of luminal diameter can usually be achieved if continued oesophageal contact with corrosive secretions can be eliminated by one of the procedures to be described.

On rare occasions, when oesophageal stricturing has progressed to an irreversible stage, because of the deposition of dense hypertrophic collagen scar, stricture resection with restoration of oesophagogastric continuity provides long-term rehabilitation of swallowing function, provided that recurrent reflux oesophagitis is prevented by alteration of the quality of secretions refluxed.

The two basic operative techniques to be described demonstrate alternative methods employed by the author when treating benign strictures of the oesophagus due to gastro-oesophageal reflux under a variety of circumstances, as follows:

1. when the stricture can be dilated adequately and an antireflux procedure can be accomplished,
2. when the stricture is intractable to mechanical dilatation, and
3. when the stricture can be dilated, but previous operation precludes the performance of an antireflux procedure.

OESOPHAGEAL DILATATION AND RESTORATION OF COMPETENCE

By uncut Collis gastroplasty with Nissen fundoplication

Preoperative assessment

All adult patients who are candidates for surgical treatment should undergo roentgenographic, manometric and endoscopic examination and preliminary oesophageal dilatation to 50 Fr size.

1

The passage of graduated Plummer dilators through the strictured oesophagus over a previously swallowed thread or an endoscopically placed wire as a guide provides valuable information about the reversibility of the stricture, as well as restoration of oesophageal function temporarily. Oesophagoscopy should be performed to define the type and severity of associated complications and to obtain cytological and biopsy material in order to rule out malignancy.

Manometric studies of oesophageal motility provide valuable information about the presence or absence of oesophageal peristalsis, along with demonstration of the specific motility disturbances.

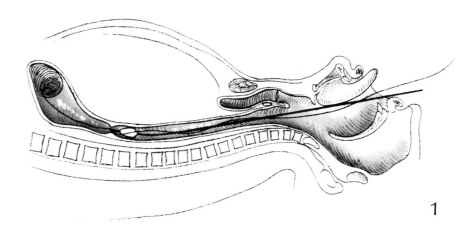

1

The operation

Prevention of aspiration of oesophageal contents into the respiratory tract during anaesthetic induction is achieved by orotracheal intubation under topical anaesthesia with the patient awake. General anaesthesia is immediately induced after the anaesthetic tube is in place and the airway has been sealed with an inflated cuff. The patient is then placed in the right lateral decubitus position (see Illustration 2) and is stabilized in position with appropriate bolsters.

2

The incision

A left thoracotomy is performed, and the pleural space is entered through the periosteal bed of the non-resected left eighth rib.

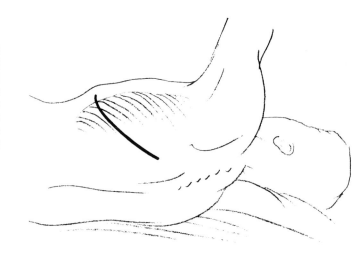

2

3

Exposure

Appropriate spreading of the intercostal incision provides easy access to the pleural cavity. After division of the inferior pulmonary ligament, the lung is retracted cephalad and the pleural leaves of the inferior pulmonary ligament are dissected anteriorly and posteriorly to expose the distal oesophagus. A Penrose drain is passed around the oesophagus and vagi to elevate the oesophagus from its mediastinal bed. The intrathoracic protrusion of proximal stomach and oesophagogastric junction is usually apparent.

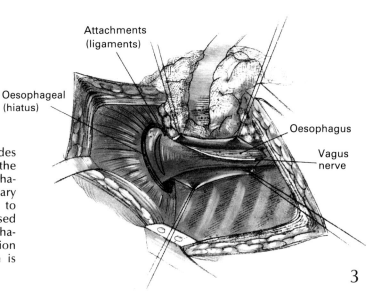

Attachments (ligaments)

Oesophageal (hiatus)

Oesophagus

Vagus nerve

3

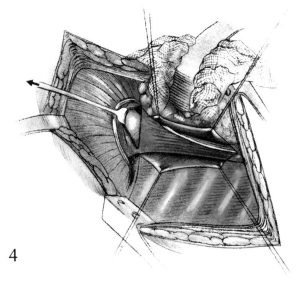

4

4

Dissection of oesophageal hiatus

A transverse incision is made in the phreno-oesophageal ligament and contiguous layers of pleura and peritoneum; a tunnel is thus created between chest and abdomen through the oesophageal hiatus. A small Richardson retractor is passed through this defect, and the oesophageal hiatus is retracted laterally.

5

Division of phreno-oesophageal ligament

By placement of the fingers of the left hand astride the attachments between the oesophagogastric junction and the crura of the diaphragm, these attachments can be safely divided; this completely frees the cardia circumferentially from all hiatal attachments.

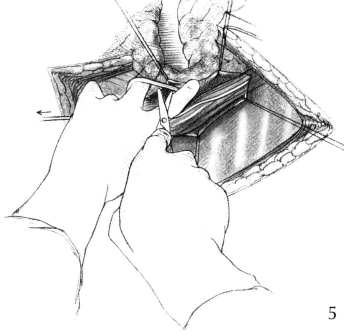

5

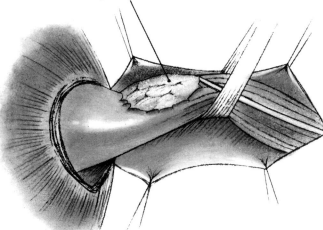

Vascular fat pad at oesophagogastric junction

Dissection of oesophagogastric fat pad

6

Vagal trunks are identified and preserved. The highly vascular fatty connective tissue at the oesophagogastric junction is carefully dissected from its lateral to its medial aspect.

6

7

The anterior vagal trunk is preserved by sweeping it medially with the fat pad. Meticulous ligation of multiple gastric nutrient vessels is required not only to reflect this fat pad, but also to clear the gastric serosa for subsequent steps of the operation.

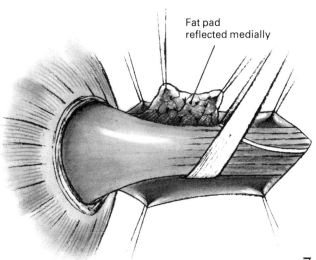

Fat pad reflected medially

7

8

Prolapse of stomach into chest

It is now possible to allow the proximal stomach to prolapse into the thorax through the oesophageal hiatus. Numerous short gastric vessels must be divided in order to bring the fundus and proximal stomach into the chest.

This freeing up of the greater curvature of the stomach is readily accomplished through the oesophageal hiatus. The gastrohepatic omentum is divided as well.

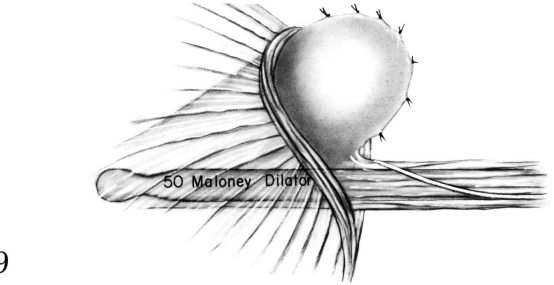

8

9

Uncut Collis gastroplasty

If the oesophagus is not shortened as a consequence of disease, an uncut Collis gastroplasty is performed. A 50 Fr Maloney dilator is advanced through the mouth down the oesophagus and into the stomach, and, as before, the oesophageal stricture is dilated. The Maloney dilator is left in place as a mandrel about which an uncut tubular extension of the oesophagus will be fashioned from the lesser curvature of the stomach. This is accurately and simply achieved by applying a TA 30 stapling device (US Instrument Co.) to the stomach at the angle of His, parallel to the lesser curvature of the stomach and the indwelling mandrel. Because the alignment pen is not used in this application, special care is required to assure that alignment of staples and crimping anvil is accurate. In addition, care must be taken in the tightening of the stapling device on the stomach so that the stomach will not be crushed, but jaw approximation will be sufficient to allow appropriate crimping of the staples when the instrument is activated.

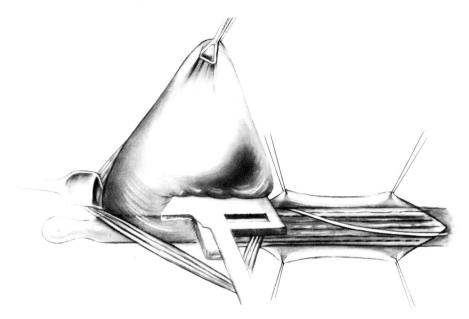

9

Nissen fundoplication

10 & 11

After the delivery of staples and removal of the stapling device, the previously mobilized fundus is now imbricated 360° around the 30 mm long uncut Collis gastroplasty tube, after the technique of Nissen. The wrap is loosely fashioned with the mandrel in place and is maintained with two rows of interrupted seromuscular silk sutures, which approximate the fundus to the Collis gastroplasty tube over its entire 30 mm length. The vagi are under the fundal wrap in their normal position. Care must be taken at each step of the procedure to avoid injury to these nerves, because accidental vagotomy is the most common cause of the 'gas-bloat' syndrome in the postoperative period. It is noteworthy that the fundoplication, as described, avoids suture placement near vagal trunks. In fact, the anchoring sutures for the plication are all actually on the stomach and not the oesophagus. Furthermore, they are on the lateral rather than the medial aspect of the neo-oesophagus tube as is the case of the classical Nissen procedure. The entire purpose of the uncut staple line and plication suture line is to establish frenula that will prevent the telescoping of the neo-oesophagus out of the fundoplication.

After the fundoplication has been completed, the reconstructed area is reduced below the diaphragm and is held in place with three interrupted horizontal mattress sutures. These sutures catch the oesophagogastric junction at the insertion of the phreno-oesophageal ligament and the superior rim of the fundoplication. They pass through the oesophageal hiatus and back into the chest through the perihiatal diaphragm, where each is tied. Crural approximation behind the oesophagus with heavy Dacron sutures is required if the hiatus is too patulous. A tight hiatus, however, should be avoided.

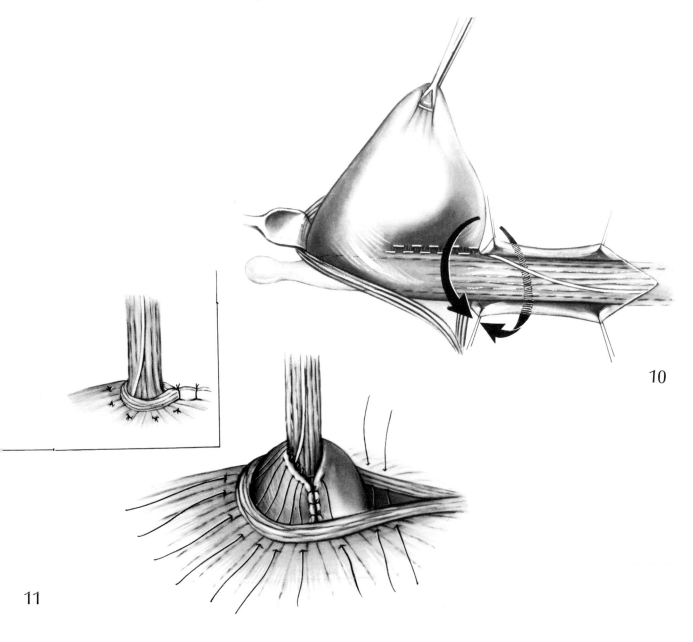

10

11

12

Partial fundoplication for amotile oesophagus

Two points deserve special mention here. First, if oesophageal peristalsis is absent, the Nissen-type 360° fundoplication, as described, may prove to be too obstructive. In patients in whom sequential peristaltic motor activity is absent on preoperative manometric study, a 270° Belsey-type plication is favoured; otherwise, the technical details of reduction and repair are identical.

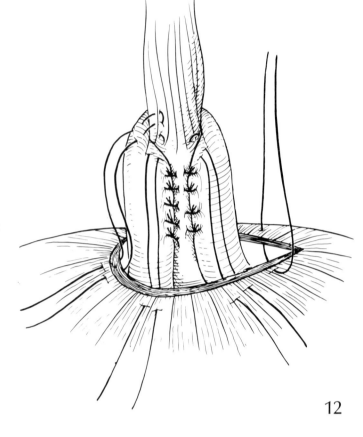

12

Cut Collis gastroplasty for shortened oesophagus

13

On rare occasions the oesophagus may be shortened cicatricially as a consequence of chronic reflux oesophagitis, and even after appropriate intrathoracic mobilization it may not be long enough to permit reduction of the stomach below the diaphragm. In this situation, it is desirable to perform an oesophageal lengthening procedure by means of the standard cut Collis gastroplasty, in which a GIA stapling device (US Instrument Co.) is used in lieu of the TA 30. Activation of the cutting blade of the GIA device not only incises the portion of stomach between the jaws of the clamp, but also lays down double parallel rows of metallic staples, a procedure effectively closing each side of the 5 cm long incision.

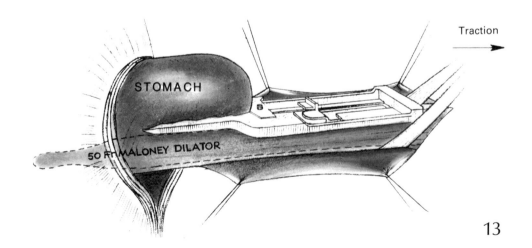

13

14

The rows of staples are buried beneath a single row of interrupted silk sutures. A Nissen or Belsey repair can then be effected around the lower end of this tubular extension of the oesophagus.

When the repair, irrespective of type, is completed, the Maloney dilator is removed, and a nasogastric tube is passed. Mediastinal pleura is loosely approximated over the distal oesophagus, and the lung is re-expanded. The chest is closed, and a single catheter is brought from the left pleural space to the outside for postoperative suction-drainage.

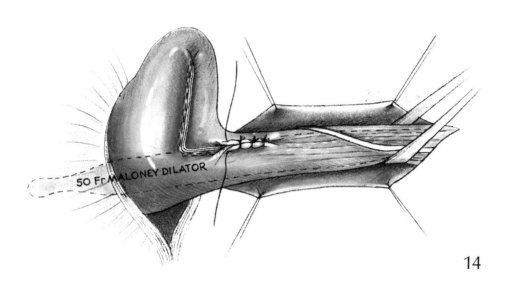

14

Postoperative care

The morning after the day of operation, the patient's oesophagus is studied fluoroscopically following ingestion of a water-soluble contrast medium (Gastrografin). If no leakage from the oesophageal or gastric suture site is evident, the chest and nasogastric tubes are removed. Oral feedings are safely progressed from a liquid to a general diet during the ensuing 48 to 72 hours. Total hospitalization is approximately 7 days.

Leakage from any site evident on radiographic examination is almost inevitably asymptomatic, localized, and confined. If this complication is observed, chest and nasogastric tube suction is continued. A subclavian central venous catheter is inserted for total parenteral alimentation, and broad-spectrum antibiotics are administered intravenously for approximately 10 days. A repeat radiographic examination is carried out at that time and almost invariably shows complete sealing of leakage sites. Oral feeding can be resumed safely after tapering off of parenteral feeding and removal of all tubes.

THE UNDILATABLE STRICTURE

Management by resection and Roux-en-Y gastric drainage procedure

On rare occasions, benign oesophageal strictures do not yield to mechanical dilatation, and it becomes necessary to resect the strictured portion of the oesophagus to restore function. Such resection removes not only the oesophageal obstruction, but also the intrinsic oesophageal sphincter. Reconstruction by oesophagogastrostomy results in permanent incompetence of the cardia with considerable risk of recurrent oesophagitis and stricture. Various procedures have been suggested to prevent this complication. One, which the author has employed with success, alters the quality of secretions present in the stomach so that they are not corrosive to the oesophagus when they reflux. Essentially, gastric achlorhydria is effected by vagotomy and antrectomy, and alkaline biliary and pancreatic reflux is prevented by means of a long-limb Roux-en-Y gastric drainage procedure.

On occasion, the effects of previous surgical procedures about the oesophageal hiatus and stomach preclude surgical restoration of gastro-oesophageal competence by standard means. Under such circumstances, if the associated oesophageal stricture proves amenable to dilatation, permanent control of oesophagitis and stricture can be obtained by similarly rendering the stomach achlorhydric and preventing biliary reflux by Roux-en-Y gastric drainage.

In either of the aforementioned circumstances, gastro-oesophageal incompetence is permanent, and bland reflux occurs without oesophageal irritation or reaction. Nonetheless, it should be apparent that special postoperative postural precautions may be required for patients who experience nocturnal respiratory aspiration.

Preoperative care

Resection of a benign oesophageal stricture caused by reflux oesophagitis should not be undertaken until a diligent preoperative attempt at dilatation over a previously placed guide has been repeatedly attempted without success.

Complete vagotomy is an essential feature of the long-limb Roux-en-Y gastric drainage procedure. Gastrojejunal stomal ulceration occurs frequently when gastric vagotomy is incomplete. If stricture resection is not contemplated and previous surgical vagotomy is to be depended on, the Hollander insulin test may be helpful in determining whether vagotomy has been complete.

In patients who are malnourished, it is usually desirable to start parenteral hyperalimentation via a subclavian vein on the day before operation and to continue such nutrition postoperatively until an adequate diet can be taken orally. Such hyperalimentation minimizes negative nitrogen balance in the postoperative patient and enhances anastomotic healing in nitrogen-depleted patients.

The operation

15

Anaesthesia, positioning, and surgical exposure of the distal oesophagus are accomplished as previously described. Access to the proximal part of the stomach and the oesophageal stricture which is necessary for resection and anastomosis is gained through a radial diaphragmatic incision that passes through the oesophageal hiatus.

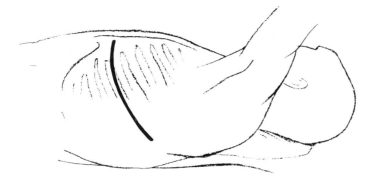

16

Resection of oesophageal stricture

Proximal transection of the oesophagus is carried out at a site well above the diseased tissue. Distally, minimal resection of the proximal portion of the stomach is effected, and the left gastric and short gastric vessels are preserved if possible. The stomach at the site of oesophageal resection is closed. Vagal trunks are resected along with the stricture.

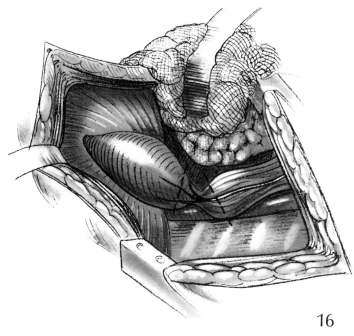

16

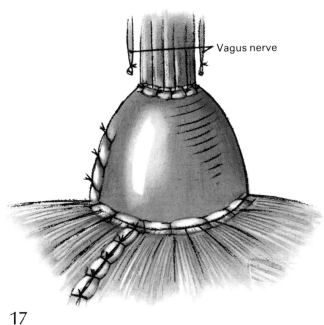

Vagus nerve

17

17

Oesophagogastrostomy

End-to-side oesophagogastrostomy is performed between the cut end of the oesophagus and the gastric fundus, which is brought into the chest. The anastomosis should be completed with a 50 Fr dilator in place. Depending on gastric mobility, several short gastric vessels may need to be divided to avoid anastomotic tension. In order to protect the anastomosis the oesophageal anastomosis should be invaginated into the stomach. The diaphragmatic incision is closed around the stomach; this creates a snug hiatus to which the stomach is anchored with sutures. The lung is re-expanded and the chest is closed and drained as previously indicated.

18

Abdominal incision

The patient is turned and placed supine on the operating table, and the abdomen is explored through an upper midline incision.

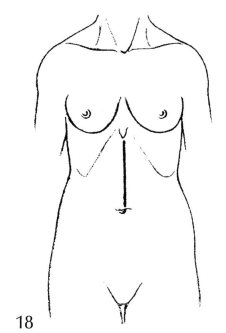

18

19

Distal hemigastrectomy (antrectomy)

If it has not been done previously, a standard distal hemigastrectomy or antrectomy is performed, with preservation of the left gastric, left gastroepiploic, and short gastric vessels. The duodenal stump is closed.

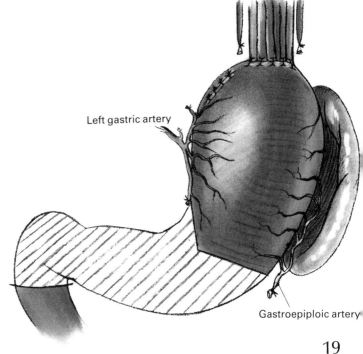

19

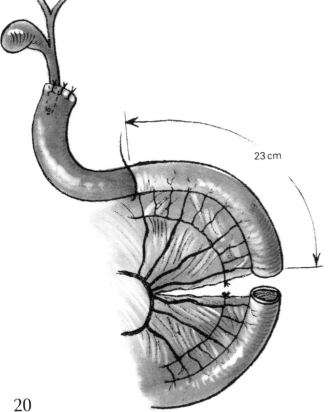

20

20

Division of jejunum

A long-limb Roux-en-Y is developed by dividing the jejunum at a point 23 cm (9 in) distal to the ligament of Treitz. The distal end of the transected jejunum is anastomosed end to end or side to end to the resected end of the stomach as a retrocolic gastric drainage procedure.

Completion of Roux-en-Y gastric drainage procedure

21

The Roux-en-Y anastomosis is completed by joining the proximal end of the transected jejunum end to side to the distal segment 45 cm (18 in) below the gastrojejunostomy. This proximal jejunal segment is approximately half the length of the long-limb gastric drainage segment, and passes behind and to the left of the latter to prevent distortion of the radian of small bowel mesentery. The 45 cm (18 in) long limb of the Roux-en-Y loop provides an effective peristaltic barrier against reflux of bile and pancreatic secretions into the stomach and oesophagus. Intersecting mesenteries are closed to prevent internal herniation.

The abdomen is closed in layers in the usual fashion, two soft-rubber Penrose drains being brought from the duodenal stump to the outside through a stab wound in the right upper quadrant of the anterior abdominal wall. A nasogastric tube is passed and threaded into the upper reaches of the long-limb Roux-en-Y segment for post-operative suction-drainage.

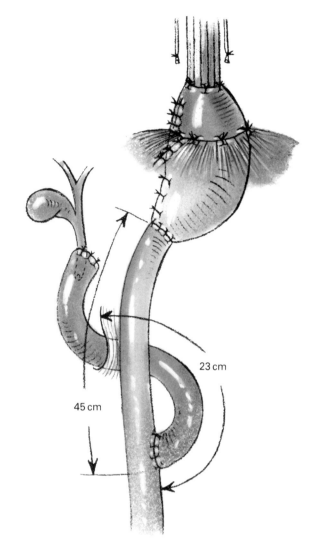

23 cm

45 cm

21

Postoperative care

Patients are kept in a slanted, head-up oesophageal bed initially. Ambulation can begin the day after operation. Nasogastric suction is usually continued until bowel function returns on the fourth or fifth day. The chest tube is removed the day after operation.

Oral feeding is not resumed until a fluoroscopic examination of the oesophagus, with use of Gastrografin, demonstrates patency without leakage at the sites of anastomosis. If leakage is apparent, the patient is not allowed oral intake; parenteral hyperalimentation is continued for 2 weeks, at which time the radiographic examination is repeated before oral feeding is begun.

Oral diet, when resumed, is rapidly advanced to solids over 4–5 days. Abdominal drains are removed by the 8th day, and patients are usually dismissed from the hospital 10 to 14 days after operation. Use of the slanted oesophageal bed is continued only if postural reflux with respiratory aspiration is experienced. Heartburn, oeso-phagitis, or recurrent stricture is not seen.

Acknowledgement

Copyright of all the illustrations in this chapter is held by the Mayo Clinic; they may not be reproduced without prior permission from the Mayo Clinic.

Operations for carcinoma of the thoracic oesophagus and cardia

John W. Jackson MCh, FRCS
Formerly Consultant Thoracic Surgeon, Harefield Hospital, Harefield Middlesex, UK

Preoperative

Indications and preparation

Age alone is not a bar to surgery for these lesions; the majority of patients are in the seventh decade and a number are over 80 years of age.

Increasing dysphagia at first to solids and then subsequently to soft foods and finally fluids leads to weight loss, inanition and dehydration.

The tumour is locally invasive and may extend beyond the normal confines of the oesophagus and stomach to become adherent to adjacent structures in the chest and abdomen. Lymph nodes are frequently involved but do not preclude a worthwhile resection; in the presence of liver or peritoneal metastases resection is of very doubtful value and alternative palliative procedures should be considered.

The prime aim of operation should be to remove the ulcerating fungating growth that lies in direct communication with the mouth and to restore swallowing. If at the same time a satisfactory cancer excision is obtained it should be regarded as a bonus. A mortality of 10 per cent is surgically acceptable and the extension of life by 1 or 2 years a real benefit to an elderly person. Operation has to be a once only procedure – there is seldom time for staged operations at this age. If dysphagia is complete operation should be carried out as soon as anaemia and dehydration have been corrected.

A careful clinical examination is essential to exclude other contraindications to radical surgery, e.g. metastases to the neck glands, liver and peritoneum. A rectal examination is carried out to exclude pelvic metastases and to assess the prostate. Severe constipation, often made worse by recent barium studies, may need attention so as to avoid faecal impaction in the postoperative period.

Investigations

Radiology

Diagnosis is established by barium swallow; if possible the distal oesophagus, stomach and cardia should be outlined in the examination. A chest X-ray is necessary to exclude carcinoma of the bronchus – the next most common cause of dysphagia – and to detect any pneumonic change due to spill from the oesophagus to the trachea. Mediastinal widening due to glands or tumour should also be looked for. Sometimes a tumour at the cardia may produce a filling defect in the fundus air bubble. If there is no fundus bubble dysphagia is absolute, but the presence of air indicates that there is a passageway.

Oesophagoscopy

Oesophagoscopy is essential to determine the level and extent of the lesion. Froth, food and other residue should be removed. Sometimes it may be possible to pass the instrument beyond the lesion into the distal oesophagus, affording temporary relief of dysphagia. Several biopsies should always be taken and the distance of the proximal and distal level of the tumour from the upper incisor teeth should be recorded. If it is not possible to get past the lesion with the oesophagoscope cautious attempts at dilatation may be made with a Moloney bougie. Perforation is an indication for emergency surgery.

Bronchoscopy

Bronchoscopy is carried out in every case to exclude primary carcinoma of the bronchus or direct or indirect involvement of the bronchial tree by the oesophageal growth. The distance of the carina from the upper incisor teeth at the time of bronchoscopy is always recorded and compared with the upper and lower level of the lesion in the oesophagus. If there is the least doubt about the appearances of the bronchial mucosa a biopsy is taken. While the patient is relaxed under the anaesthetic the abdomen should be palpated to feel for and exclude any mass in the stomach, liver secondaries, ascites or a barium-loaded bowel.

Preoperative treatment

It may be possible to improve the patient's swallowing temporarily by removing impacted food or fungating tumour at the time of oesophagoscopy. Usually dehydration and electrolytic imbalance need to be corrected by intravenous therapy. Anaemia should be corrected by blood transfusion. With intravenous alimentation there is rarely any need for a feeding gastrostomy or jejunostomy. It is usually better to proceed to surgery.

Simple dental treatment should be carried out during this period – scaling and the removal of loose teeth which might be dislodged at operation. Oral candidiasis is common and antifungal agents may be required.

Chest infection, often associated with oesophageal spill-over, may call for a period of treatment with physiotherapy and antibiotics.

Generally these patients do not benefit by having their operations deferred.

The operations

The oesophagus may be replaced by stomach, colon or small intestine. If the growth is confined to the oesophagus the author uses stomach and if the cardia and lower oesophagus are involved jejunum is preferred. An upper partial gastrectomy with oesophagogastric anastomosis may be justified in the elderly if the stomach is not grossly involved or where metastases indicate a poor prognosis. The procedure will restore swallowing and rid the patient of the alimentary part of his tumour. The use of colon is described in the chapter on 'Colon replacement of the oesophagus', pp. 355–369).

OESOPHAGECTOMY WITH GASTRIC REPLACEMENT (IVOR LEWIS)

Anaesthesia

The patient is anaesthetized and a double lumen tube inserted so that the right lung can be excluded from the circuit for part of the operation.

An intravenous drip, using a central venous pressure line, is set up. The bladder is catheterized and the catheter left in for 24–48 h. Urinary output is recorded half hourly during the operation and at regular intervals in the post-operative period.

Stage 1: Abdominal

1

The incision

With the patient supine laparotomy is made using an upper midline incision or a transverse incision midway between the xiphoid process and umbilicus, dividing the rectus muscles. This affords good access to the pylorus and to the spleen and cardia.

The abdomen is explored to exclude metastases or other disease. If growth is palpable at the cardia a left-sided approach may be preferred and the incision can be extended into the chest along the eighth rib. Alternatively, the abdomen can be closed (after mobilization of the stomach) and the patient turned, with resection and anastomosis through a left thoracotomy.

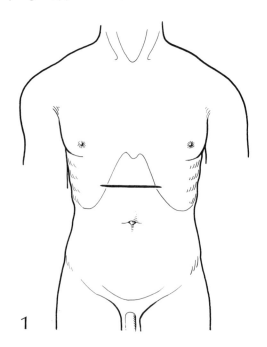

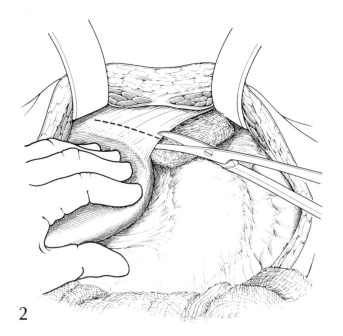

2

Division of the left triangular ligament should be carried out at an early stage. The ligament is brought into view by placing a swab or pack behind it before dividing it with scissors. The left lobe of the liver may now be retracted downwards so as to reveal the oesophageal hiatus.

3

The stomach, omentum and transverse colon are delivered into the wound. An opening is made in the gastrocolic omentum on the greater curve below the short gastric vessels, so as to gain access to the lesser sac. The gastrocolic omentum is divided or separated from the colon, preserving the right gastroepiploic arch. The short gastric and left gastric vessels are divided using forceps and ligature or the Auto Suture LDS instrument. It is important not to tie or clip too close to the greater curve of the stomach. The spleen is not removed as a set part of the operation but if it is in the way or bleeds it should be removed. The gastrohepatic omentum is opened and frequently carries a sizeable hepatic branch from the left gastric artery, which may be divided provided there is an adequate main hepatic artery. The right gastric vessels are preserved and the left gastric pedicle is cleared from above and from behind within the lesser sac; the artery and vein are tied separately close to the coeliac axis. Any enlarged glands are removed and sent for histological examination. The oesophageal hiatus is defined by sharp dissection. The phreno-oesophageal ligament is divided and the oesophagus mobilized above and below the hiatus. It is not necessary to enlarge the hiatus. The mediastinum is explored through the hiatus using finger and swabs. Pyloroplasty is only carried out if the pylorus is small or scarred. A patulous pylorus or overzealous pyloroplasty may induce biliary reflux to the gastric remnant and cause oesophagitis above the oesophagogastric anastomosis postoperatively.

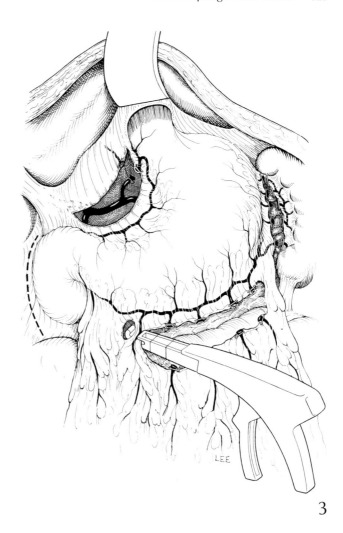

3

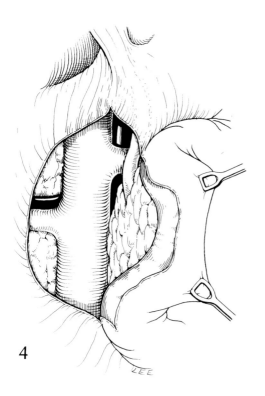

4

4

The peritoneum lateral to the duodenum may be divided to improve mobilization of the pylorus and if extra length is required it may also help to mobilize the duodenum and the head of the pancreas.

When haemostasis is satisfactory the viscera are replaced and the abdomen closed.

Stage II: Thoracic

Anaesthesia

If a double lumen endotracheal tube has been inserted at the time of induction it is a distinct advantage to exclude the right lung from the anaesthetic circuit for at least part of this stage of the operation.

5

Position of patient and incision

The patient is turned on to the left side and secured to the table. A right thoracotomy is carried out along the upper border of the sixth rib.

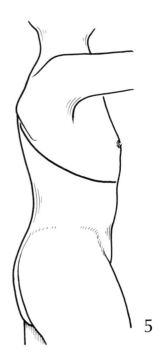

6

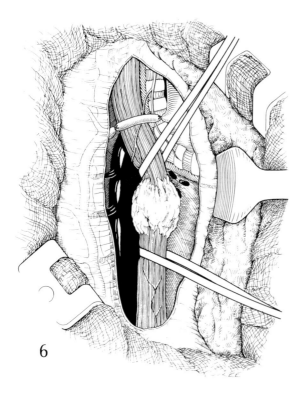

The lung is freed to the hilum, retracted anteriorly and allowed to collapse. The lesion in the oesophagus is inspected and palpated. The azygos vein is ligated and divided and the mediastinal pleura opened along the length of the oesophagus.

Tapes are passed around the oesophagus above and below the tumour. Using sharp dissection in front of the oesophagus the pericardium, lower trachea and both main bronchi are separated from the oesophagus taking the subcarinal and mediastinal lymph nodes with the oesophagus. A plane is then opened posteriorly between the oesophagus and the spine and aorta. The tumour may be densely adherent to any one of these structures as if by direct extension, and it must be separated by a process of sharp dissection, stealth and persuasion. Clean and intact mobilization is not always possible. Occasionally the oesophageal lumen is entered but it is essential to avoid the disaster of entering the aorta or the tracheobronchial tree. The thoracic duct may be seen or divided inadvertently, resulting in the escape of chyle into the mediastinum. The divided ends must be sought, and tied, clipped or oversewn. Otherwise it should be removed along with any associated lymph nodes. One or two sizeable vessels from the aorta may need to be ligated or secured with a suture.

7

As soon as the oesophagus and its tumour are free in the mediastinum the stomach is delivered into the chest through the oesophageal hiatus; its initial presentation is noted so as to avoid subsequent rotation – the greater curve should lie towards the mediastinum. The pylorus may present through the hiatus. The upper oesophagus is mobilized to the base of the neck.

A Petz clamp or other stapling instrument is applied obliquely across the stomach below the cardia, preserving the lateral part of the fundus.

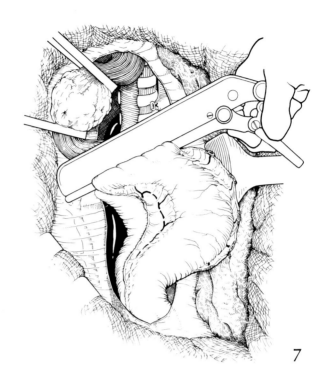

7

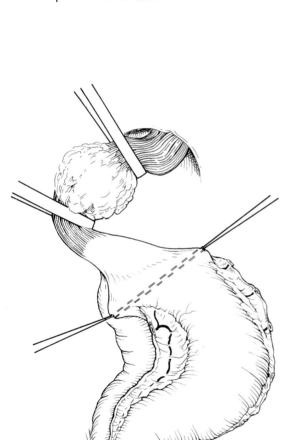

8

8

The stomach is divided with diathermy or a knife between the rows of staples.

9

The stapled stomach edge is oversewn with a continuous suture of 2/0 chromic catgut. The suture is tied and the ends held in forceps.

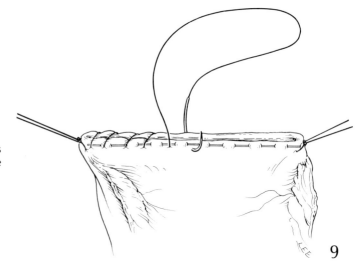

9

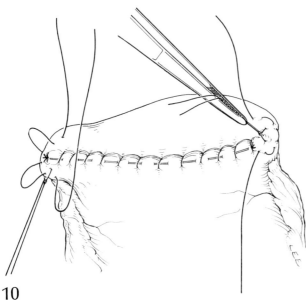

10

10

The TA 90 Auto Suture instrument inserts two rows of overlapping staples in close approximation and these do not need to be oversewn, but the line of staples should be invaginated by a continuous Lembert suture of chromic catgut so as to ensure serosal apposition and prevent contact and contamination of the mediastinum by the divided mucosa.

Several seromuscular bites (4 or 5) of a non-absorbable suture (3/0 linen) encircle the ends of the catgut suture (or staple) line in an open horseshoe formation.

11

The catgut knot and the end of the catgut suture line are invaginated and the linen suture tied as the catgut is cut close to its knot.

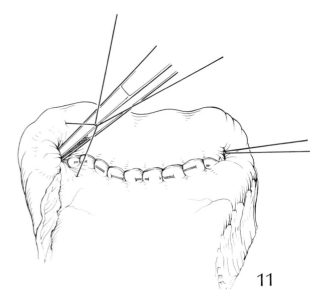

11

12

Interrupted seromuscular mattress stitches of linen are now placed over the intervening segment.

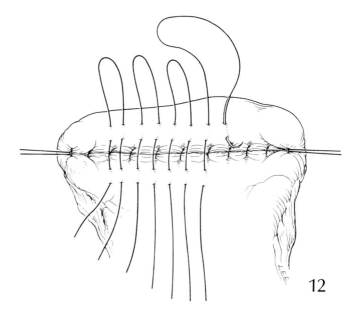

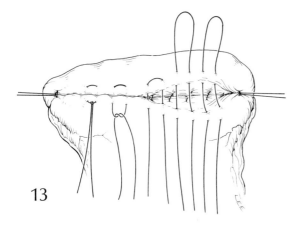

13 & 14

The sutures are tied and serosal apposition is secured over the whole length of the suture line.

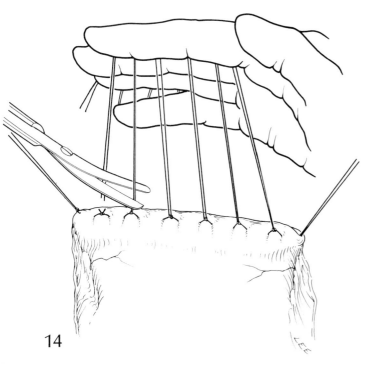

15

The stomach is laid in the oesophageal bed and its highest point, usually the fundus, should reach the root of the neck – indeed if the oesophageal tumour is high, anastomosis can be effected in the neck by a separate cervical incision after the chest is closed (*see* chapter on 'Colon replacement of the oesophagus', pp. 355–369).

A site is chosen near the fundus of the stomach for anastomosis with the oesophagus. It should be away from the suture line closing the upper end of the stomach so as to avoid leaving a bridge of ischaemic tissue.

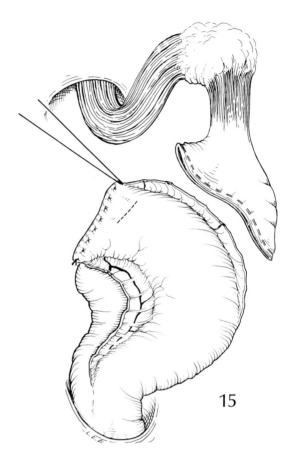

15

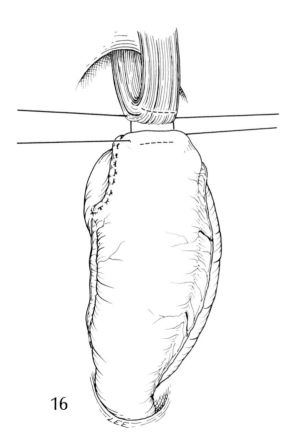

16

16

Two seromuscular (3/0 linen) stitches are placed between the oesophagus above the proposed site of section and on either side of the place chosen for the gastric stoma.

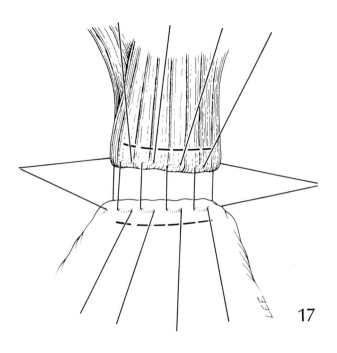

17

Four or five seromuscular stitches are inserted between these to bring the oesophagus and stomach together without tension or tearing. The outer stitches are clipped or preserved, the inner cut.

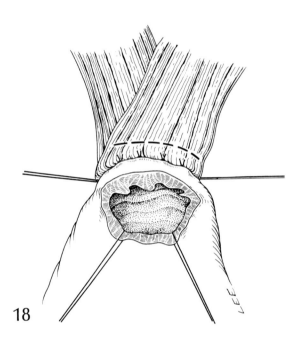

18

The stomach is opened with scissors or diathermy along the line chosen for the stoma and excess gastric contents removed with gentle suction. Haemostasis is secured. Two 3/0 Ethibond stay sutures are placed in the free edge of the stomach opening so as to divide it into three equal parts and held in mosquito forceps.

19

The oseophagus is divided with a knife at a point level with the stoma. Free bleeding should occur and clamps are not used here. A clamp may be applied to the distal oesophagus to avoid spillage. The specimen is removed.

Two stay sutures of 3/0 Ethibond are inserted on the free edge of the divided oesophagus to match those on the stomach and are held in mosquito forceps. These hold the oesophagus and the gastric stoma open.

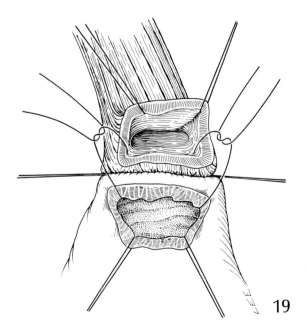

20

A row of interrupted, all-layers stitches is applied between the stomach and oesophagus posteriorly. The knots are tied on the mucosa.

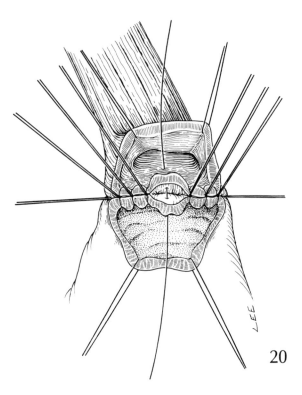

20

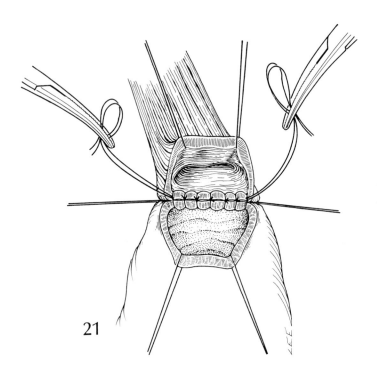

21

21

The end stitches are preserved and held in forceps with a loop for easy identification, and the remainder are cut.

22

A nasogastric tube with a radiopaque marker line is passed down the oesophagus by the anaesthetist to the anastomosis and its tip advanced through the stomach towards the pylorus so that it lies near the pylorus with the side-holes in the stomach to prevent distension of the elongated tube-like stomach.

Closure of the front row of the anastomosis commences at each angle using a series of interrupted Connell all-layers stitches. Each stitch starts and finishes on the outside of the stomach or oesophagus with a loop on the mucosa so as to invert the mucosa.

When tied, the knots of this row are outside the lumen of the anastomosis.

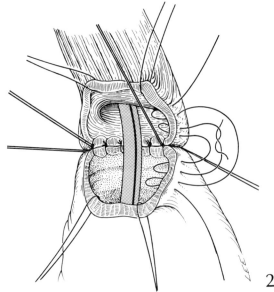

22

23

After two or three of these stitches have been placed near each angle the internal angle stitches held in *Illustration 21* are cut and the 3/0 Ethibond stay sutures removed. Further Connell stitches close the middle third. The stitches clipped and preserved in *Illustration 17* are retained.

24

A row of interrupted seromuscular stitches, two bites on the stomach and one transversely on the oesophagus, so as to pick up its outer longitudinal muscle, draws a cuff of stomach up over the previous layer and hides it from sight.

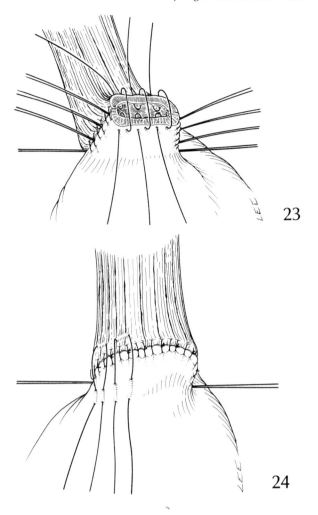

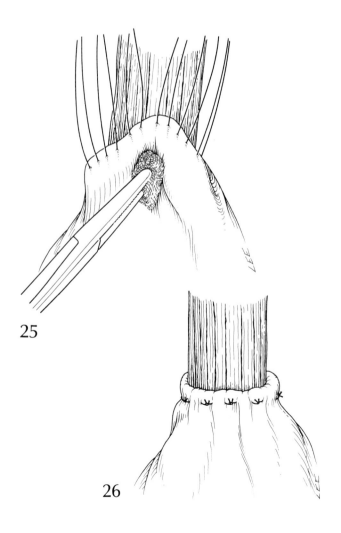

25

When tying these stitches the stomach is eased up over the oesophagus with a swab or pledget to avoid tension and promote inversion.

26

The anastomosis is now complete. Additional stitches are rarely indicated.

There should be no tension, and any redundant stomach in the chest may be returned to the abdomen. The anastomosis and the tube of stomach take their place in the mediastinum in the bed of the excised oesophagus.

The pleura is loosely closed over the anastomosis.

A basal intercostal drain (36 Fr) is inserted posteriorly to drain the costodiaphragmatic sulcus; its tip may be fixed in position by a catgut stitch. It should not encroach on the stomach or anastomosis. A separate mediastinal drain (32 Fr) may be placed at the same time if there is uncertainty about the viability of the stomach or the anastomosis or fear of a chylous leak. The tip is positioned and secured with a loop of catgut.

The lung is now reinflated and the chest closed.

TOTAL GASTRECTOMY WITH JEJUNAL REPLACEMENT, ROUX-EN-Y

The aim of this operation is to remove the entire stomach and as much as possible of the oesophagus above the tumour (10–12 cm) along with the left gastric glands, sometimes taking spleen and pancreas back to the portal vein.

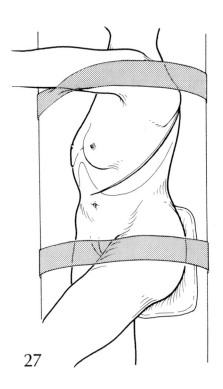

27

Anaesthesia

The patient is anaesthetized and a double lumen tube inserted so that the left lung can be excluded from the anaesthetic circuit for part of the operation.

An intravenous drip, using a central venous pressure line, is set up. The bladder is catheterized and the catheter left in for 24–48 h. Urinary output is recorded half hourly during the operation and at regular intervals in the post-operative period.

Position of patient and incision

27

The patient is secured on the operating table in a semi-lateral position with the pelvis at 45° and the chest nearly vertical to facilitate access to the chest and the abdomen.

The full incision extends from the midline anteriorly between the xiphoid and the umbilicus obliquely across the costal margin and along the seventh or eighth ribs, to the interval between the tip of the scapula and the spine.

The abdomen is opened first between the midline and the costal margin, dividing the left rectus muscle. The extent and operability of the lesion are assessed. Free fluid, peritoneal seedlings, liver and pelvic metastases indicate that a palliative procedure is all that can be achieved. Fixation near the hiatus or involvement of coeliac axis glands are unfavourable signs but need not constitute a bar to resection and a trial mobilization may be deemed worthwhile.

Once it has been decided to proceed, the skin incision is continued over the costal margin, dividing the latissimus dorsi and serratus muscles as far as the trapezius. The periosteum on the entire length of the upper border of the seventh or eighth rib is stripped, the pleura opened and a chest spreader inserted. The costal margin is cut and the musculophrenic vessels secured.

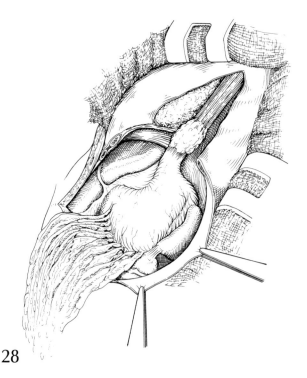

28

28

The diaphragm is divided circumferentially, leaving a short cuff attached to the rib cage. The anaesthetist allows the left lung to become deflated and retracted forwards so as to expose the oesophagus. The pulmonary ligament is divided and the mediastinal pleura opened along the oesophagus which is now separated from the back of the pericardium anteriorly and the aorta posteriorly. Several large aortic oesophageal vessels may require ligation. The thoracic duct is not so frequently seen from this side but may require ligation. The oesophagus is mobilized with as much fat and as many glands as possible to the level of the aortic arch and the left main bronchus. If the right pleural cavity is opened the pleura must be repaired, otherwise bowel might herniate into the right chest.

29

The lienorenal ligament is divided and the perinephric space entered so as to mobilize the spleen. A decision must now be made whether to preserve or remove the spleen, bearing in mind the possible benefits with respect to cancer clearance against the possible problem of post-splenectomy sepsis. If the spleen has to be removed the splenic artery and veins are dissected out, tied and divided. Otherwise the short gastric vessels are divided, preserving the spleen. The stomach and omentum are now separated from the colon as far as the pylorus, usually in an avascular plane (see p. 000). Lesser sac adhesions are divided and mobilization completed from the pylorus to the hiatus. Sometimes the oesophagus may be mobilized without dividing the hiatus. If the tumour is adherent at the hiatus the diaphragm should be divided to this point and the lesion mobilized by including part of the muscle of the hiatus and crura. The left gastric vessels are cleared and divided close to the coeliac axis. The gastrohepatic omentum is divided, taking care to ligate the hepatic branch of the left gastric artery.

If the tumour is adherent to the tail of the pancreas but the lesion is otherwise operable, the tail of the pancreas should be mobilized with the spleen and the splenic vessels and divided close to the superior mesenteric vein (see p. 000). The splenic and left gastric arteries are ligated flush with the coeliac axis.

The pancreas is transected, the pancreatic duct (or ducts) ligated and the raw surface excluded from the peritoneal cavity. If in doubt a drain should be left in. Partial pancreatectomy increases the morbidity of the operation and should only be carried out if the pancreas is invaded by tumour.

Before dividing the pylorus, the right gastric and gastroepiploic vessels and closing the duodenum, it is wise first to prepare the jejunum for the Roux-en-Y reconstruction. Occasionally a suitable length of jejunum cannot be obtained and a decision will then have to be made as to whether to interpose a segment of colon between the oesophagus and the duodenum (see chapter on 'Colon replacement of the oesophagus', pp. 000–000) or to fashion a tube from the greater curve of stomach.

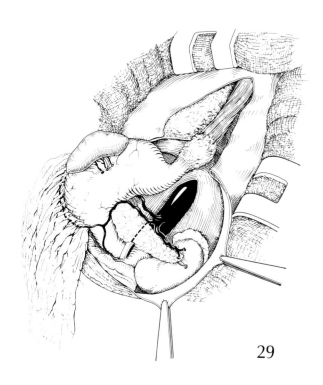

29

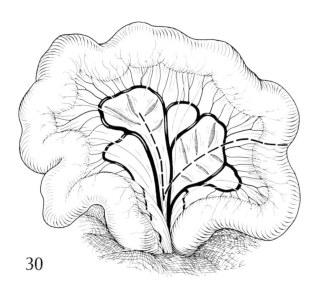

30

30

The jejunum below the duodenojejunal flexure is inspected and a loop selected where the mesentery is beginning to lengthen and the vascular pattern becomes more easily discernible. The vessels in the mesentery may be more readily displayed by turning off the room and overhead lights and transilluminating it with a beam from a horizontal spot lamp. From the proposed point of division the arteries and veins are tied and divided individually so as to preserve the vascular arcades to a length of distal jejunum. The pulsations close to the bowel are observed as each major vessel is clamped. With patience and by making radial slits on either side of the mesentery a loop 25–30 cm long is made available. The small bowel is then divided between non-crushing clamps and the ends covered and returned to the abdomen while the oesophagogastric excision is completed.

31

The right gastric and gastroepiploic vessels are now secured and the pylorus mobilized as far as the duodenum. The duodenum is divided between Payrs crushing clamps (or with the TA 30 or GIA Auto Suture instruments).

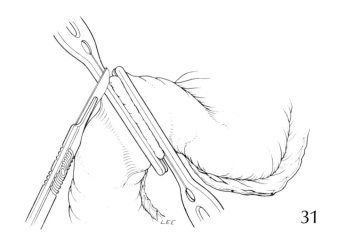

31

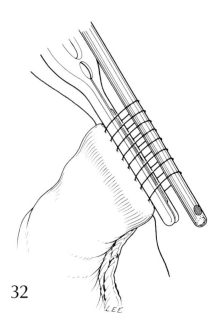

32

32

If a Payrs clamp is used the crushed duodenal stump must be oversewn with catgut. A metal rod (usually the sucker tube) placed over the Payrs clamp helps to form a series of open loops which facilitate removal of the Payrs clamp.

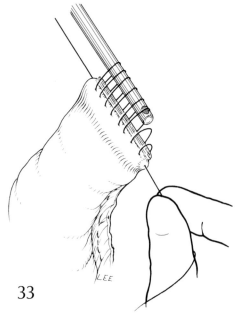

33

33

On removal of the clamp the sucker tube is withdrawn as the loops are tightened.

The sutured (or stapled) stump is then invaginated as follows.

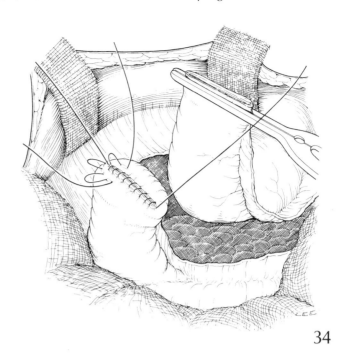

34

34

A four-bite seromuscular horse-shoe suture is placed at each corner and tied.

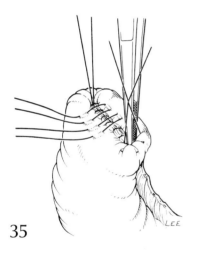

35

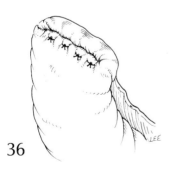

36

35 & 36

Three or four interrupted seromuscular sutures are now placed over the intervening segment.

The entire stomach tumour and lower oesophagus, and if necessary the spleen and tail of the pancreas, are now free. The oesophagus is mobilized in the mediastinum to above the level of the inferior pulmonary vein and sometimes to the aortic arch. The distal jejunum is drawn up posteriorly through the transverse mesocolon and the oesophageal hiatus to lie in the oesophageal bed.

End-to-end anastomosis is effected between the oesophagus and the jejunum below the aortic arch by the method described for oesophagogastric anastomosis (see Illustrations 16–26). Occasionally it may be necessary to shorten the jejunal loop because of redundancy or uncertainty about the blood supply to the end. If extra length is required an end-to-side anastomosis may provide an extra 3–4 cm.

A nasogastric tube is passed from the mouth down the upper oesophagus across the anastomosis as previously described.

37

The tip of the nasogastric tube is located below the opening in the mesocolon at the site of the end-to-side jejunojejunal anastomosis which is now effected using the same principles as in oesophagogastric anastomosis. This completes the Roux-en-Y. The mediastinal pleura is repaired and the jejunum and the anastomosis buried in the mediastinum. The oesophageal hiatus and the opening in the mesocolon are closed around the jejunal segment and the free edges of the mesentery are attached to the peritoneum so as to prevent internal herniation.

The diaphragm and costal margin are repaired with non-absorbable sutures. The chest is drained and the abdomen and chest wall closed.

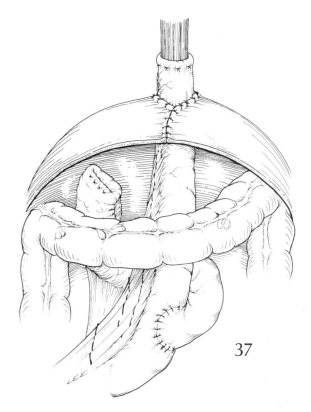

37

Postoperative care and complications

Blood transfusion is continued to match the estimated blood loss. During the operation the patient may lose imperceptibly a considerable volume of fluid from the exposed viscera in the chest and abdomen and this must be replaced intravenously. Central venous pressure should be recorded and maintained at $10–14\,cmH_2O$. Haemoconcentration must be avoided. A steady flow of urine is a satisfactory index of adequate fluid replacement.

Antibiotics are administered if indicated.

The nasogastric tube is allowed to siphon into a bag and may be aspirated occasionally. As soon as bowel sounds return, oral feeding is begun with sips of water, tea or ice cream and progressively increased. Warm and cold feeds each stimulate peristalsis.

The chest drain is removed as soon as drainage is minimal and the chest X-ray satisfactory, and often before commencing feeding. It is not left longer 'just in case of a leak at the anastomosis'.

Leaks from the anastomosis become less common with experience. They should be suspected when there is undue pain or fever or if a pleural effusion develops and they must be confirmed by Gastrografin swallow as immediate resuture is the only hope of salvation. Some surgeons insist on a satisfactory Gastrografin swallow before commencing oral feeding.

Barium studies are necessary if dysphagia develops postoperatively: sometimes the anastomosis will need dilatation and this may have to be repeated but usually an adequate diet maintains a satisfactory lumen. If dysphagia returns or persists after 3 months local recurrence is probable.

When a total gastrectomy has been carried out macrocytic anaemia may eventually develop and it is wise to commence injections of vitamin B12 while the patient is in hospital and advise that they be repeated monthly.

Postgastrectomy dumping may occasionally be experienced. If so, the patient is advised to take extra nourishment between the three main meals of the day; a lump of sugar or a piece of chocolate may reverse early symptoms.

An alteration in bowel habit – more frequent stools – is common and a fatty stool may be experienced after the Roux-en-Y operation, but this usually settles. Diarrhoea may be controlled by codeine phosphate tablets 30 mg hourly until the diarrhoea stops and then less frequently; but first, and always, a rectal examination should be performed to exclude spurious diarrhoea due to impacted faeces or barium.

Further reading

Jackson, J. W., Cooper, D. K. C., Guvendik, L., Reece-Smith, H. The surgical management of malignant tumours of the oesophagus and cardia: a review of the results in 292 patients treated over a 15 year period (1961–75). British Journal of Surgery 1979; 66: 98–104

McKeown, K. C. Trends in oesophageal resection for carcinoma, with special reference to total oesophagectomy. Annals of the Royal College of Surgeons of England 1972; 51: 213–239

Ong, G. B. Unresectable carcinoma of the oesophagus. Annals of the Royal College of Surgeons of England 1975; 56: 3–14

Illustrations by Leslie Arwin, Kathleen E. Sweeney and Gillian Lee

Transhiatal oesophagectomy

Mark B. Orringer MD, FACS
Professor and Head, Section of Thoracic Surgery;
University of Michigan, Ann Arbor, Michigan, USA

History

The technique of transhiatal (or blunt) oesophagectomy, whereby the oesophagus is resected through abdominal and cervical incisions without the need for thoracotomy, was developed before the availability of endotracheal anaesthesia permitted safe transthoracic operations[1–3]. Until recently it was mainly used to resect a *normal* thoracic oesophagus concomitantly with laryngopharyngectomy for pharyngeal or cervical oesophageal carcinoma, the stomach being used to restore continuity of the alimentary tract[4–11]. Transhiatal resection for diseases of the intrathoracic oesophagus has hitherto been uncommon[12, 13]. Based on a personal experience with more than 250 patients, however, we have come to believe that there is seldom an indication for opening the thorax in patients requiring oesophageal resection for either benign or malignant disease[14–17].

Principles and justification

The necessity for a combined thoracoabdominal procedure in a debilitated patient, whose nutritional and pulmonary status have been compromised by impaired swallowing, and the disastrous results of disruption of an intrathoracic oesophageal anastomosis are major contributing factors to the morbidity and mortality rates of oesophageal replacement.

With appropriate mobilization, the stomach will reach to the neck in virtually every patient[18]. There are several benefits in performing a total thoracic oesophagectomy with a cervical anastomosis:

1. Regardless of the level of the oesophageal tumour, the maximum surgical margin possible is obtained, minimizing suture line tumour recurrence.
2. Postoperative death from mediastinitis and sepsis, resulting from anastomotic disruption, is virtually eliminated.
3. Significant gastric reflux is the exception, in contrast to its frequent occurrence when an intrathoracic oesophagogastric anastomosis has been performed.

The physiological insult of a combined thoracic and abdominal operation can be dramatically reduced by the technique of transhiatal oesophagectomy without thoracotomy for both benign and malignant disease. The obvious criticism of this technique is that it ignores two basic principles of surgery – adequate exposure and haemostasis. The surgeon, however, quickly learns to assess resectability by palpation; it is important not to persist with 'blunt' dissection if there is any excessive fixation of the intrathoracic oesophagus to adjacent tissues such as the membranous trachea or aorta. Measured intraoperative blood loss is well within accepted limits, averaging approximately 1 litre.

The abdominal approach not only provides adequate exposure for oesophagectomy but also permits exposure of all portions of the gastrointestinal tract used for oesophageal substitution; if for any reason the stomach is found unsuitable, the colon can readily be mobilized.

Preoperative

Preoperative preparation

1. Vigorous pulmonary physiotherapy, including deep breathing exercises and incentive spirometry, is given for up to 14 days. Smoking is forbidden and antibiotics administered if indicated.
2. In patients with severe weight loss secondary to severe oesophageal obstruction, nasogastric tube feeding, through a tube placed after dilatation of the benign or malignant stricture at oesophagoscopy is given for up to 14 days, ensuring 2000–3000 calories/day (8.4–12.6 kJ/day).
3. Intravascular volume is invariably depleted in these patients; one unit of blood is therefore transfused for every 4–5 kg of weight loss.

4. Dental consultation is undertaken for repair or removal of carious teeth, as poor oral hygiene can be a factor in the severity of infection should a cervical anastomotic leak occur.
5. Where extensive gastric scarring and shortening resulting from previous ulceration or caustic ingestion might preclude use of the entire stomach for oesophageal replacement, the colon is prepared.

Anaesthetic management

1. Use of a double-lumen endotracheal tube permits one-lung anaesthesia and better exposure through a limited thoracotomy on the rare occasions when a transthoracic approach is found to be necessary, but standard endotracheal intubation is used routinely.
2. Continuous intraoperative monitoring of intra-arterial pressure is necessary to detect hypotension, which may result from cardiac displacement during transhiatal oesophagectomy or from blood loss. A well secured radial artery catheter is advantageous.

   The patient's arms are placed at the sides, not extended on arm boards, to allow the surgeon and his assistant greater access to abdomen, chest and neck. If the anaesthetist indicates that hypotension is severe or has been prolonged, the surgeon must stop the dissection long enough to allow cardiac output to recover.
3. The bladder is catheterized and urinary output is monitored.

The operation

The patient is positioned supine with the head turned toward the right on a soft ring and the neck is extended by a small folded sheet placed beneath the scapulae. The operative field extends from the mandibles to the pubis and anterior to both midaxillary lines. The arms are padded and placed at the patient's side. If there is unusual concern that a transthoracic exposure may be required for the oesophagectomy, the appropriate side should be elevated on a folded blanket, the arm bent with the hand placed in the small of the back, and the operating table rolled toward that side to flatten the patient and provide exposure for a standard upper midline abdominal incision.

After the peritoneal cavity has been entered, the left lobe of the liver is mobilized by dividing the triangular ligament, and the liver is padded and retracted laterally to gain exposure of the diaphragmatic hiatus. Use of a self-retaining table-mounted upper abdominal retractor greatly facilitates the operation. The stomach is assessed for its suitability as an oesophageal replacement. Extensive gastric scarring and shortening from prior ulcer disease or the sequelae of caustic ingestion preclude use of the entire stomach for oesophageal replacement. In such cases, the colon, which has been prepared preoperatively, is mobilized.

1 & 2

Gastric mobilization is begun by gently retracting the greater omentum downward and away from the stomach to facilitate identification of the gastroepiploic vessels. The course of the right gastroepiploic artery from the pyloroduodenal area to the mid greater curvature, where it generally terminates as it enters the stomach or divides into smaller branches which anastomose with the left gastroepiploic artery, is identified. The lesser sac is entered through an avascular area of the omentum, opposite the point of convergence of the right and left gastroepiploic vessels at the midportion of the greater curvature of the stomach. The omentum is divided between right-angled clamps applied at least 2 cm below the right gastroepiploic artery to ensure that this vessel is not injured during gastric mobilization. After separating the omentum from the lower half of the greater curvature of the stomach, the surgeon may facilitate identification of the left gastroepiploic vessels along the high greater curvature by inserting his hand behind the remaining attached omentum and retracting it downward. Great care must be taken at this point to avoid injury to the spleen. For this reason, the remaining gastrocolic and greater omentum are divided as close to the stomach as possible without injuring it.

Once mobilization of the omentum from the stomach has been completed, attention is directed to the lesser curvature. The filmy gastrohepatic omentum is incised, and the left gastric artery is divided between the clamps as close to the stomach as possible and ligated. When large coeliac lymph nodes from metastatic oesophageal carcinoma are present, cure is not possible, and no attempt is made to resect the involved glands, unless they are readily separable from the adjacent vessels. The right gastric artery is carefully identified and protected during mobilization of the lesser curvature of the stomach. A pyloromyotomy which extends from 1.5 cm on the stomach through the pylorus and on to the duodenum for 0.5–1 cm is performed, so eliminating the need not only for a gastric suture line in the abdomen which would follow pyloroplasty, but also for a suture line at a right angle to the axis of the elongated stomach. The site of the pyloromyotomy is marked with metal clips for future roentgenographic localization and is covered with adjacent omentum secured in place with several fine sutures. A generous Kocher manoeuvre is carried out to gain maximum upward reach of the mobilized stomach to permit the pylorus to reach from its usual position in the right upper quadrant of the abdomen almost to the xyphoid process in the midline.

Peritoneum overlying the oesophagogastric junction is next incised and the oesophagogastric junction is encircled with a rubber drain. As the drain is retracted downward by one hand, thereby tensing the oesophagus, the other hand is inserted through the diaphragmatic hiatus and blunt, gentle mobilization of the lower 5–10 cm of oesophagus from the mediastinum is carried out. When oesophagectomy is being performed for benign disease or for tumours which do not involve the distal oesophagus, the oesophagogastric junction is divided with the GIA surgical stapler. A rubber drain is sutured to the lower oesophagus with No. 1 silk sutures. This drain, rather than

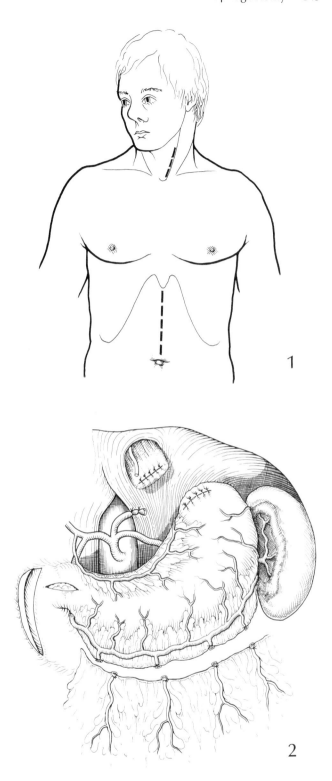

the stomach, can then be used for subsequent traction on the oesophagus to minimize trauma to the organ that will replace the oesophagus. The gastric staple suture line at the cardia is oversewn with a running 3/0 polypropylene inverting Lembert suture.

3

With the mobilized stomach delivered from the peritoneal cavity and placed upon the anterior chest, it can be seen that the gastric fundus, rather than the divided cardia, reaches most superiorly. The high lesser curvature of the stomach may be tethered by fibroareolar tissue and the distal branches of the divided left gastric artery, preventing free extension of the gastric fundus to the neck through either the posterior or anterior mediastinum.

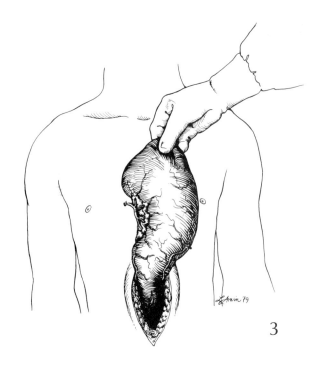

3

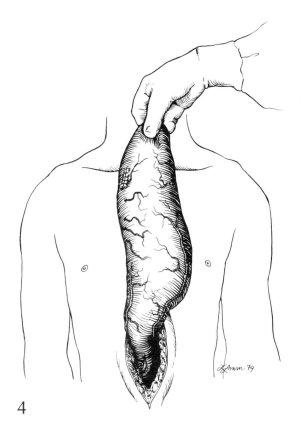

4

4

By carefully removing this tissue from the stomach with fine-tipped haemostats and ties, additional cephalad reach of the fundus is gained. The right gastroepiploic artery, however, must be carefully protected. In most patients, with the stomach placed on the anterior chest wall, the gastric fundus will reach 2–4 cm above the level of the clavicles. One is therefore assured of an adequate gastric length to reach to the neck, as repositioning the stomach into the posterior mediastinum, which is the shortest, most direct route between the cervical oesophagus and the abdomen, will gain an additional 2–3 cm of cephalad reach. After the gastric mobilization is completed, the stomach is returned to the abdomen, a jejunostomy inserted and the oesophageal dissection begun.

5

While downward traction is applied to the oesophageal rubber drain by the left hand, the right hand is inserted behind the oesophagus through the diaphragmatic hiatus, which is progressively dilated one finger at a time, until the entire hand and forearm can be inserted into the posterior mediastinum. A surgeon whose glove is larger than a size 7 may have difficulty unless the lateral crus of the hiatus is incised, but this is not routine. Transhiatal oesophagectomy must be performed as a midline dissection, with the volar aspect of the fingers closely applied to the oesophagus to minimize the chance of entry into the pleural cavities or of injury to the tracheobronchial tree, particularly in the region of the carina. After 5–10 cm of distal oesophagus have been mobilized, attention is turned to the neck.

A 5 cm long oblique cervical incision parallel to the anterior border of the left sternocleidomastoid muscle is made (see Illustration 1). This incision is kept short intentionally, extending inferiorly no further than the suprasternal notch, and cervical dissection is kept to a minimum, so that in the event of a postoperative anastomotic leak, the small wound can be opened in its entirety yet heals rapidly. The platysma and omohyoid fascial layers are incised and, using narrow thyroid retractors, the sternocleidomastoid muscle and carotid sheath and its contents are retracted laterally and the larynx and trachea medially. The recurrent laryngeal nerve is identified and protected. The middle thyroid vein or inferior thyroid artery may be divided and ligated as necessary. The dissection is carried directly posterior to the prevertebral fascia, which is followed bluntly with the index finger into the superior mediastinum. An oesophageal stethoscope or 40 Fr bougie in the oesophagus facilitates identification and mobilization of the cervical oesophagus. The plane between the trachea and oesophagus is developed by sharp dissection, always keeping the recurrent laryngeal nerve in view to avoid injury to it. The cervical oesophagus is mobilized from adjacent tissues circumferentially, being particularly careful not to injure the posterior membranous trachea, and is encircled with a rubber drain. With upward traction on this drain, blunt dissection of the upper oesophagus from the mediastinum is carried out, again dissecting in the midline and keeping the finger against the oesophagus at all times. The upper thoracic oesophagus generally may be mobilized almost to the level of the carina through this approach. Division of the cervical oesophagus is performed using the GIA surgical stapler, and a rubber drain to be used for traction is sutured to the distal end with heavy silk.

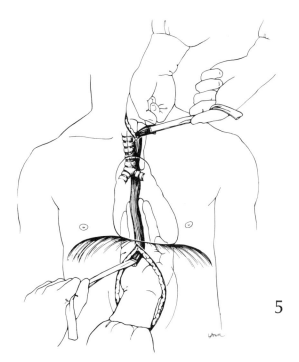

5

6

Blunt dissection of the oesophagus from the posterior mediastinum may be facilitated by a small gauze square held in sponge forceps and introduced through the cervical incision into the superior mediastinum. This 'sponge stick' may be guided along the prevertebral fascia and into the inferior mediastinum either by the surgeon's or the assistant's hand inserted from below through the diaphragmatic hiatus. Perioesophageal attachments and vagal fibres may be gently swept away from the oesophagus with this sponge. Once the 'sponge stick' inserted through the cervical incision can be felt by the hand inserted from the abdomen, mobilization of the posterior oesophagus from the prevertebral fascia has been achieved. During this and subsequent portions of the transhiatal oesophagectomy, careful continual monitoring of intra-arterial blood pressure is necessary to avoid prolonged hypotension which can result from cardiac displacement.

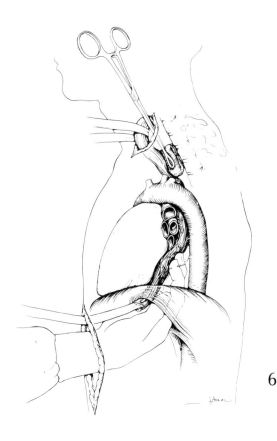

6

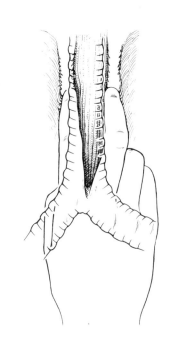

7

7

Circumferential mobilization of the upper 5–8 cm and the lower 8–10 cm of the intrathoracic oesophagus is readily achieved under direct vision through the cervical and abdominal incisions, respectively. The truly 'blind' part of the transhiatal oesophagectomy involves the oesophagus which is immediately adjacent to the lower trachea and carina and the subaortic area. In these areas, the greatest care must be exercised during the dissection. After elevating the oesophagus away from the spine posteriorly (see Illustration 6), the anterior oesophagus is similarly mobilized by sweeping away any attachments to the pericardium or posterior membranous trachea. If the fingers of one hand inserted through the cervical incision along the anterior upper oesophagus meet those of the other hand inserted from below along the anterior lower oesophagus, then the anterior oesophageal dissection has been completed, leaving only the lateral attachments to be divided. The right hand can then be inserted through the diaphragmatic hiatus anterior to the oesophagus and advanced into the superior mediastinum until the index and middle fingers can feel the area of upper oesophagus which has been circumferentially mobilized and the lateral attachments. With posterior pressure against the prevertebral fascia in this area and keeping the oesophagus trapped between the index and middle fingers, a gentle downward raking motion of the hand will generally avulse any small remaining perioesophageal attachments. If at any point in the transhiatal oesophagectomy a pleural tear is recognized, a chest catheter should be inserted at once and connected to suction. This is not a serious complication if recognized and treated promptly.

8

At times, the entire upper oesophagus is freed down to the level of the carina, and the lower oesophagus is similarly mobile up to this point, yet, fibrotic attachments between subcarinal nodes and adjacent oesophagus prevent completion of the dissection. By reaching up into the superior mediastinum through the diaphragmatic hiatus and delivering the upper oesophagus and its attached rubber drain down into the abdomen, one can form a horseshoe of the now entirely intra-abdominal thoracic oesophagus, which is anchored by a few remaining attachments. Narrow, deep retractors placed at either side of the diaphragmatic hiatus permit visualization of these fibrous bands so that direct clamping, division and ligation can be performed. In most instances, however, this horseshoe manoeuvre is not required and the completely mobilized oesophagus is delivered into the cervical or abdominal wound, drawing its attached rubber drain through the posterior mediastinum. Haemostats are placed across the cervical and abdominal ends of the transmediastinal rubber drain, the oesophagus is detached from the drain and removed from the field.

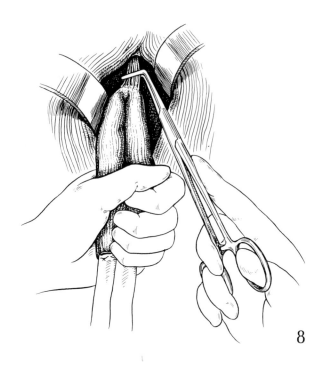

8

9

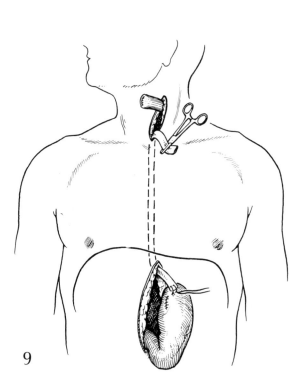

9

In order to ensure an adequate posterior mediastinal tunnel for the stomach, after removing the oesophagus, the entire hand and forearm of the surgeon are inserted through the diaphragmatic oesophageal hiatus and posterior mediastinum until 3 or 4 fingers are visible in the cervical incision. During this procedure the blood pressure must be watched carefully. A 28 Fr Argyle Saratoga sump catheter is then inserted through the cervical incision and into the posterior mediastinum until it is felt within the diaphragmatic hiatus from the abdominal incision. The upper abdomen and lower mediastinum are irrigated with saline solution, and the sump catheter is used to evacuate both the fluid and blood from the abdomen and mediastinum. The stomach is then again delivered on to the anterior chest wall, and the area of the gastric fundus which will extend most cephalad is identified (see Illustration 4). The abdominal end of the transmediastinal rubber drain is secured to the gastric fundus at this site with two 3/0 cardiovascular sutures. The mediastinal sump catheter is removed, and the stomach is carefully positioned through the diaphragmatic hiatus and into the posterior mediastinum by a combination of gentle traction on the cervical end of the rubber drain and guidance through the abdominal incision. As the fundus appears in the cervical incision, it is gently grasped and pulled into the wound while a hand inserted into the mediastinum from the abdomen continually pushes the stomach upward. This hand should also be used to ascertain that the stomach has not been twisted during its positioning in the chest.

10

The gastric fundus, now in the neck, should reach well behind the divided cervical oesophagus. In the abdomen, the pylorus should rest just below the hiatus. The gastric fundus is sutured to the prevertebral fascia behind the divided cervical oesophagus with two 3/0 polypropylene sutures (*see Illustration 11b*). These sutures anchor the stomach in the neck so that the cervical oesophagogastric anastomosis which will subsequently be performed on the anterior surface of the fundus will be under no tension.

To avoid contamination of the abdomen by intraoral contents, the cervical oesophagogastric anastomosis is not begun until the abdominal incision is closed completely and excluded from the field. Before closing the abdomen, however, a final inspection for bleeding, particularly in the area of the spleen, is made; the edge of the diaphragmatic hiatus is 'tacked' to the anterior gastric wall with two or three 3/0 silk sutures to prevent intrathoracic herniation of bowel and a feeding jejunostomy is inserted. No abdominal or mediastinal drains are used routinely.

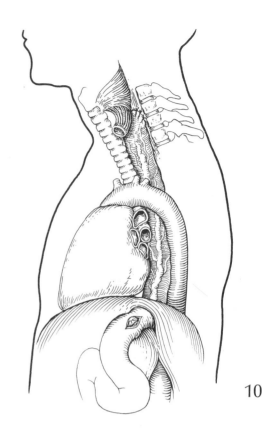

10

11a–d

A single layered end-to-side anastomosis between the cervical oesophagus and gastric fundus is performed using interrupted absorbable 4/0 Dexon. The cervical oesophagus, which has been divided and closed previously with the GIA surgical stapler (*a*), is retracted superiorly. After suspending the gastric fundus from the prevertebral fascia (*b*), a 2 cm vertical incision is then made in the stomach (*c*). The cervical oesophageal staple line is cut away obliquely, leaving the anterior oesophageal wall at least 1 cm longer than the posterior wall (*d*). It is essential not to discard too much oesophagus so that an adequate length is available to ensure a tension-free anastomosis.

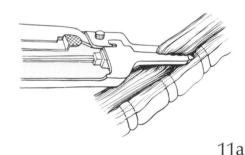

11a

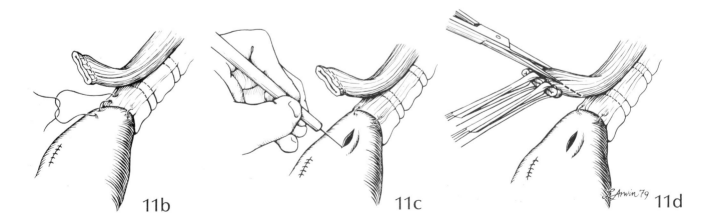

11b

11c

11d

12.a–g

The anastomosis is divided into four quadrants. Beginning at the apex of the gastric incision and the midpoint of the posterior oesophageal wall (a), sutures are placed and secured to adjacent drapes so that the tied knots will be on the inside of the anastomosis. Four to six sutures are placed in each posterior quadrant, beginning medially and working laterally (b and c). Each suture traverses all layers of both the oesophagus and stomach obliquely, passing 2–3 mm from the cut edge of the mucosa and 4–5 mm from the cut edge of the muscle or serosal layers, respectively. The sutures are placed 3 mm apart. The sutures of both posterior quadrants are tied from the most lateral to medial and all sutures are cut except the two corner stitches (d).

A sump nasogastric tube is passed through the anastomosis and into the stomach by the anaesthetist. This tube is used postoperatively for decompression of the intrathoracic stomach. The anterior quadrant sutures are then placed, beginning laterally from each corner stitch and working toward the midline, and alternating from one quadrant to the other, tying the knots on the inside and cutting the sutures sequentially (e). When there is room for only three or four final sutures, inversion of the last segment of the anastomosis is ensured by placing modified Gambee stitches (far-near-near-far; outside-in, inside-out, outside-in, inside-out) (f). These are the only anastomotic sutures with knots tied on the outside (g).

Metal clip markers are placed on either side of the anastomosis for future roentgenographic localization. The cervical wound is irrigated and closed very loosely over a small rubber drain with three to five interrupted absorbable sutures. A portable chest roentgenogram is obtained in the operating room at the conclusion of the operation, and chest tubes are inserted as required for pneumothorax prior to endotracheal extubation.

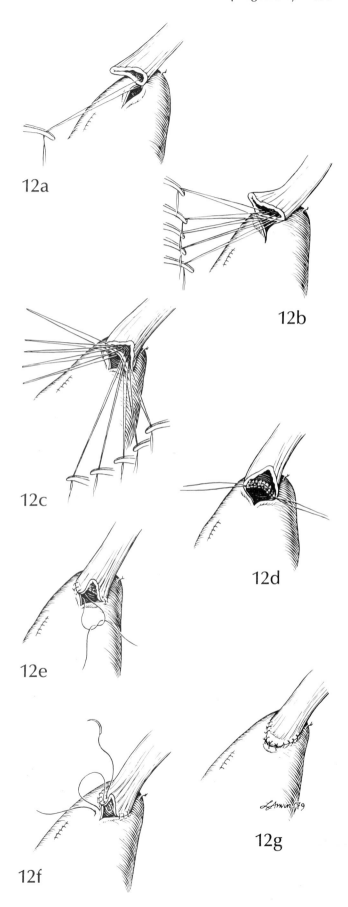

12a

12b

12c

12d

12e

12f

12g

13

Transhiatal oesophagectomy with a limited proximal gastrectomy, utilizing the remaining stomach for a cervical anastomosis, is applicable in patients with localized tumours of the oesophagogastric junction. If the tumour is limited to the oesophagogastric junction and adjacent stomach, the entire greater curvature of the gastric fundus, including that point which ordinarily reaches most cephalad to the neck (*), may be preserved while still obtaining a 4–6 cm gastric margin distal to the neoplasm. A proximal hemigastrectomy for such a tumour wastes valuable stomach (stippled area) that can be used for oesophageal replacement and contributes little to the cancer operation.

With tumours involving the oesophagogastric junction, the surgeon must determine at abdominal exploration if mobilization of the tumour from the diaphragmatic hiatus is possible and if uninvolved oesophagus above the tumour can be reached from the abdominal approach. Mobilization of the thoracic oesophagus and division of the cervical end should not be performed unless the surgeon is satisfied that there is an adequate gastric margin distal to the tumour so that gastric division preserving the entire greater curvature is possible. If, in error, the entire thoracic oesophagus is mobilized first and the cervical end divided, and then the tumour is found to be so large that a proximal hemigastrectomy is required to resect it, the surgeon will find that there is insufficient gastric length to reach to the neck.

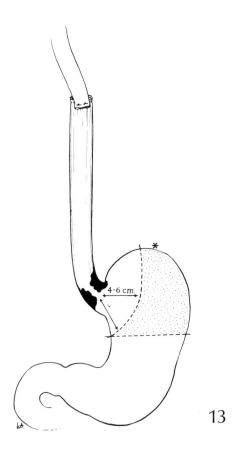

13

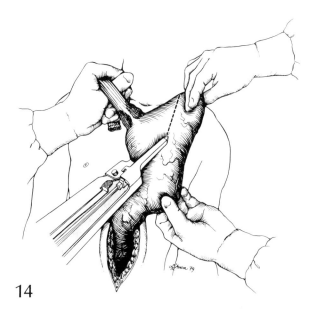

14

14

When an oesophagogastric junction tumour is resected, the stomach should not be divided until the entire oesophageal dissection has been completed. The mobilized upper oesophagus is divided in the neck, a rubber drain is sutured to its cervical end and the oesophagus is delivered downward through the posterior mediastinum and diaphragmatic hiatus. After the thoracic oesophagus and stomach have been placed on the anterior abdominal wall, the stomach is divided with the GIA surgical stapler, applied well away from palpable tumour. The gastric suture line is oversewn with a running 3/0 polypropylene Lembert stitch. The greater curvature gastric 'tube' is then sutured to the posterior mediastinal rubber drain and positioned in the chest and neck as described above to allow a cervical oesophagogastric anastomosis.

Postoperative care

Despite the magnitude of the operation, transhiatal oesophagectomy with cervical oesophagogastric anastomosis is far better tolerated physiologically than the traditional combined thoracic and abdominal approach, as it is essentially an upper abdominal procedure. Although some patients may require mechanical ventilatory assistance the night of operation if the procedure has been prolonged, the average operative time of 3–4 h for transhiatal oesophagectomy generally permits endotracheal extubation the afternoon or evening of operation. However, the patient should be *fully* conscious before being extubated, to ensure adequate ventilation, which may be compromised by postoperative splinting from incisional pain as well as by recurrent laryngeal nerve paresis secondary to cervical or mediastinal dissection.

Pre- and postoperative effort is directed at early ambulation. By the second or third day after operation, 5 per cent dextrose and water is begun via a jejunostomy feeding tube at a rate of 30 ml/h. Postoperative ileus beyond 24–48 h is *rare* after this procedure and the gastrointestinal tract can be used quickly as a route for nourishment. The nasogastric tube is removed when drainage is consistently below 100 ml/8 h, usually by the third postoperative day. If fluids via the jejunostomy tube are well tolerated, a standard tube feeding diet is instituted as soon as possible, diarrhoea being carefully controlled with diphenoxylate (Lomotil) or paregoric as required. Generally within the first 4–5 days after operation, the intra-arterial catheter, cervical wound drain, Foley urethral catheter, intravenous lines and nasogastric tube have been removed, allowing unimpeded ambulation as well as respiratory physiotherapy. Oral liquids are begun once removal of the nasogastric tube has been tolerated well for 24 h. Diet is advanced progressively as tolerated to a mechanical (dental) soft diet, and as oral intake is increased, jejunostomy feedings are concomitantly decreased and then discontinued. A routine postoperative barium swallow examination, to evaluate the anastomosis and emptying of the intrathoracic stomach through the pyloromyotomy (both marked by metal clips), is obtained on the tenth postoperative day. The jejunostomy tube is removed 4–6 weeks after operation.

Any fever above 38°C (101°F) 48 h after operation is regarded as indicative of an anastomotic leak and warrants an immediate contrast study. As the metal clip markers placed at operation define the level of the anastomosis, a limited amount of contrast material is necessary to delineate precisely the area in question. Unexplained postoperative fever following an oesophageal operation is *never* attributed to pulmonary complications, urinary tract sepsis or any other cause *until* an anastomotic leak has been conclusively excluded with a contrast study of the anastomosis. If an anastomotic disruption is diagnosed, the small cervical wound is opened in its entirety and packed gently; closure of the fistula within 7–10 days is usual.

Recurrent laryngeal nerve paresis following this operation may be the result of traction on the nerve either during construction of the cervical anastomosis or during the superior mediastinal dissection at the level of the aortic arch. Secondary cervical dysphagia from cricopharyngeal dysfunction may be quite disturbing and necessitate prolonged jejunostomy tube feedings and passage of oesophageal bougies (46 Fr or larger) until the hoarseness and dysphagia resolve, generally within 4–8 weeks of operation.

Personal results

During the past 8 years, I have performed transhiatal oesophagectomy without throacotomy in 270 patients: 86 with benign disease and 184 with carcinomas at various levels of the oesophagus (40 pharyngo-oesophageal or cervicothoracic, 8 upper third, 61 middle third, and 75 distal third). Oesophageal resection and reconstruction were performed in a single stage in 265 patients, and the oesophageal substitute was positioned in the posterior mediastinum in the original oesophageal bed in 261 patients. Continuity of the alimentry tract was restored by anastomosing the pharynx or cervical oesophagus to stomach (249 patients) or to a colonic graft (19 patients). Colon was utilized only in patients with a history of a prior gastric resection for peptic ulcer disease or gastric stenosis from caustic ingestion.

Patients with pharyngeal or cervicothoracic oesophageal malignancies are a subset of patients with unusually high morbidity and mortality related to prior radiation therapy to the operative field and the need for an anterior mediastinal tracheostomy. Among the 230 patients with beign or malignant disese of the intrathoracic oesophagus, there have been 15 hospital deaths (6.5% mortality), none being the direct result of the technicalities of oesophagectomy. Average measured intraoperative blood loss has been approximately 1 000 ml. No patient in the entire series has required a thoracotomy for intrathoracic haemorrhage either during the operation or in the acute postoperative period. Approximately two-thirds of the patients have required intraoperative placement of a chest tube because of entry into one or both pleural cavities during the oesophagectomy. Transient hoarseness due to left recurrent laryngeal nerve injury ocurred in 35 of our initial 134 patients. Since adopting a policy of avoiding placement of retractors against the tracheo-oesophageal groove during the cervical portions of the operation, this complication has occurred only three times in our last 136 patients. Other complications have included anastomotic leak (14 patients = 6%), chylothorax (5 patients = 2%), and membranous tracheal tear (4 patients = 1.7%).

The average hospitalization for these patients is 14 days after operation, and 75% have been discharged within 10 days. The functional results of oesophageal substitution using the stomach have been very good, and the actuarial survival of our patients undergoing transhiatal resection for carcinoma has been comparable to that reported by others in patients undergoing more radical transthoracic oesophagectomy[20]. Our results support our contention that a thoracic incision is seldom required to resect the oesophagus for either benign or malignant disease. Transhiatal oesophagectomy without thoracotomy is a safe, well tolerated operation, the dangers of which can be minimized by careful technique and experience.

Acknowledgements

Illustrations 3, 4, 11a–d, 12a–g and 14 are reproduced by courtesy of Little, Brown and Company[19] and Illustrations 5, 6 and 13 are reproduced by courtesy of C.V. Mosby Company[14].

References

1. Denk, W. Zur Radikaloperation des Öesophaguskarzinoms. Zentralblatt für Chirurgie 1913; 40: 1065–1068

2. Turner, G. G. Carcinoma of the oesophagus – the question of its treatment by surgery. Lancet 1936; 1: 67–72

3. Turner, G. G. Carcinoma of the oesophagus – the question of its treatment by surgery. Lancet 1936; 1: 130–134

4. Ong, G. B., Lee, T. C. Pharyngogastric anastomosis after oesophagopharyngectomy for carcinoma of the hypopharynx and cervical oesophagus. British Journal of Surgery 1960; 48: 193–200

5. Le Quesne, L. P., Ranger, D. Pharyngolaryngectomy with immediate pharyngogastric anastomosis. British Journal of Surgery 1966; 53: 105–109

6. Harrison, D. F. N. Surgical management of cancer of the hypopharynx and cervical oesophagus. British Journal of Surgery 1969; 56: 95–103

7. Leonard, J. R., Maran, A. G. Reconstruction of the cervical esophagus via gastric anastomosis. Laryngoscope 1970; 80: 849–862

8. Stell, P. M. Esophageal replacement by transposed stomach: following pharyngolaryngo-esophagectomy for carcinoma of the cervical esophagus. Archives of Otolaryngology 1970; 91: 166–170

9. Akiyama, H., Hiyama, M. A simple esophageal bypass operation by the high gastric division. Surgery 1974; 75: 674–681

10. Taw, J. L. Pharyngo-gastric anastomosis in a kyphotic patient with carcinoma of the cervical oesophagus. Australian and New Zealand Journal of Surgery. 1973; 42: 377–380

11. Mappes, G., Haas, E. Geschlossener transmediastinaler Durchzug des Magens als einzeitiger totaler Osophagusersatz beim Hypopharynx–und zervikalen Osophagus–Karzinom (English Abstract). Deutsche Medizinische Wochenschrift 1975; 100: 1066–1068

12. Kirk, R. M. Palliative resection of oesophageal carcinoma without formal thoracotomy. British Journal of Surgery 1974; 61: 689–690

13. Thomas, A. N., Dedo, H. H. Pharyngogastrostomy for treatment of severe caustic stricture of the pharynx and esophagus. Journal of Thoracic and Cardiovascular Surgery 1977; 73: 817–824

14. Orringer, M. B., Sloan, H. Esophagectomy without thoracotomy. Journal of Thoracic and Cardiovascular Surgery 1978; 76: 643–654

15. Orringer, M. B., Orringer, J. S. Esophagectomy without thoracotomy – a dangerous operation? Journal of Thoracic and Cardiovascular Surgery 1983; 85: 72–80

16. Orringer, M. B., Sloan, H. Anterior mediastinal tracheostomy – indications, techniques, and clinical experience. Journal of Thoracic and Cardiovascular Surgery 1979; 78: 850–859

17. Orringer, M. B. Transhiatal esophagectomy without thoracotomy for carcinoma of the thoracic esophagus. Annals of Surgery 1984; 200: 282–288

18. Orringer, M. B., Sloan, H. Substernal gastric bypass of the excluded thoracic esophagus for palliation of esophageal carcinoma. Journal of Thoracic and Cardiovascular Surgery 1975; 70: 836–851

19. Orringer, M. B., Sloan, H. Esophageal replacement using stomach substernally and after blunt oesophagectomy. In: Nyhus, L. M., Baker, R. J. eds. Mastery of Surgery. Boston: Little, Brown and Co., 1984: 426–439

20. Skinner, D. B. En bloc resection for neoplasm of the esophagus and cardia. Journal of Thoracic and Cardiovascular Surgery 1983; 85: 59–71

Illustrations by Lesley Skeates

Colon replacement of the oesophagus

Hugoe R. Matthews FRCS
Consultant Thoracic Surgeon, East Birmingham Hospital, Birmingham, UK

Introduction

The oesophagus is the only part of the gut that is both long and relatively straight. Removal of any part of it produces a gap which has to be filled by a replacement or reconstructive procedure, if alimentary continuity and the capacity to swallow are to be restored. Very occasionally reconstruction may be possible by end-to-end oesophageal anastomosis, but in most cases it will be necessary to use some other part of the gut, namely stomach, jejunum or colon. With the development and wider use of conservative operations for reflux stricture the need for colon replacement has declined, but it remains a very important method of reconstruction, particularly in unusual and difficult cases. The operation is lengthy and complicated and needs to be performed expertly, but it provides an excellent replacement for the oesophagus over long periods of time.

Indications

Colon is chosen for reconstruction for one of two reasons.

In patients in whom all three viscera (stomach, jejunum, colon) may be used, the colon is preferred in the expectation that it will give the best long-term functional result. The performance of successful colon grafts over 20 years or more has been well established in cases of oesophageal atresia, and colon should be favoured in young patients with a potentially long life ahead of them. Such patients are also more likely to tolerate the increased duration and complexity of this procedure without adverse effects.

In patients in whom the stomach or jejunum cannot be mobilized sufficiently to bridge the gap left by oesophageal resection, colon has to be selected as the only available method of reconstruction. This applies when the stomach is affected by disease or previous surgery (e.g. partial gastrectomy) and when a sufficient length of jejunum cannot be obtained because of an inadequate blood supply to the graft.

Indications for the operation therefore include:

1. oesophageal atresia, where primary anastomosis is impossible or has proved unsuccessful;
2. gastro-oesophageal reflux with complications (e.g. stricture, short oesophagus, penetrating ulcer) which cannot be treated by a more conservative operation;
3. corrosive strictures of the oesophagus;
4. malignant tumours of the oesophagus, particularly those requiring laryngo-oesophagectomy;
5. benign tumours which are extensive, diffuse or locally recurrent;
6. motility disorders (e.g. spasm or achalasia) where symptoms are severe and previous operations have failed;
7. oesophageal injury, where the oesophagus has had to be removed or repair has failed.

It should be stressed that this list is not exhaustive or exclusive – other cases certainly occur for which colon reconstruction is appropriate.

Prerequisites

It is important to remember that colon cannot be used for reconstruction unless three basic requirements are met.

1. It must be free of any significant disease, e.g. diverticulitis, colitis or carcinoma. A barium enema must be obtained well in advance of operation in any patient with a history or clinical suspicion of colonic disease. If the investigation is left until just before operation, barium retention may lead to constipation and a heavily loaded colon, which would be unsuitable for a graft. In some centres a barium enema is performed routinely in every case that might require a colon graft, but this is unnecessary, particularly in children and young adults, and anyway does not guarantee the suitability of the organ for grafting.
2. It must be possible to isolate a segment of sufficient length with a satisfactory arterial and venous blood supply. This means that the marginal connections of the arterial arcades must be intact and patent, and that the vessels must be capable of being visualized and isolated at operation. If the mesocolon is thick and fatty, or the vessels are atherosclerotic, then it may be impossible to prepare a satisfactory graft.
3. It must be suitably prepared with respect to its faecal content. If the colon is distended with hard, soft or liquid faeces it cannot be used as a graft. Ideally it should contain no faeces, or small hard masses which can be removed easily. This is achieved by confining the patient to liquids only for 5 days before operation and encouraging him to open his bowels whenever he feels the urge. One glycerine suppository may be given not less than 24 hours before operation. Vigorous bowel preparation, as for the diseased colon, is quite inappropriate for the normal colon: enemas, washouts, cathartics and oral antibiotics may all result in an inflamed, oedematous colon that is unsuitable for grafting.

It follows that the final decision regarding the suitability of colon for reconstruction can only be made during the course of the operation. This, means that before embarking on operation the surgeon must have an alternative plan, in case the colon proves unsuitable; also, the oesophagus must not be devitalized or resected until the availability of a suitable substitute has been confirmed by exploration and dissection.

Methods

1a, b & c

Colon can be used for reconstruction in a variety of ways. It can be used to replace either a part or the whole of the oesophagus, or the oesophagus plus laryngopharynx. The segment forming the graft can be taken from the right (a), transverse (b) or descending (c) portions of the colon, and the vessels either left attached to their usual origins, or divided, so as to form a 'free' graft with anastomosis to an adjacent artery and vein at the new site.

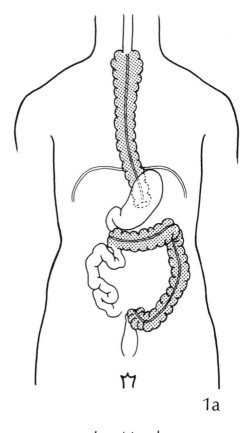

1a

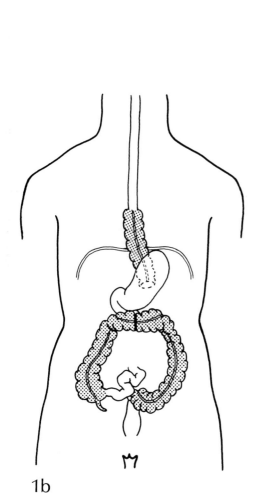

1b

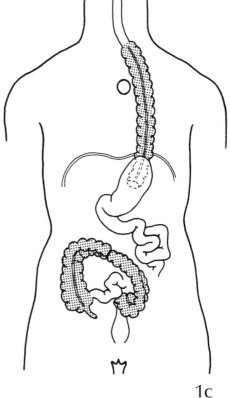

1c

2

In addition to actual replacement of the excised oesophagus, colon can be used to bypass a diseased area, with the original oesophagus being left in place. This can be done as a definitive operation, or as a first stage in order to improve the patient's condition so that the oesophagus can be resected later.

Whether used as a replacement or bypass, the graft can be placed in one of four different positions in the body.

In the mediastinal position (see *Illustration 1*) the graft is placed in the same position as the excised oesophagus with the anastomosis in the chest or neck. This is the shortest route between the oesophagus and the distal gut and probably offers the best arrangement for providing unobstructed passage of food.

In the transpleural position (see *Illustration 1c*) the graft is placed in one or other pleural cavity, but outside the mediastinum. Anastomosis may be in the chest or neck. When in the neck, it will be necessary to create a tunnel through the thoracic inlet through which the graft is passed.

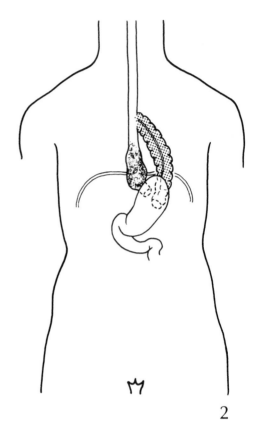

2

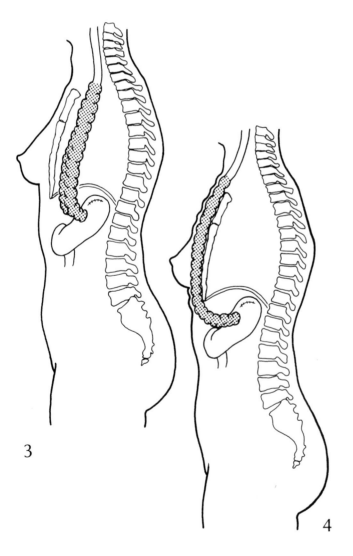

3

4

3

In the retrosternal position the graft is placed in a tunnel in the anterior mediastinum between the pericardium and the back of the sternum, with anastomosis in the neck. A greater length of colon is required but thoracotomy is avoided.

4

In the subcutaneous position the graft is placed in a tunnel between the skin and the front of the sternum, again with anastomosis in the neck. This avoids any possibility of contaminating the pleura but requires an even longer segment of colon.

Finally, the surgical approach may be through various incisions, including laparotomy, right or left thoracotomy, left thoracolaparotomy and right, left or bilateral neck incisions, or any combination of these. The choice of approach is determined by the location of the lesion and the type of reconstruction intended.

Common to all these alternatives, however, is the fact that the success of the operation depends almost entirely on the preparation of a segment of colon with a vigorous blood supply and of sufficient length so that anastomoses can be made without tension. The detailed account that follows is limited to one method, which will serve well for the majority of cases, but the principles of preparation of the graft will apply whichever part of the colon and whichever route are being used.

Essentially the method described below, developed by Belsey[1], utilizes an isoperistaltic graft formed from the left transverse and descending colon, with the blood supply based on the left colic artery. This has a number of significant advantages, including a reliable blood supply, less disparity between the size of the oesophagus and the colon and good access to both oesophagus and colon through a single left thoracoabdominal incision.

Preoperative

Before operation patients should be in the best possible state, both physically and mentally, so that the risk and effects of any complications are minimized. The time required for preparation will obviously depend on the condition of the patient and the urgency of the problem. Ideally patients should be ambulant, active and in good general health. Those who are bedridden, listless and apathetic are likely to have a more complicated recovery.

In addition to oesophageal studies, routine investigations should include the haemoglobin concentration, biochemical profile, lung function tests, chest radiograph and electrocardiogram, in order to identify potential problems. Smoking must be stopped at least one week before operation and all patients instructed by an experienced physiotherapist in the breathing and coughing techniques that will be required after operation. The bowel is prepared as described above.

Conditions which can be corrected prior to operation must be dealt with, but those which cannot be treated will have to be ignored. Anaemia, dehydration, uraemia and severe malnutrition may all require attention; any associated medical disorders (e.g. diabetes) must be treated as effectively as possible. Nutrition should be improved perorally wherever possible, by dilatation or even temporary endoscopic intubation, rather than by prolonged intravenous or nasogastric tube feeding, which are generally undesirable. A preliminary gastrostomy complicates the operation. It should be reserved for patients with an undilatable obstruction with severe respiratory complications, which must be treated before operation is possible.

The operation

Anaesthesia

Premedication and anaesthetic technique are the responsibility of the anaesthetist, but one-lung anaesthesia should be provided with a Robertshaw or Gordon-Green tube whenever possible. This greatly improves access to the oesophagus and minimizes handling and retraction of the lung. A central venous line is desirable for blood volume control, and a urinary catheter should be inserted if operation is likely to be prolonged unduly. Arterial pressure monitoring is required only for high-risk cases. Prophylactic intravenous or intramuscular antibiotics are given soon after induction, in order to provide high blood levels during operation.

Position and incision

5

For the standard operation the patient is positioned as shown. An incision is made starting at the left linea semilunaris, at or just inferior to the level of the umbilicus, and continuing up over the costal margin, then along the line of the seventh rib, to end at the angle of the ribs posteriorly. Latissimus dorsi and the abdominal wall muscles are divided in the line of the incision, and the serratus anterior divided obliquely about 1 cm from its origin on the ribs. The muscles of the sixth intercostal space are divided along the upper border of the seventh rib using diathermy and the cartilaginous costal margin cut with a scalpel. The pleura is opened and the diaphragm incised circumferentially over a distance of approximately 15 cm, about 1–2 cm from its origin on the ribs, leaving the phrenic nerve undamaged.

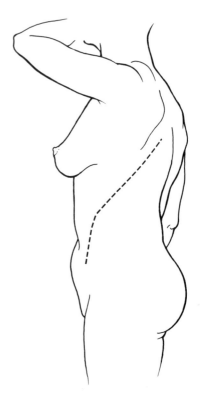

5

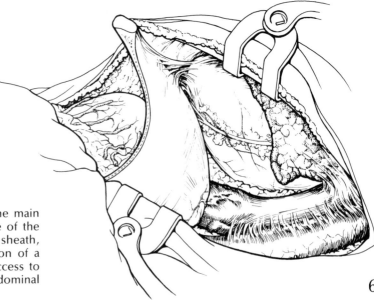

6

The peritoneum is then opened in the line of the main incision, from the centre of the abdominal edge of the diaphragmatic incision to the edge of the rectus sheath, giving a 'T'-shaped abdominal exposure. Insertion of a large, racheted chest retractor gives excellent access to the whole of the left chest and the necessary abdominal organs.

6

Exploration of the oesophagus

7

The oesophagus is explored first, in order to determine that resection is necessary and possible, and the level at which the anastomosis has to be performed, unless this is already known. The ipsilateral lung is collapsed by the anaesthetist and the mediastinal pleura incised from below the aortic arch to the diaphragm. The lower oesophagus is then dissected free from the mediastinum (taking all adjacent connective tissue if a carcinoma is present) and encircled with a tape for retraction. In cases of stricture the level and severity of obstruction is identified by the passage of flexible mercury bougies via the mouth. It is important at this stage that dissection does not proceed to the point where the oesophagus is devitalized, in case there is no suitable organ available for reconstruction.

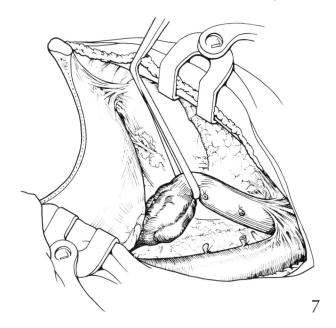

7

8

Mobilization of the colon

Having established that resection is required the colon is examined to check that it is free from disease and determine that its vascular connections and faecal content make it suitable for grafting. It has to be mobilized extensively, first so that the graft will reach the desired level, and, second, in order to permit secure re-anastomosis of the colon after its division. This mobilization should extend from the right half of the transverse colon to the descending left colon, the precise limits being determined by the length of graft required. The process is begun by the separation of the greater omentum from its attachment to the anterior border of the colon. This is done by scissor dissection in the relatively bloodless plane adjacent to the colonic wall; any adventitious vessels which are encountered are ligated and divided, but the vessels in the mesocolon must be preserved meticulously. The left colon is mobilized by division of its lateral peritoneal reflection in the left paracolic gutter, care being taken to avoid damage to the ureter. The whole segment is further freed from its connective tissue attachments by a combination of sharp and blunt dissection, so that it can be lifted out of the wound, remaining attached only by the mesocolon containing the middle and left colic vessels and their branches.

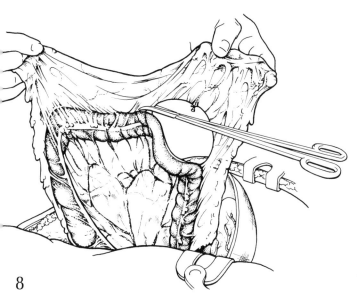

8

9

Selection of the graft segment

Now the points at which the bowel is to be divided must be determined in order to provide a graft of sufficient length for the reconstruction. Some surgeons formally measure the length required, but in general it is wise to be generous – surplus can always be trimmed but a short graft cannot be made longer. For lower oesophageal reconstruction only a short segment of colon is required, extending approximately from S_1 to S_2, with the vessels eventually being divided at S_3. For complete oesophageal reconstruction the additional length is obtained mainly from the right transverse colon, so that the graft extends from approximately L_1 to L_2, with the vessels being divided at L_3.

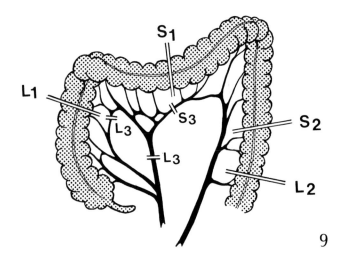

9

10

Isolation of the graft blood supply

When the colon has been lifted out of the wound and transilluminated from behind so that the vessels are clearly visible, the mesocolon is divided from its root up to the points at which the bowel is to be divided. During this manoeuvre the vascular arcades adjacent to the colon wall and any other small vessels are ligated and divided, but the branches of the middle colic vessels which go to the graft are left intact. Where the colon is to be cut, it is cleared of fat and connective tissue over a distance of 1–2 cm to facilitate later anastomosis.

Small bulldog clamps are then applied to occlude any branches of the middle colic vessels which go to the graft segment, in order to test the adequacy of its blood supply, which is now based entirely on the left colic vessels. If the graft remains pink and healthy and with visible pulsation in the vessels at its proximal end, then it will be suitable for reconstruction. If it shows signs of ischaemia then the blood supply is restored by removing the clamps from the middle colic vessels and an alternative method of reconstruction will have to be found.

10

Excision of the oesphagus

11

Leaving the clamps in place on the middle colic vessels, the diseased oesophagus can now be excised. Any necessary dissection is completed and a strong transfixion suture is placed through the whole wall of the oesophagus just above the diseased area. This is tied securely and the end cut long for later retraction. A further ligature is tied around the oesophagus beyond this (to avoid spillage) and the oesophagus divided transversely between the two.

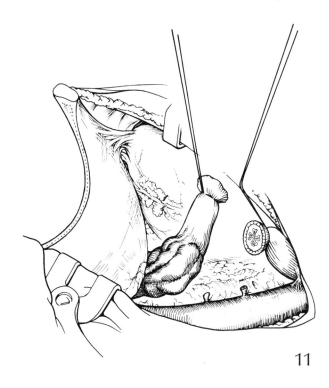

11

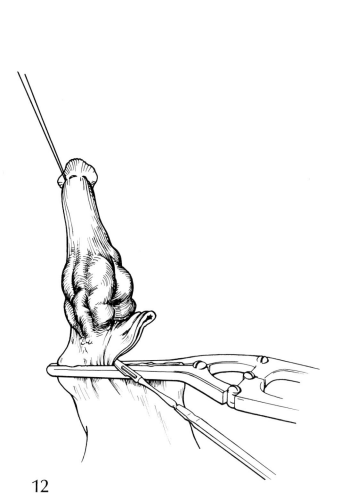

12

12

The lower oesophagus is then drawn down through the hiatus and the cardia exposed and cleaned so that it can be divided and closed securely, but extensive mobilization is not necessary. A Payr's crushing clamp is applied across the desired line of section at the cardia and the lower oesophagus cut off proximal to it. The cardia is closed with two layers of continuous sutures, using catgut and silk.

13

Because the stomach is now denervated a pyloromyotomy is performed routinely to prevent troublesome postoperative gastric stasis. Using fine, angled Pott's scissors a 1–2 cm incision is made longitudinally across the pylorus on its posterior aspect, dividing all the circular muscle fibres until the mucosa bulges outwards freely. Some surgeons omit this step altogether; others simply dilate the pylorus digitally, or with various instruments, through a small gastrotomy, but there is general agreement that a formal pyloroplasty is not required unless the duodenum is ulcerated or scarred.

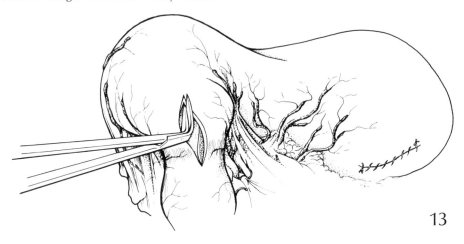

13

14

Separation of the graft

Attention is now redirected to the graft segment. Assuming that it continues to look healthy, the bulldog clamps are removed and the vessels are finally ligated and divided at the same point. Two bowel clamps are then placed across the colon, at each point where it is to be divided, and the colon divided between them. If crushing clamps are used, the colonic ends must be trimmed before subsequent anastomosis; if non-crushing clamps are used, there is no need to trim the ends but care must be taken not to damage the blood supply to the ends of the colon. The graft segment is now completely separated except for its vascular attachments. It is placed temporarily in a corner of the operative field, where it will not be damaged or kinked, and covered with a swab moistened in saline.

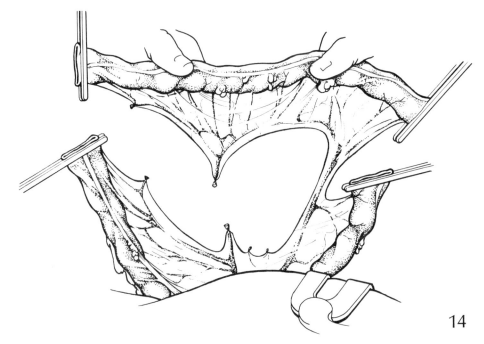

14

15

Colocolic anastomosis

Large bowel continuity is now restored by end-to-end anastomosis of the divided colon. The two ends of the mobilized colon are lifted out of the wound and swabs placed round them to avoid contamination of the peritoneum. The ends are approximated with a stay suture, the clamps removed and any adjacent faeces evacuated with small swabs which are immediately discarded. Anastomosis is then performed (our own preference is for interrupted sutures of 36 gauge atraumatic monofilament stainless steel wire, which are placed 3 mm apart). The knots are initially placed on the inside of the colon, but must be placed on the outside for the last few sutures. On completion, the bowel is returned to the abdomen where the anastomosis should lie comfortably and without tension. No attempt is made to close the mesocolon.

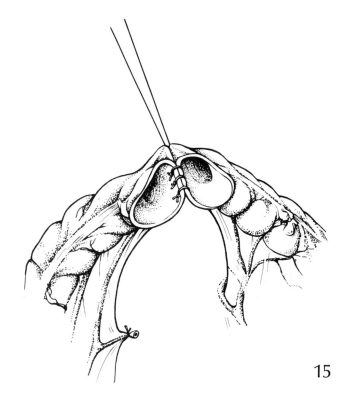

15

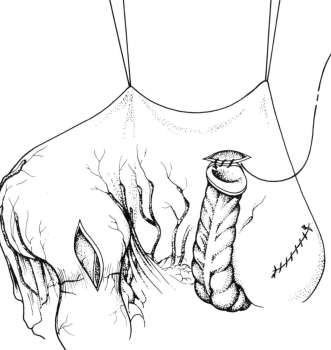

16

16

Gastrocolic anastomosis

Two stay sutures are placed in the margin of the greater curvature of the stomach and elevated in order to expose the posterior wall of the body of the stomach. An incision corresponding in size to the distal end of the graft is made in the mid-portion of the stomach, for end-to-side anastomosis of the graft. The siting of this anastomosis is important: there must be a considerable length of colon below the diaphragm which can be compressed by the weight of the abdominal organs, in order to prevent gastro-oesophageal reflux – particularly in the recumbent position. If the graft is joined to the cardia or fundus, reflux is liable to occur.

The distal end of the graft and the gastric wall are approximated by suture, the bowel clamp removed and faeces evacuated as before. A one-layer anastomosis is then performed, using continuous 36 gauge wire and providing a lumen sufficient to allow the passage of a normal sized bolus of food.

17

Oesophagocolic anastomosis

The proximal end of the graft is passed through the oesophageal hiatus and positioned in the mediastinum so that it will reach to the level of anastomosis without tension. The oesophagus is elevated by traction on the transfixion suture and the oesophagus and colon approximated by a stay suture at the intended point of anastomosis. The bowel clamp is removed and faeces dealt with as before. The oesophagus is then incised transversely, posteriorly over a short distance, through healthy, well-vascularized tissue, proximal to the transfixion suture. End-to-end anastomosis of the colon and oesophagus is begun posteriorly with a single layer of continuous wire sutures. The oesophagus is divided progressively as the suturing proceeds. Finally the piece of oesophagus containing the transfixion suture is excised completely and the anastomosis completed anterolaterally. This technique involves an open anastomosis but avoids retraction of the oesophagus during suturing or the use of clamps on the oesophagus, which may damage the blood supply.

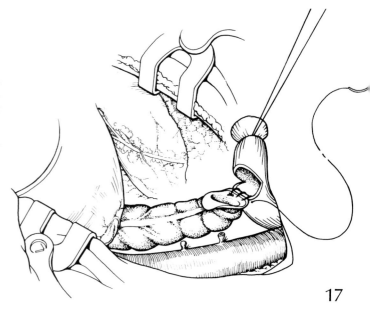

17

Variations

18

If oesophageal bypass, rather than replacement, is being performed, the proximal end of the colon is anastomosed end-to-side to a lateral vertical incision in the wall of the oesophagus.

19

If total oesophagectomy is being performed, the proximal end of the colon is closed securely by suture and also attached firmly to the transfixed end of the oesophagus by sutures. The oesophageal remnant and graft segment are then drawn upwards deep to the aortic arch and positioned in the apex of the chest ready for delivery and anastomosis in the neck.

Closure of the incision

Haemostasis is achieved before closing the incision and the graft and anastomoses examined to make sure that there is no evidence of leakage or ischaemia. The left lung is inflated and the diaphragm and deep layers of the abdominal wall are closed with continuous synthetic absorbable sutures. A large fenestrated intercostal drain (e.g. size 32 Argyle) is inserted in the pleura through a separate stab incision, sutured to the skin and connected to an underwater seal. To diminish postoperative incisional pain the intercostal nerves adjacent to the incision may be injected with local anaesthetic or frozen with the cryoprobe. Finally the ribs, muscle layers of the chest wall and abdomen, subcutaneous tissues and skin are closed using continuous synthetic absorbable sutures.

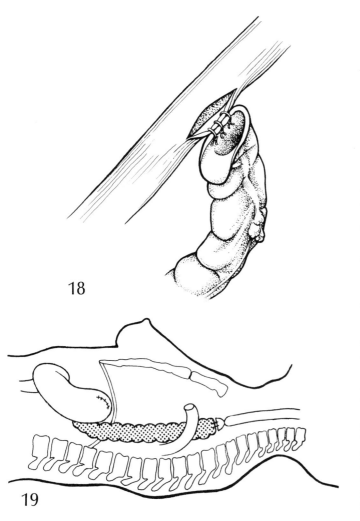

18

19

RECONSTRUCTION IN THE NECK

20

A separate cervical incision is necessary for reconstructions which require an anastomosis in the neck. After the chest has been opened it is usually better for the neck exposure to be performed as a separate operation, after the patient has been repositioned on his back and redraped. The incision is then made on the same side as the thoracotomy. If the approach has been entirely through a laparotomy, however, the cervical exposure can be made at the same time.

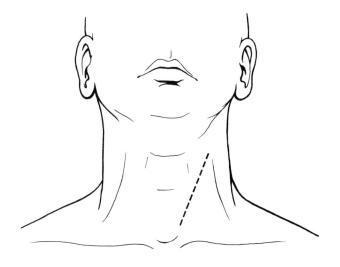

20

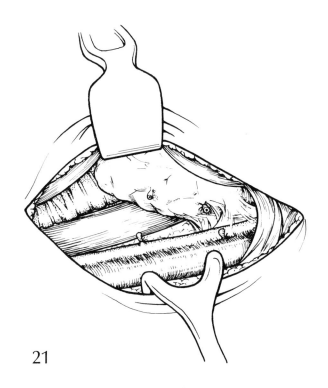

21

21

An oblique incision 10 cm long is made in the right or left side of the neck along the anterior border of the sternomastoid muscle, extending upwards and backwards from the suprasternal notch. The platysma is divided in the line of the incision and the sternomastoid retracted laterally. The omohyoid muscle is divided and the middle thyroid vein and inferior thyroid artery isolated, ligated and divided, preserving the recurrent laryngeal nerve. The thyroid gland is then retracted medially and the carotid and jugular vessels retracted laterally, giving access to the lateral wall of the oesophagus.

22 & 23

If the oesophagus is being resected, its proximal stump is delivered, together with the attached proximal end of the graft, and end-to-end anastomosis performed, as already described. If a bypass is being performed, the upper end of the graft is retrieved and the upper oesophagus is mobilized by a combination of sharp and blunt dissection and encircled with a tape, so that sufficient access is obtained for a lateral oesophagotomy and end-to-side anastomosis of the colon. On completion of the anastomosis the superficial muscular layers and skin are closed without drainage.

22

23

24

For laryngo-oesophagectomy a much larger exposure is required, consisting of an 'H'-shaped incision, with the horizontal limb approximately at the level of the crico-thyroid membrane. Upper and lower flaps are raised to allow wide excision of the primary tumour and the cervical lymph nodes bilaterally. The upper trachea is divided clear of the growth and a terminal tracheostomy fashioned through a separate stoma in the lower flap, followed by end-to-end anastomosis of the colon and pharynx.

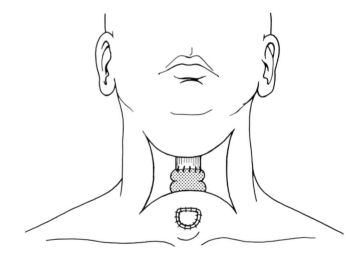

24

Postoperative care

After operation the patient should be awake and cooperative. He is usually admitted to the intensive care unit for the first night, but this is for careful observation of respiration and circulation rather than vigorous therapy. Pulse, blood pressure, central venous pressure, peripheral temperature, urine output, ECG and blood gases are monitored and chest radiographs obtained. Intravenous analgesics are given in small doses as required, provided they do not compromise the patient's respiration or his ability to cooperate with chest physiotherapy. Routine artificial ventilation should not be required. Any lost blood volume is replaced, but intravenous fluid administration should be restricted to maintenance requirements (e.g. 2 litres per 24 hours for a normal adult) and should consist of 5 per cent dextrose solution, as saline administration may lead to sodium retention and tissue oedema.

Nasogastric tubes are neither necessary nor desirable, and oral liquids are normally commenced by the second or third day, when bowel sounds are present. The patient then progresses to free fluids, sloppy diet and minced diet over a period of about one week. Intravenous nutrition is required only if prolonged complications prevent an adequate oral intake. The chest drain is removed when it has ceased to function – normally on the second or third day.

Complications

Clearly all the complications that may be associated with a laparotomy or thoracotomy can occur after colon reconstruction, but only those which relate specifically to the use of colon will be discussed here. Despite the complexity of the procedure serious complications are surprisingly infrequent, but they do occur and may be fatal.

Early complications

Early complications are related to the blood supply of the graft or the healing of the various anastomoses.

Graft infarction

This is caused by an inadequate arterial or venous blood supply and is liable to be fatal even if treated promptly by re-operation. The patient develops a tachycardia, with signs of shock and toxaemia which are resistant to treatment. There is a foul smell in the chest drain. It is important to realize that in the early stages the bowel wall may maintain its integrity, even though it is devitalized, so that there is no obvious alimentary leak from the chest. X-ray contrast studies may show no abnormality. Exploration is required early if the condition is even suspected. The dead graft is excised, the stomach closed and a terminal oesophagostomy fashioned in the neck. If the patient survives, an alternative method of reconstruction is performed at a later date.

Anastomotic breakdown

This may vary from complete separation of the two ends to a localized leak from some point on the circumference of the anastomosis. It is caused by local ischaemia of the tissues, tension on the anastomosis or poor surgical technique. Treatment will depend on the severity and site of the breakdown.

Oesophagocolic anastomosis Complete separation requires reoperation. The anastomosis can be refashioned if there is adequate tissue, but if there is not, a terminal oesophagostomy is constructed, the proximal end of the graft closed and further reconstruction performed later. Limited leaks can usually be expected to heal, provided there is no distal obstruction. They are therefore treated conservatively, with no oral intake, intravenous nutrition, antibiotics and chest drainage if necessary. Serial radiographic contrast studies are used to follow the progress of healing.

Gastrocolic anastomosis Leakage at this anastomosis is rare but would require re-operation in order to avoid a generalized peritonitis. Normally there should be sufficient colon below the diaphragm to permit re-anastomosis if necessary.

Colocolic anastomosis Dehiscence or leakage at this site leads to a faecal peritonitis and requires immediate re-operation, with the construction of a terminal colostomy and closure or exteriorization of the distal end of the colon. If the patient survives, the colon is re-anastomosed later.

Late complications

Late complications may include anastomotic strictures, stasis or poor motility in the graft and reflux of gastric content into the residual oesophagus.

Anastomotic strictures are treated by dilatation or refashioning procedures, according to their site and severity. Delayed passage of food through the graft is not amenable to surgical correction, though 'redundant' colon is sometimes excised from the distal end of the graft in the hope of improving symptoms. These are not generally severe, but, if they are, a different form of reconstruction may have to be considered.

Reflux of gastric content into the graft itself should have no adverse effect on the colonic mucosa, but if there is no valvular mechanism below the diaphragm, the refluxed material may reach the remaining oesophagus and cause the typical changes of reflux oesophagitis. If these are severe, operation is required to mobilize the colon below the diaphragm and re-implant it into the stomach in such a way as to provide a compressible segment that will form an effective antireflux barrier.

Reference

1. Belsey, R. Reconstruction of the esophagus with left colon. Journal of Thoracic and Cardiovascular Surgery 1965; 49: 33–55

Pulsion intubation of the oesophagus

I. Barnett Angorn FRCS(Ed), FRCS
Professor of Surgery, University of Natal, Durban, South Africa

Introduction

Peroral pulsion intubation is used almost exclusively for the palliation of dysphagia due to malignant obstruction of the oesophagus and cardia. The technique is preferable to traction intubation which requires laparotomy and gastrotomy with an increase in morbidity and a prolongation of hospital stay. Pulsion intubation permits correction of protein–energy malnutrition with minimal dietary modification, and relief can be obtained from the sequelae of pulmonary aspiration or oesophagorespiratory fistula.

Preoperative

Indications

Pulsion intubation to relieve dysphagia may be required:

1. In neoplastic strictures of the oesophagus, usually squamous carcinoma in the following circumstances.
   (a) Medical contraindications to surgery or radiotherapy.
   (b) Clinically detectable organ invasion or distant dissemination.
   (c) Dysphagia due to tumour recurrence following surgery or radiotherapy.
   (d) Malignant strictures longer than 6 cm involving the upper thoracic oesophagus (20–32 cm from the incisor teeth). These tumours are invariably unresectable.
   (e) Demonstrable oesophagotracheal or oesophagobronchial fistula.
   (f) Unresectability established at laparotomy or thoracotomy.
   (g) The development of an anastomotic stricture following surgery or a fibrous stricture following radiotherapy.
2. Where unresectable tumours of the stomach invade the cardia and lower oesophagus.
3. Where the oesophagus is compressed or invaded by intrathoracic tumours.
4. In patients with benign oesophageal strictures, where surgery is contraindicated and repeated dilatation is hazardous or ineffective.

Contraindications

Failure of the cricopharyngeal sphincter to close over the proximal end of the tube causes gagging and will preclude intubation of high lesions.

Intubation in the presence of jaw fixity, ankylosis of the cervical spine or thoracic spinal deformity can be facilitated by using the fibreoptic endoscope and a flexible introducer.

Preparation of patient

Anteroposterior and lateral chest X-rays (1.8 m films) following a barium swallow will indicate the level of obstruction, the length of the stricture and the alignment of the oesophageal axis. Dentures should be removed and loose teeth extracted. Food and fluids are withheld for 12 h before intubation. Fluid contents are aspirated and food residues removed by oesophageal wash-outs.

Equipment

Both the rigid and flexible oesophagoscope should be available. The 35 cm rigid Negus oesophagoscope allows adequate biopsy and dilatation of lesions of the upper thoracic oesophagus.

The flexible instrument is preferred for lesions of the distal oesophagus and cardia. Introduction of a guide-wire into the stomach via the biopsy channel under direct visual or radiological control permits safer dilatation of distal strictures.

1a & b

Bougies

Graduated neoplex oesophageal bougies (a) can be passed via the rigid oesophagoscope for dilatation under vision.

Alternatively the solid but flexible Celestin dilator (b) can be passed over a guide-wire. Each dilator is 75 cm long with a central channel. The dilating complex is 20 cm long and has an external diameter covering the range of either 4–12 mm (in 2 mm steps) or 4–18 mm (first step of 8 mm, followed by 2 mm steps).

2a & b

Tubes

The Procter-Livingstone tube (a) is preferred. It is an armoured soft latex rubber tube with an internal diameter of 12 mm and an outer diameter of 18 mm. The proximal end is expanded to fit snugly above the tumour and prevent food passing between the tube and the oesophageal wall. Three lengths are available: 10 cm, 15 cm and 19 cm. An attractive alternative is the Celestin pulsion tube (b) with a distally sited flange to prevent cephalad displacement. This tube can be inserted with a special balloon introducer stiffened by the use of a mandril.

3

Position of patient

The patient lies supine on the operating table, the head supported on a grommet ring. The table break permits flexion and extension of the cervical spine.

Anaesthesia

General anaesthesia using a high dose Fentanyl technique allows rapid induction and reversal of anaesthesia. An endotracheal tube should be inserted after preliminary bronchoscopy.

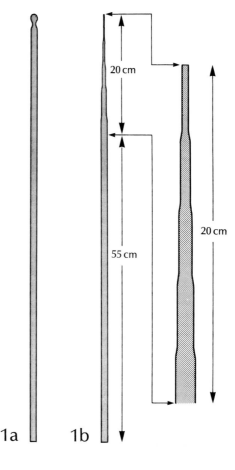

1a 1b

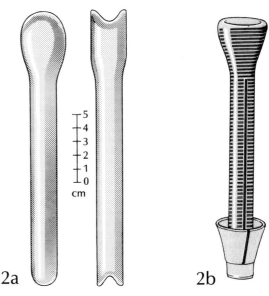

2a 2b

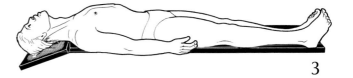

3

The operation

Endoscopy

Bronchoscopy is first performed to identify compression of the tracheobronchial tree, tumour invasion or the presence of a fistula. Tracheobronchial secretions are aspirated. The well lubricated oesophagoscope is then advanced under direct vision as far as the stricture, from which biopsies are taken.

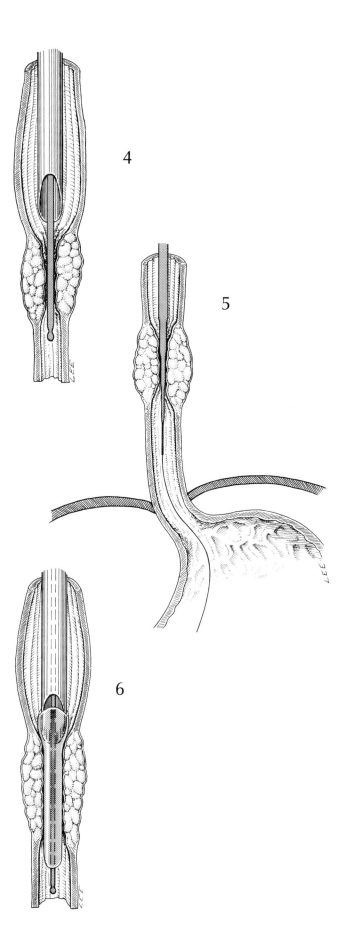

4

4

Stricture dilatation using the rigid oesophagoscope

Dilatation is achieved by the sequential passage of graduated bougies to 40 Fr gauge. To avoid perforation of the oesophagus or stomach, the bougie should only traverse the length of the stricture. Longitudinal rupture of a tumour during dilatation does not increase morbidity as the tube effectively tamponades any mural defect.

5

5

Stricture dilatation using the flexible endoscope

An Eder–Puestow guide wire is passed through the stricture via the biopsy channel of the endoscope. A generous length of wire should be advanced into the stomach to avoid withdrawal during removal of the dilator. After withdrawal of the endoscope the Celestin dilator is threaded over the guide wire until the maximum diameter of the dilating complex traverses the stricture. The wire is firmly held by an assistant to prevent curling or displacement.

6

Intubation

A 20 Fr gauge bougie is passed through the dilated stricture and left *in situ*. A lubricated tube of appropriate length is inserted over the bougie, through the stricture, using the rigid oesophagoscope as a 'pusher'. The expanded proximal end of the tube rests on the upper shoulder of the stricture. The bougie and oesophagoscope are removed after verifying that the tube is correctly sited.

6

Postoperative care

Patients must be nursed in the semi-sitting position and carefully observed, particularly for evidence of respiratory obstruction, aspiration pneumonia and oesophageal perforation.

Routine contrast studies will confirm the position and patency of the tube. In the absence of complications oral feeding can be begun immediately.

Complications

Haemorrhage

Major haemorrhage is uncommon, and usually ceases spontaneously. Fatal haemorrhage is associated with aortic disruption.

7

Oesophageal perforation

Perforation occurs during bouginage either at the junction of normal oesophagus and the upper end of the tumour or near the cardia where the oesophagus deviates to the left. The tube may project through the perforation into the mediastinum. Emergncy treatment should include oesophageal bypass.

Tube migration

Proximal migration is commoner than distal migration. Patients complain of dysphagia and contrast studies confirm the diagnosis. Tube removal and replacement is well tolerated.

Tube obstruction

Tube obstruction can result from food impaction, tube migration or failure of a short tube completely to traverse the stricture. Oesophagoscopy and contrast studies will aid in identifying the nature of the obstruction.

Respiratory

Intubation of bulky tumours may produce tracheal compression, necessitating removal of the tube for the relief of respiratory obstruction.

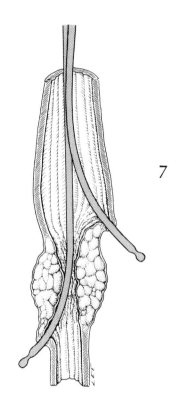

7

Bronchial aspiration should be treated by bronchoscopic suction. Atelectasis and bronchopneumonia may follow, requiring physiotherapy and antimicrobial agents.

Further reading

Atkinson, M., Ferguson, R., Parker, G. C. Tube introducer and modified Celestin tube for use in palliative intubation of oesophagogastric neoplasms at fibreoptic endoscopy. Gut 1978; 19: 669–671

Celestin, L. R., Campbell, W. B. A new and safe system for oesophageal dilatation. Lancet 1981; 1: 74–75

Hegarty, M. M., Angorn, I. B., Bryer, J. V., Henderson, B. J., Le Roux, B. T., Logan, A. Pulsion intubation for palliation of carcinoma of the oesophagus. British Journal of Surgery 1977; 64: 160–165

Index

375